Animal Andrology: Theories and Applications

Animal Andrology: Theories and Applications

Editor

Arundhati Nimbalkar

scitus
academics

Animal Andrology: Theories and Applications

Edited by **Arundhati Nimbalkar**

ISBN: 978-1-68117-043-5

Library of Congress Control Number: 2015935438

SCITUS Academics LLC,
www.scitusacademics.com
Box No. 4766, 616 Corporate Way,
Suite 2, Valley Cottage,
NY 10989

Printed in United States of America on Acid Free Paper ∞

Contents

Preface

Andrology is the medical specialty that deals with male health, particularly relating to the problems of the male reproductive system and urological problems that are unique to men. It is also known as "The science of Men". It is the counterpart to gynaecology, which deals with medical issues which are specific to the female reproductive system. However unlike gynecology, which has a plethora of medical board certification program worldwide, andrology has none. Andrology has only been studied as a distinct specialty since the late 1960s: the first specialist journal on the subject was the German periodical Andrologie now called Andrologia, published from 1969 onwards. Understanding animal andrology is fundamental to optimizing genetic breeding traits in domestic and wild animals. This book provides extensive coverage of male reproductive biology, discussing the essentials of sperm production, harvest and preservation before covering the applications to a range of animals including cattle, horses, pigs, small ruminants, camelids, cats and dogs, poultry and exotic species. It also examines the laboratory procedures that provide the basis of general fertility research.

Editor

Chapter 1

Advances in Stem Cell Therapy for Erectile Dysfunction

Ching-Shwun Lin

Knuppe Molecular Urology Laboratory, Department of Urology, School of Medicine, University of California, San Francisco, CA 94143-0738, USA

ABSTRACT

Stem cell (SC) therapy for erectile dysfunction (ED) has been investigated in 35 published studies, with one being a small-scale clinical trial. Out of these 35 studies, 19 are concerned with cavernous nerve (CN) injury-associated ED while 10 with diabetes mellitus- (DM-) associated ED.

(Adipose-derived SCs ADSCs) were employed in 18 studies while bone marrow SCs (BMSCs) in 9. Transplantation of SCs was done mostly by intra cavernous (IC) injection, as seen in 25 studies. Allogeneic and xenogeneic transplantations have increasingly been performed but their immune-incompatibility issues were rarely discussed. More recent studies also tend to use combinatory therapies by modifying or supplementing SCs with angiogenic or neurotrophic genes or proteins. All studies reported better erectile function with SC transplantation, and the majority also reported improved muscle, endothelium, and/or nerve in the erectile tissue. However, differentiation or engraftment of transplanted SCs has rarely been observed; thus, paracrine action is generally believed to be responsible for SC's therapeutic effects. But still, few studies actually investigated and none proved paracrine action as a therapeutic mechanism. Thus, based exclusively on functional outcome data shown in preclinical studies, two clinical trials are currently recruiting patients for treatment with IC injection of ADSC and BMSC, respectively.

INTRODUCTION

Erectile dysfunction (ED) is a term recommended by a panel of experts in 1992 to replace the term "impotence" [1]. These experts also defined ED as an inability of the male to attain and/or maintain penile erection sufficient for satisfactory sexual performance. Although not life threatening by itself, ED is a strong predictor of high-mortality diseases such as coronary artery disease and cardiovascular disease [2–5]. ED does directly and negatively impact the quality of life of the afflicted men and their spouse [6–11]. In a 1999 report the worldwide prevalence of ED was estimated to be 152 million men in 1995 and predicted to increase to 322 million men by 2025 [12]. While the majority of ED cases can be treated with currently available medications or devices, approximately 20% of the overall ED patient population remains unresponsive to treatment [13], and in certain patient populations, such as those having diabetes mellitus (DM) or having undergone radical prostatectomy (RP), the failure rates are even higher, at 40% [14–16]. Moreover, regardless of their therapeutic efficacy or inefficacy, all current treatment options treat only the symptoms, not the underlying causes, and most of them need to be taken by or administered to the patient when having an erection which is perceived as necessary. Thus, current research efforts are geared toward finding long-term solutions that can reverse the pathogenesis of ED and thereby restore the patient's ability to achieve natural penile erection. One of such research efforts is the investigation of stem cells (SCs) as therapeutic agents, and in this review article I will summarize and discuss all available relevant data in this field of research.

ERECTILE FUNCTION

Penile erection is a physiological process that involves the expansion and elongation of a paired cylindrical structure called corpora cavernosa (singular: corpus cavernosum, CC) that run the length of the penis [17]. Inside each CC is a maze of miniscule chambers called sinusoids that are collapsed and occupy a minimal amount of space when the penis is in the flaccid state. When a man is sexually aroused, blood enters the sinusoids, resulting in their expansion and thus penile erection. When sexual stimulation subsides, blood exits the sinusoids, and the penis returns to the flaccid state.

The cycle of sinusoidal expansion and collapse is locally controlled by smooth muscle cells (SMCs, or CSMCs as pertaining to CC), which form a multilayered structure as part of the sinusoidal wall [18, 19]. When CSMCs are in a contracted state, blood flow into the sinusoids is kept at a minimum; when CSMCs transit to a relaxed state, blood flow into the sinusoids is increased, resulting in sinusoidal expansion. The cycle of CSMC contraction and relaxation is in turn controlled by two other tissue components inside the CC, namely, the cavernous endothelial cells (CECs) and the cavernous nerves (CNs). CECs are located as a single layer of cells alongside the CSMCs inside each sinusoid, and together, CECs and CSMCs form the wall that defines each sinusoid [18, 19]. CNs, which arise from neurons in the inferior hypogastric plexuses in humans or in the major pelvic ganglia (MPG) in the rat [20, 21], track throughout the CC and end in the vicinity of CSMCs [18, 19]. Sexual stimulation causes CNs to release nitric oxide (NO), which enters nearby CSMCs, triggering their relaxation [22–24]. The subsequent increase of blood flow into the sinusoids induces shear stress on the CECs, triggering their release of NO. This CEC-derived

NO is believed to permit a sustained CSMC relaxation that is essential for a satisfactory intercourse [25–29].

The paired CC is enveloped in a dense fibrous sheath called tunica albuginea (TA). During erection, the increased blood flow into the sinusoids causes CC to expand and compress against the TA. Being a sturdy and resilient structure, the TA permits CC expansion, but with increasing resistance. As the tension between the expanding CC and the resisting TA increases, so does the overall penile rigidity. Furthermore, the compression of CC against TA causes the closure of subtunical veins that otherwise would allow the escape of blood from the sinusoids. Such a venous occlusive mechanism ensures that the CC remains fully engorged and the penis fully erect until the cessation of sexual stimulation [17].

NO, which is critical for triggering CSMC relaxation, is formed within CECs and CNs by nitric oxide synthase (NOS) that catalyzes the conversion of L-arginine and oxygen to L-citrulline and NO [30]. While performing the same function in NO production, the endothelial NOS (eNOS) and the neuronal NOS (nNOS) are encoded by two separate genes [30]. More importantly, from a technical standpoint, eNOS and nNOS are sufficiently different in their protein sequences so as to permit the generation of their specific antibodies [31, 32]. In ED research, including many studies that will be discussed in this review, these antibodies have proven to be highly valuable for the assessment of ED-related changes in the cavernous endothelium and nerves.

NO enters CSMCs by diffusion, and once inside, it activates the soluble guanylyl cyclase, which then catalyzes the conversion of GTP to cGMP [22, 23]. When cGMP concentration is sufficiently high, activation of cGMP-dependent kinase (also known as protein kinase G, PKG) occurs, and this leads to the phosphorylation of several downstream targets (e.g., ion channels), causing CSMCs to relax and thus penile erection [22, 23]. When sexual stimulation ceases, cGMP production is also halted. Meanwhile, existing cGMP is hydrolyzed by phosphor diest erases (PDEs), most notably, PDE5 [33, 34]. When cGMP concentration drops below a threshold level, PKG is deactivated and its downstream targets dephosphorylated, thereby returning CSMCs to the contracted state and the penis to the flaccid state [22, 23].

ERECTILE DYSFUNCTION

The worldwide prevalence of ED was estimated to be 152 million in 1995 and predicted to be 322 million by 2025 [12]. ED can be classified as psychogenic, organic, or mixed psychogenic/organic [17]. The organic type of ED is further classified into neurogenic, vasculogenic, cavernous, hormonal, drug-induced, and systemic disease-related [17]. For all published SC-for-ED studies, only the neurogenic, vasculogenic, and cavernous types are relevant. Specifically, in concern with neurogenic and vasculogenic types, the relevant studies focused on CN injury-associated and DM-associated ED, respectively. And, in concern with cavernous type of ED, which loosely defines local tissue abnormalities, there have been two TA injury-related SC-for-ED studies.

The majority of organic types of ED can be treated with intracavernous (IC) injection of erectogenic agents, transurethral prostaglandin suppository, vacuum device, and/or PDE5 inhibitors (PDE5Is) [35]. In particular, PDE5Is are currently the most prescribed treatment because of their ease of use (as orally taken pills) and overall proven efficacy [35]. However, in a recent study of 327 ED patients who were prescribed PDE5Is by their physicians, only 148 (45.3%) were still using the medication during a 3-year follow-up period, while 160 (48.9%) had discontinued and 19 (5.8%) never took the medication [36]. Thus, among those who had taken PDE5Is, more than half (52%; 160/308) had decided not to continue. When asked to choose among 11 reasons for discontinuation, 38% of the dropout patients selected "noneffectiveness." Other significant reasons chosen were "concerns about the cardiovascular safety of PDE5Is" (15.7%), cost (13.7%), and "lack of spontaneity" (8.7%). When categorized by specific ED types, patients who were diabetic had the highest discontinuation rate (28/36; 78%), followed by patients whose ED was caused by treatments such as RP (37/56; 66%) [36]. such high dropout rates for these two types of ED are not entirely unexpected, as an earlier study already identified them as least responsive to PDE5I treatment [14]. These two types of ED therefore will be discussed in detail in the following two sections. For other types of ED that have been investigated as SC treatment targets, only the TA injury-associated ED will also be discussed in detail in a separate section. The reasons are as follows: (1) it is necessary to clarify whether TA injury can truly cause ED, (2) hyperlipidemia-associated ED has been investigated in only one SC-for-ED study, (3) aging-associated ED is related to the normal process of aging, not to any specific disease, and (4) these latter two types of ED are usually responsive to PDE5I treatment.

DIABETES-ASSOCIATEDED

In an official document titled "National Diabetes Statistics, 2011," the National Institute of Health of the USA reports that DM affects 25.8 million people, or 8.3% of the general population in the USA, and among residents 65 years of age and older, 10.9 million (26.9%) had DM in 2010 [37]. In a peer-reviewed publication that analyzed prior epidemiological studies totaling 370 country-years and 2.7 million participants, Danaei et al. [38] reported that the number of people with DM worldwide increased from 153 million in 1980 to 347 million in 2008. Furthermore, in a forward-looking projection, the International Diabetes Federation estimated that by 2030 the number of people with DM worldwide will be 552 million [39]. Thus, the global diabetes epidemic is alarmingly real.

DM is associated with a large assortment of complications, including ED. For men with DM, 50–75% have ED, regardless of age [40]. Diabetic men also tend to incur ED 10–15 years earlier and are 3 times more likely to have ED than nondiabetic men [41, 42]. Importantly, both the severity of ED and the impact on quality of life by ED are significantly greater in diabetic than in nondiabetic men [43, 44]. DM-associated ED is also highly refractory to PDEI treatment, with only 44% success rate, compared to 85% for hypogonadal ED patients [14]. Diabetic ED patients also ranked the highest in terms of discontinuation of treatment with PDE5Is (at a dropout rate of 28/36 or 78%) [36]. Thus, the identification of an effective treatment for DM-associated ED is one of the most important objectives of current ED research efforts.

DM is a systematic disease that affects every part of the body. In the penis, it is associated with reduced contents of all three key components for erectile function, namely, CN, CEC, and CSMC [45–49]. The reduction of CEC content is likely due to DM-induced apoptosis in CEC as demonstrated by immunohistochemical analysis of CC samples between diabetic and nondiabetic patients [50]. This clinical histological finding has recently been corroborated by a basic science study, which identified mitochondrial fragmentation and cellular apoptosis in CECs cultured in high glucose medium [32, 51]. Histological analysis of CC samples also identified a significantly higher apoptotic index in the CSMC of diabetic versus nondiabetic rats [52]. Similarly, the reduced penile CN content has been shown to be due to apoptotic cell death of nNOS-positive neurons in the MPG of diabetic rats [48]. Thus, how to prevent and/or reverse these pathological processes is critically important for the effective treatment of DM-associated ED. In this regard, SC therapy has been considered promising, due to SC's well-known regenerative capacity.

POSTPROSTATECTOMY AND POSTRADIOTHERAPYED

Prostate cancer is the most common malignancy in men, with estimated numbers of new cases and related deaths being 217,730 and 32,050, respectively, in the USA in 2010 [53]. As prostate cancer is usually locally confined (~80% of cases), the most common treatments have been RP or external beam radiation therapy (RT) [54]. However, despite being highly effective, these treatments often incur after treatment complications, such as ED [55, 56]. In a recent study of 1655 men treated with RP or RT, the reported incidence of ED ranges from 60.8% to 93.9%, depending on treatment choice and assessment time (2, 5, or 15 years after treatment) [57].

It is generally agreed that post-RP ED is caused by inadvertent injury to the CNs, which run alongside the prostate. However, despite the introduction of nerve-sparing RP 30 years ago, ED remains a frequent consequence of such surgeries [58, 59]. Therefore, it is now commonly believed that, although leaving the CNs intact, nerve-sparing RP still causes subtle changes that are not obvious to the surgeons [55, 60]. These changes cause CNs to undergo Wallerian degeneration and eventually lose their connection to the corpora cavernosa [56, 61]. Alternatively, the surgery-incurred insults may temporarily prevent the CNs from releasing NO into the CC, and without NO-induced engorgement, the penile tissue becomes hypoxic and its CSMC replaced by collagens [56, 60, 61]. In support of this theory, a reduced smooth muscle to collagen ratio has been observed in the penis of CN injury animal models [62–66] and in CC biopsies of RP-treated patients [67].

RP and RT are used to treat prostate cancer at comparable rates [54]; they are also associated with posttreatment ED at similar rates [57]. However, while RP-associated ED has been intensively investigated at the basic science level, RT-associated ED is rarely studied [49]. Nevertheless, three independent studies have found that radiation over the lower abdomen in the rat caused reductions in erectile response and in CN and CSMC contents [49, 68, 69]. Thus, post-RP and post-RT ED appear to share a common pathological mechanism, that is, treatment-induced CN injury followed by CSMC atrophy.

Similar to other types of ED, post-RP and post-RT ED are most commonly treated with PDE5Is [56]. However, as its name indicates, a PDE5I inhibits PDE5, which, by breaking down cGMP, terminates the NO-activated erectile signaling pathway [23, 33]. Therefore, when CNs are injured, as in the situation with RP or RT-treated patients, their ability to release NO into CC is compromised, and if there is no NO release into CC, erection would not occur, regardless whether PDE5 is inhibited or not. This dependence on a functional CN may explain why PDE5Is have a low success rate (~43%) in treating post-RP ED [14] and a high discontinuation rate (~66%) in post-RP ED patients who were nevertheless prescribed with PDE5Is [36]. Thus, it is obvious that the effective treatment of post-RP and post-RT ED requires repair of the damaged CN, and this has been the goal of the majority of SC-for-ED studies, especially those published in the past two years.

PEYRONIE'S DISEASE-ASSOCIATEDED

The estimated prevalence of PD varies greatly among different studies, with the highest being up to 7.1% of men in the general population [70]. PD is characterized by the presence of a fibrous plaque (or plaques) in the TA that causes pain and deformity (curvature, narrowing, and shortening) in the erect penis [70]. PD therefore negatively impacts the patient's sexual function and partner relationship [71]. However, in popular media, such as the Internet, PD patients' sexual dysfunction is often incorrectly defined as a type of "erectile dysfunction," despite the fact that most PD patients are able to achieve erection. Nevertheless, in serious scientific publications, PD is frequently described in the Introduction section as a disease that directly causes ED, with reference to a study by Lopez and Jarow [72]. In that study, 76 out of 95 (80%) PD patients were determined as having concomitant ED, and 36% and 59% of these PD+ED patients were further identified as having abnormal arterial blood flow and veno-occlusive dysfunction, respectively. Thus, the authors concluded that, when compared to abnormal arterial blood flow, veno-occlusive dysfunction was the principal cause of ED in PD patients. However, it should be noted that the study never examined whether PD (TA plaque) caused veno-occlusive dysfunction or ED. In another study that evaluated 143 PD patients, only 27 (19%) were found to have concomitant ED, and 22 (including 4 diabetics) of the 27 PD+ED patients were found to have veno-occlusive dysfunction [73]. So, on one hand, these two studies disagree sharply in the prevalence of ED among PD patients (80% versus 19%), but on the other, they do agree that veno-occlusive dysfunction is the principal cause of ED in PD patients. Importantly though, neither study provides evidence that PD (TA plaque) caused veno-occlusive dysfunction or ED. In fact, in an earlier study only 18 out of 62 PD patients (29%) were found to have concomitant ED, and 17 out of these 18 PD+ED patients were further identified as having some underlying diseases (such as DM) that contributed to their ED [74]. Therefore, none of these three studies provides evidence that PD (TA plaque) is a direct cause of ED in PD patients. Finally, in the only animal study that attempted to answer why PD patients suffer from ED, PD was simulated in the rat by injection of transforming growth factor- (TGF-) into the TA (to induce fibrosis) or by surgical incision in the TA (to cause trauma) [75]. Six weeks later both groups of rats were found to have altered TA histology and lowered erectile response when compared to sham-treated rats. Therefore, this study appears to have obtained evidence that TA abnormalities can cause ED, but the question remains whether treatment of PD can result in the restoration of erectile function.

Plaque excision followed by patch grafting is a common surgical procedure for the correction of penile deformities in PD patients [76]. However, in spite of its proven efficacy, postsurgical complications such as ED can occur [77]. Therefore, various approaches, including the use of novel graft materials, have been investigated toward minimizing the occurrence of these complications [76]. In a recent animal study, porcine small intestine submucosa (SIS), which has already been used for TA reconstruction in PD patients, was seeded with adipose-derived stem cells (ADSCs) and then grafted into incised rat TA to see if ADSC seeding can reduce the incidence of postsurgery ED [78]. In another recent animal study [79] ADSC was injected into the TA of TGF--induced PD rats to see if ADSC can reduce the severity of ED. Further discussion on these two studies will be given in "Animal Models" subsection.

CURRENT STATE OF STEM CELL THERAPY FOR ERECTILE DYSFUNCTION

The first SC-for-ED study was published in 2004, and since then, up to November 2013, there have been a total of 34 additional studies in this field of research (Table 1). While 15 of these studies were published between 2004 and 2011, 20 were published after 2011. Thus, it is evident that an accelerated pace of publication occurred at the start of 2012. In any event, among all 35 studies, 19 chose CN injury-associated ED as the disease target, and 18 employed ADSC as the therapeutic cell type (Table 1). While the disease target preference reflects clinical needs (i.e., post-RP and post-RT ED as described earlier), the cell type choice is most likely due to ADSC's abundant tissue source, ease of isolation, and proven therapeutic efficacy across all medical disciplines (see details under "adipose-derived stem cell").

Table 1: Number of published stem cells for erectile dysfunction studies

Years	**2004–2011**	**2012-2013**	**2004–2013**
Number of studies			
Total	**15**	**20**	**35**
Disease model			
Aging	2	1	3
CN injury	7	12	19
Hyperlipidemia	1	0	1

T1DM	2	6	8
T2DM	2	0	2
TA injury	0	2	2
SC type			
ADSC	5	13[a]	18
BMMNC	1	0	1
BMSC	4	5	9
EPC[b]	1	0	1
ESC	1	0	1
SkMSC	2	1	3
Testis SC	0	1	1
UCBSC	1	0	1

As clinical trial of SC therapy for ED is not yet approved in most countries, there has been only one published clinical SC-for-ED study and it involved only 7 type 2 DM (T2DM) patients [80]. While that study was carried out in Korea, two clinical trials have been approved in France and the USA and are currently recruiting patients. The French trial (Identifier: NCT01089387) is a phase I-II trial and will test the safety and benefit of IC injection of autologous bone marrow mononucleated cells (BMMNC) in post-RP ED patients. The US trial (Identifier: NCT01601353) will evaluate the safety and treatment efficacy of IC injection of autologous ADSC in patients with organic ED.

In addition to the above-mentioned research and clinical trials, SC's therapeutic potential has also inspired several business opportunities. By searching the Internet with "stem cell erectile," one can find many "treatment centers" that offer autologous ADSC treatment for ED at prices of several thousand US dollars. While most of these businesses are located in developing countries such as the Philippines and Thailand, some indicate their presence in the USA. This is surprising because for-profit SC treatment of any disease is illegal in the USA, and criminal convictions have been handed down on cases that involved treating patients with SCs. Therefore, at issue are probable fraudulent advertisements. In any event, SC therapy for ED remains largely in the preclinical investigational stage, and this is what will be discussed in the following sections.

ANIMAL MODELS

All but one preclinical SC-for-ED studies used rats as animal models; the singular exception used mice (Tables 2, 3, and 4). Aging animal models were used in 3 studies (Table 2), and they were rats between 20 and 30 months of age. Hyperlipidemia rat model was used in one study (Table 2), and it was established by feeding with a commercially formulated high-fat diet (mainly 2% cholesterol and 10% lard) for 5 months. The high cost of this diet and the lengthy time requirement are hindering factors for this model's widespread usage. TA injury animal models were used in two studies (Table 2), and they were established by two different procedures. In the earlier study, a 0.5 cm incision was made through both lateral sides of the rat's TA, and a SIS graft seeded or not seeded with ADSCs was then interpositioned into the incision and sutured. As such, this animal model should probably be called a TA reconstruction rather than a TA injury ED model. In the later study, TA injury was induced by injection of 50g of TGF- into the TA, and one day later, ADSC was injected into the same site as a treatment for the injured TA. Thus, as far as treatment target is concerned, this is an acute TA injury, not PD, animal model, because PD is characterized clinically as a chronic disease.

Table 2: Published studies of stem cell therapy for noncavernous nerve injury, nondiabetic erectile dysfunction

Publication year	First author	Animal model	Stem cell type	Modification/ supplementation*	Transplantation route	Reference
2007	Bivalacqua	Aging rat	Allogeneic BMSC	eNOS transduction	IC	[81]
2008	Nolazco	Aging rat	Mouse SkMSC	None	IC	[82]
2010	Abdel Aziz	Aging rat	Allogeneic BMSC	None	IC	[83]
2010	Huang	Hyperlip-idemia rat	Autologous ADSC	None	IC	[84]
2012	Ma	TA injury rat	Autologous ADSC	None	SIS graft	[78]
2013	Castiglione	TA injury rat	Human ADSC	None	Intratunical	[79]

For enhancing stem cell's therapeutic efficacy.

*Table 3: Published studies of stem cell therapy for diabetic erectile dysfunction

Publication year	First author	Patients/ animal model	Stem cell type	Modification/ supplementation*	Transplantation route	Reference
2010	Bahk	T2DM patients	Allogeneic UCBSC	None	IC	[80]
2010	Garcia	ZDF rat	Autologous ADSC	None	IC	[85]
2011	Gou	STZ rat	Allogeneic EPC#	VEGF transfection	IC	[86]
2011	Qiu	STZ rat	Allogeneic BMSC	None	IC	[87]
2012	Qiu	STZ rat	Allogeneic BMSC	VEGF transduction	IC	[88]
2012	Sun	STZ rat	Allogeneic BMSC	None	IC	[89]
2012	Nishimatsu	STZ rat	Allogeneic ADSC	None	IC	[90]
2012	Ryu	STZ mouse	Syngeneic SVF	None	IC	[91]
2013	He	STZ rat	Allogeneic BMSC	KCNMA1 transduction	IC	[92]
2013	Liu	STZ rat	Human ADSC	VEGF transduction	IC	[93]

*For enhancing stem cell's therapeutic efficacy.

#Possibly BMMNC.

Table 4: Published studies of stem cell therapy for cavernous nerve injury erectile dysfunction

Publication year	First author	CN injury method#	Stem cell type	Modification/ supplementation*	Transplantation route	Reference
2004	Bochinski	Crush	Allogeneic ESC	BDNF transduction	IC or intra-MPG	[94]
2006	Kim	Transection	Allogeneic SkMSC	None	IC	[95]
2009	Fall	5-mm resection	Allogeneic BMMNC	None	IC	[96]
2010	Albersen	Crush	Autologous ADSC	None	IC	[97]
2010	Kendirci	Crush	Allogeneic BMSC	p75LNGFR selection	IC	[98]
2011	Lin	5-mm resection	Autologous ADSC	None	Nerve graft	[99]
2011	Woo	Transection	Allogeneic SkMSC	None	IC	[100]
2012	Fandel	Crush	Autologous ADSC	None	IC	[101]
2012	Kim	Crush	Allogeneic BMSC	BDNF transduction	Intra-MPG	[102]
2012	Kovanecz	5-mm resection	Mouse SkMSC	Oral sildenafil	IC	[103]

2012	Piao	Crush	Human ADSC	BDNF PLGA	CN scaffold	[104]
2012	Qiu	Radiation	Allogeneic ADSC	None	IV	[105]
2012	Qiu	Crush	Autologous SVF	None	IC	[106]
2013	Jeong	Crush	Human ADSC	BDNF PLGA Oral udenafil	CN scaffold	[107]
2013	Kim	Crush	Human ADSC	NGF hydrogel	CN scaffold	[108]
2013	You	Not described	Human BMSC	None	IC + Periprostatic	[109]
2013	You	Stretch	Human ADSC	None	IC + Periprostatic	[110]
2013	Choi	Crush	Human testis SC	None	Periprostatic	[111]
2013	Ying	Crush	Autologous ADSC	None	IC	[112]

*For enhancing stem cell's therapeutic efficacy.

#All performed in rats.

Type 1 DM (T1DM) animal models were used in 8 studies (Table 3), and they were all established by intraperitoneal injection of streptozotocin (STZ). The ease of this DM-induction procedure is certainly the main reason why this animal model is frequently used in research despite the fact that only 5% of DM patients are type 1. On the other hand, only one study has used T2DM animal model—the Zucker Diabetic Fatty (ZDF) rat. The high cost (>$300 per rat) of this mutant rat is probably prohibitory for most researchers to consider its usage, especially when knowing that STZ-induced DM animal models are well accepted as clinically relevant.

CN injury models were used in 19 SC-for-ED studies (Table 4), and their purposes were to simulate postradical prostatectomy (post-RP) or postradiation therapy (post-RT) ED. To simulate post-RP ED, the investigator performs a lower abdominal incision and, with the aid of a dissecting microscope, identifies the two branches of CN, which arise from the MPG and course proximally on both sides of the prostate and distally alongside the urethra toward the penis. An injury is then applied at a location 2–5 mm from the MPG. The types of injury can be crush, freezing, transection, or resection. Crush is commonly done by applying a hemostatic clamp to the CN so as to simulate accidental nerve contusion or traction that occurs during nerve-sparing RP. Freezing is commonly done by applying a cryoprobe to the CN so as to offer another way of preserving nerve structural continuity. Both transection (a simple cut) and resection (removal of a CN segment) can be considered as representing nonnerve sparing RP, but transection is more likely to allow nerve reconnection than resection is. Thus, among all types of experimental CN injuries, resection is the most severe. In the majority of SC for CN injury ED studies, crush is most frequently used (11/19, Table 4).

While hundreds of studies have employed post-RP ED animal models, only 5 studies have worked with post-RT ED models [68, 69, 105, 113, and 114]. These studies used similar procedures but with slightly different dosage, duration, and frequency of radiation. In the study by van der Wielen et al. [114], a 3 mm thick lead shield with a 3 cm 4 cm window was placed on the rat to confine the radiation to the lower abdomen. Radiation was then delivered at 7.4 Gy for 5 consecutive days. This protocol was initially adopted in our recently published study [105], but after getting a 50% death rate, we modified it by using a lead shied with a smaller window (2.5 cm 3 cm) and delivering radiation at a smaller dosage (4 Gy/day for 5 days). These modifications resulted in no death, yet achieving the goal of inducing ED in the irradiated rats. Thus, some adjustments appear to be necessary for each research group to produce the optimal post-RT ED animal model.

STEM CELL BASICS

SCs can be classified according to their differentiation potential into pluripotent and multipotent, where pluripotent signifies the potential to differentiate into all cell types, whereas multipotent, some but not all cell types. SCs can also be classified according to their source into embryonic (ESC) and adult (ASC), where embryonic indicates the inner cell mass of a blastocyst, whereas adult, various tissues of a developed or developing individual. In terms of differentiation potential, ESC is pluripotent whereas ASC multipotent. However, many studies, including several in ED field, have stated that SCs isolated from adult tissues are pluripotent. This misunderstanding is a result of accepting in vitro differentiation data that were generated by using nonphysiological conditions and nonspecific cell markers (see below for further details). Furthermore, even if in vitro evidence is acceptable, there is no possibility to demonstrate ASC's differentiation into "all" cell types. As such, it is prudent to define ASCs as multipotent. In any event, depending on their tissue origin or the tissue type they can differentiate into, ASCs can be further classified into hematopoietic, neural, epithelial, and mesenchymal. Because mesenchymal SCs (MSCs) are by far the most frequently used cell types in SC-for-ED research, some of their characteristics relevant to ED research are discussed below.

MSCs have the potential to differentiate into mesenchymal tissues, such as bone, cartilage, and fat. They were first identified in the bone marrow but have now been shown to exist in virtually all postnatal tissues, including skeletal muscle and adipose tissue [115, 116]. MSCs have also been consistently localized to the vicinity of blood vessels, and, therefore, the term "perivascular" has been used to denote MSC's tissue location [115, 116]. While "perivascular" can mean near but outside of blood vessels, our investigation of the tissue location of ADSCs indicated that they reside in the capillaries and in the adventitia of blood vessels [117]. Thus, in that paper's Discussion section we proposed the term "vascular stem cells (VSCs)" to denote ADSCs. Since then, several other research groups and a more recent study of ours have confirmed the adventitial localization of ADSCs [118–122]. Thus, based on these ADSC studies and many other MSC studies, we have recently redefined MSCs as VSCs, and we also defined VSCs as "cells that reside within the blood vessel wall and can differentiate into all of the cell types that constitute a functional blood vessel" [123]. Based on this definition, VSCs can differentiate into pericytes, smooth muscle, and endothelial cells, which are then assembled into mature blood vessels, during angiogenesis or neovasculogenesis within any particular tissue. Additionally, during normal tissue cycling and in times of tissue injury, VSCs can also differentiate into tissue-specific cells (e.g., adipocytes) so as to maintain tissue homeostasis and to replace lost cells.

MSC's multipotent differentiation potential is what initially attracted interests to this field of research. However, up to this date, it remains controversial whether cellular differentiation is truly responsible for MSC's therapeutic efficacy. First, it is important to know that virtually all claims of MSC's differentiation potential are based on in vitro evidence. In fact, the International Society for Cellular Therapy (ISCT) recommended using chemical or immunohistochemical (IHC) staining of cultured MSCs as a means to demonstrate their differentiation potential [124]. As such, while numerous MSC studies have fulfilled this in vitro criterion, relatively few have investigated whether MSCs do indeed differentiate into particular cell types after transplantation into a host. In the few studies that did conduct such investigations, the results are either utterly negative or kind-of positive [125]. Such difficulties in recognizing MSC's in vivo differentiation potential are mainly due to the lack of specific MSC markers and the unreliability of current cell-tracking labels, as discussed in our recent review article [126].

The ISCT also recommended that MSCs be verified by flow cytometric analysis for expression of cell surface markers [124]. Specifically, ≥95% of the population must express CD105, CD73, and CD90, and ≤2% of the population must not express CD45, CD34, CD14 or CD11b, CD79a or CD19, and HLA class II. However, all three recommended positive markers, CD105, CD73, and CD90, are expressed in a wide variety of cells while one of the recommended negative marker, CD34, has proven to be highly useful for the identification and isolation of several MSC types, particularly, ADSCs [127]. In fact, CD34+ bone marrow cells were used to generate the Stro-1 monoclonal antibody [128, 129], which has since been used in hundreds of studies for the identification and isolation of a wide variety of MSC types [130, 131]. As such, the ISCT-recommended MSC criteria are in need of a revision.

The scarcity of evidence supporting cellular differentiation as a therapeutic mechanism has prompted considerations for alternative explanations, and presently the leading theory is that MSCs exert therapeutic effects through secretion of paracrine factors [125, 132–134]. Specifically, MSCs have been shown to secrete trophic and immunomodulatory factors that have the potential to (1) stimulate local tissue regeneration, (2) modulate local and systematic inflammatory responses, and (3) mobilize host cells, particularly bone marrow SCs (BMSCs), as repair cells for injured tissues. However, while gaining increasing acceptance, the paracrine theory raises an obvious question: Why not just use the paracrine factors as therapeutic agents? The answer may lie in the fact that MSCs are live cells and therefore capable of responding to host tissue needs, and their paracrine repertoire is obviously much larger and more diverse than single factors. Nevertheless, just like cellular differentiation, paracrine action as a mechanism for MSC's therapeutic effects remains largely unproven. Further details, especially those relevant to SC-for-ED studies, will be discussed in the "Therapeutic Mechanism" section.

STEM CELLS USED IN PUBLISHED ERECTILE DYSFUNCTION STUDIES

Embryonic Stem Cell

ESC has been used in only one SC-for-ED study, and it is the first SC-for-ED study (published in 2004) [94]. The study was conducted in our laboratory and was a very challenging task mainly because of the difficulty in establishing rat ESC in culture [135–137]. In any event, while we finally succeeded in establishing the culture and demonstrated its therapeutic efficacy, ethical concerns about using embryos as a source of therapeutic cells and the emergence of MSCs as substitutes led us to begin exploring ADSC as a more clinically feasible therapeutic agent. Subsequently, we published our first ADSC paper in 2006 [138], and since then we have focused entirely on ADSC as a promising therapeutic agent.

Bone Marrow Stem Cell

Because MSCs were first identified and isolated from bone marrow, many published studies, including several SC-for-ED studies, have simply used the term "MSCs" to denote BMSCs. However, MSCs have now been isolated from many nonbone marrow tissues [115, 116]; therefore, "BMSCs" should be used as a more discriminative term for bone marrow-derived MSCs. In any event, BMSCs have been investigated in thousands of studies, including 9 SC-for-ED studies, with overall proven therapeutic efficacy. However, it should be noted that in preclinical studies that use small animals as cell donors, the isolation of BMSCs is commonly done after sacrificing these animals. Therefore, transplantation of BMSCs in such studies is mostly allogeneic and sometimes xenogeneic. This would of course raise immunocompatibility issues, but such issues are rarely addressed. In any event, for clinical applications, which are likely to employ autologous transplantation, the preparation of BMSCs requires bone marrow aspiration and several weeks of cell culture/expansion [139].

Bone Marrow Mononuclear Cell

A preclinical ED study employed BMMNCs to treat CN injury ED [96]. The cells were harvested from donor rats and injected into ED rats without characterization; therefore, their relevance to SC research cannot be determined with certainty. However, the authors hinted at such relevance by stating in the paper's Introduction that "bone marrow is a well-established source of multipotent stem cells, including mesenchymal stem cells, endothelial progenitor cells, and hematopoietic stem cells." Furthermore, while heterogeneous in cell composition, BMMNCs can be reasonably expected to contain some SCs. Thus, despite lacking experimental evidence for SC relevance, the study is included for discussion in this SC-focused review article. More importantly, this preclinical study apparently provided the scientific basis for the afore-mentioned French clinical trial (Identifier: NCT01089387) that is currently recruiting patients.

Endothelial Progenitor Cell

Endothelial progenitor cell (EPC) has been used or claimed to have been used in one SC-for-ED study [86]. However, EPC is concerned with several outstanding issues that are important to both ED and non-ED research; therefore, despite being used in only one SC-for-ED study, EPC will be discussed at a disproportional length.

EPC was first reported as circulating blood cells that display endothelial-specific cell surface markers [140]. In recent years, both its relevance to ED and its identity as a SC type have been controversial. In regard to its ED relevance, several studies have shown that ED patients had a reduced number of circulating EPC [141–145], and another study even suggested that boosting EPC number through dietary supplementation could enhance erectile function [146]. However, three studies from another research team have found the opposite; that is, ED patients had higher numbers of circulating EPC [147–149]. These latter studies thus suggested that the discrepancy might be due to differences in the immunophenotypes that were used to evaluate the identity of the isolated EPCs. However, the actual reason is more likely due to uncertainties about what EPC really is [150, 151]. For example, it has been shown that EPC might be monocytes contaminated with platelet microparticles [152], or they might be injured or senescent vascular endothelial cells that slough into the bloodstream [153]. Regardless, accumulating evidence has shown that different EPC subsets are in fact various hematopoietic lineage cells; thus, it has been suggested that the term EPC be retired [154, 155].

In the one and only EPC-for-ED study, the so-called EPCs were isolated from the bone marrow, not the expected circulating blood. Furthermore, in the study's Methods section, the isolated bone marrow cells were called "mononuclear cells," and the cited studies also suggest that the cells were BMMNCs. One of these studies is titled "Endothelial progenitor cells: identity defined?" [156], and another study concludes: "the adult EPCs we find so far may be mononuclear/macrophages." [157] Thus, despite being called EPCs, the cells used in this ED study are likely BMMNCs.

Umbilical Cord Blood Stem Cell

Umbilical cord blood SC (UCBSC) has been used in only one SC-for-ED study, and it is a clinical study, the only published clinical study [80]. However, umbilical cord blood is known to contain both hematopoietic and mesenchymal SCs [158], and based on the following considerations, the UCBSC in this study is most likely MSC. First, the cells were provided by a company (also partaking in the study) that commercializes umbilical cord blood-derived MSCs. Second, one of the described characteristics of these cells was their being CD34−. Third, MSC's characteristics were addressed extensively in the report's discussion. Forth, in a recent study in which the same company was involved, the cells were clearly described as umbilical cord blood-derived MSCs [159].

Skeletal Muscle-Derived Stem Cell

Three ED studies have used skeletal muscle-derived stem cells (SkMSCs) as treatment cells. The first study isolated such cells from rats [95] while the two more recent studies from mice [82, 103]. These cells were all used to treat ED in rat models; therefore, the transplantation was xenogeneic in the two more recent studies. In one of these two studies [82], the reason for choosing mice over rats as cell donor was "these (mouse) MDSCs are the only ones prepared by this method that have been extensively characterized as stem cells." However, rat SkMSCs isolated by the same method (see below) were described in the ED study by Kim et al. [95] that was published 2 years earlier. And, several urology-related papers that employed rat SkMSCs were also published earlier, including two that were published 7 years earlier [160, 161]. In any event, the same group of researchers still used mouse SkMSCs to treat ED in rats in their more recent study [103], this time giving no reason.

The cell isolation method used in all three SkMSC-for-ED studies is termed "preplating," meaning the selection of SkMSCs through several rounds of cell seeding (plating) in plastic cell culture flasks. Only cells that do not adhere in one particular round are seeded in the next round, because early adhering cells (1st and 2nd rounds) have been shown to be more fibroblastic whereas late adhering cells (5th and 6th rounds) more myogenic [160, 161]. Thus, for clinical applications, which are likely to employ autologous transplantation, the preparation of a sufficient number of SkMSCs requires several weeks of cell seeding, culturing, and expansion [162].

Adipose-Derived Stem Cell

ADSC is now the most frequently used cell type in SC-for-ED research, with 18 studies versus 9 for the second-place BMSC. The principal reasons for such an increased interest in ADSC are (1) its overall proven similarities with BMSC, (2) its overall proven therapeutic efficacy across medical disciplines, (3) its abundant tissue source, (4) its ease of isolation, and (5) the availability of automated isolation devices.

The first demonstration of adipose-derived stromal cells as SCs is generally credited to a study published in 2001 by Zuk et al. [163]. But, the fact is that one year earlier Halvorsen et al. [164] already showed that such cells could be induced to express adipocyte- and osteoblast-specific proteins. Nevertheless, Zuk's study is far more thorough in the experimental approach and far more convincing in the outcome data; thus, it indeed deserves being commonly referred to as the first ADSC paper. Still, it should be pointed out that in 2001, there were 5 other ADSC publications [165–169], and they too need to be acknowledged as pioneering studies in this field of research.

The isolation of ADSC involves a centrifugation step that results in the separation of the stromal vascular fraction (SVF) from the rest of the adipose tissue homogenate. The SVF, which appears as a pellet in the centrifuge tube, contains endothelial cells, smooth muscle cells, pericytes, fibroblasts, mast cells, and preadipocytes [170]. Culturing of SVF cells under standard conditions (i.e., in Dulbecco modified essential medium) eventually (within 2-3 passages) results in the appearance of a relatively homogenous population of mesenchymal cells that are now commonly called ADSC (or ASC, which is recommended by the International Fat Applied Technology Society but can be confused with ASC for adult stem cells). Thus, the relationship between SVF cells and ADSCs is similar to that between BMNNCs and BMSCs, as discussed earlier.

While cultured ADSCs have been used in most SC-for-ED studies, uncultured SVF cells have been increasingly tested as therapeutic agents. The reasons are mainly the emergence of machines that can rapidly process a human lipoaspirate into SVF cells and reports that such cells are as effective as ADSCs in experimental therapies. However, when considering cell dosage for transplantation, it is important to know that, from one gram of fat, the SVF pellet contains approximately 250,000 cells, but only 2% of these cells can adhere to plastic culture dish and be further propagated to become the eventual ADSC [171].

Testis-Derived Stem Cell

A recently published study demonstrated the isolation of SCs from human testis [111]. These cells were positive for CD34 and localized to the testicular stroma; therefore, they are most likely MSCs. However, while it would seem more logic to use these cells for infertility treatment, the study chose CN injury ED instead. In any event, the authors stated that these cells might represent a promising new autologous cell source for clinical use. But, it remains to be seen whether patients will be willing to sacrifice portions of their testicles for the treatment of their ED.

STEM CELL MODIFICATION

A few studies have tested SCs that were transduced or transfected with genes known to encode proteins that positively regulate erectile function [81, 86, 88, 92–94, 102]. Transfection with plasmids results in cells that only transiently express the transfected gene while transduction requires using a viral vector and a lengthy process to select for positively transduced cells [172]. Therefore, the implementation of transfected or transduced SCs in clinical trials will require preclinical demonstration of highly significant benefits when compared to their untransfected counterparts. Whether this has been accomplished in ED research will be discussed in the "main therapeutic outcomes" section.

STEM CELL LABELING

For the purpose of tracking SCs after their transplantation, various compounds or genes have been used as cell labels. However, every label has its shortcomings, as discussed in detail in our recent review [126]. Briefly, the use of LacZ gene, which encodes bacterial -gal, is hampered by endogenous expression of -gal in mammalian tissues. The use of GFP gene, which encodes a green fluorescence protein, is troubled by autofluorescence in mammalian tissues. DAPI, a DNA labeling dye, binds DNA noncovalently; therefore, it can leak from transplanted cells to host cells. Dil, a cell membrane labeling dye, binds to cell membrane noncovalently; therefore, it can also leak from transplanted cells to host cells. BrdU is a thymidine analog, and its detection requires harsh treatment of tissue samples. Therefore, cellular proteins can no longer be detected by IHC or immunofluorescence (IF) due to loss of antigenicity. EdU is a newer thymidine analog that requires no special tissue treatment for detection; therefore, costaining by IHC or IF for cellular proteins is feasible. However, similar to the situation with BrdU, long-term detection of transplanted cells is possible only if the cells are relatively quiescent, as the label gets diluted with each round of cell replication.

IMMUNOCOMPATIBILITY

In preclinical studies that employ rats or mice as disease models, transplantation of SCs is most commonly allogeneic. This is due to the following: (1) allogeneic transplantation requires SC isolation from as few as one animal whereas autologous transplantation requires SC isolation from each test animal and (2) vital tissues such as bone marrow and skeletal muscle cannot be harvested in sufficient quantities for autologous SC preparation without seriously harming the animals. In the case with ADSC, despite its more abundant harvestable tissue source than BMSC or SkMSC, increasingly more studies are conducting xenogeneic transplantation, nonetheless, and the donor species has been exclusively humans [173]. The reason is obviously the high availability of adipose tissues that are removed from millions of patients who elect to undergo liposuction or lipectomy. In any event, whether allogeneic or xenogeneic, studies that performed such transplantations usually do not talk about the immunocompatibility issue [173]. Thus, it cannot be certain whether the investigators were unaware of or chose to ignore such issues. The immunocompatibility issue can actually be addressed easily by citing certain published studies that focused on MSC's immunogenicity. For example, we have recently published a review article on MSC's immunocompatibility issues [173], and although the MSC in question is ADSC, the discussion is actually applicable to all MSCs. This review article itself or some of its referenced studies can be cited to explain why MSCs can be transplanted allogeneically or xenogeneically in immunocompetent recipients without the use of immunosuppressants. Briefly, MSCs have been rather consistently shown to possess immunosuppressive and immunomodulatory properties, and there is also convincing evidence that MSCs do not express major histocompatibility complex-II and therefore elicit no immune reaction when transplanted allogeneically or xenogeneically. For concerns that animal studies may not translate into human outcomes, a recently published phase 1/2 clinical study [174] can be a helpful reference. In this study, 30 patients with ischemic cardiomyopathy were equally randomized into an allogeneic and an autologous groups for transendocardial BMSC injection. The resulting findings are (1) a satisfactory safety profile for both groups, (2) improvement in structural and functional cardiac measures for both groups, and (3) low (3.7%) alloimmune reactions in patients receiving allogeneic MSCs.

STEM CELL TRANSPLANTATION

IC injection of erectogenic agents is a well-established method to induce erection in ED patients; therefore, in the first SC-for-ED study we tested whether IC injection of SCs could treat CN injury ED in rats [94]. Meanwhile, because CNs originate from MPG, we also tested intra-MPG injection of SCs. As the results showed that both transplantation routes were equally effective in treating CN injury ED, and due to the fact that IC injection is easier to perform than intra-MPG injection, IC injection has become the preferred method for the transplantation of SC into CN-injury and other types of ED animal models (25 out of 35 studies). However, it should be pointed out that CN injury causes pathological changes in the MPG; therefore, for treating CN injury, IC injected SCs need to be able to migrate to the MPG and/or release soluble factors that can reach the MPG via blood flow. Such therapeutic mechanisms have received supports from our studies that showed (1) IC injected ADSCs can migrate to the MPG in response to CN injury

[101,175], (2) cultured ADSCs abundantly secrete CXCL5 cytokine, and (3) CXCL5 possesses both angiogenic and neurotrophic properties [176, 177].

As intra-MPG injection is less clinically feasible than IC injection, it has not been used again until recently in which CN injury ED was the treatment target [102]. While positive outcomes were reported, no reason was given as to why choosing this more difficult injection method. In any event, the same group of researchers also tested other transplantation methods in three additional CN injury ED studies. Specifically, SCs were applied to the injured CNs and then covered with a scaffold material of either poly (lactic-co-glycolic acid) (PLGA) or hydrogel [104, 107, 108]. While positive outcomes were observed, it is presently unknown whether this scaffold approach is better than IC injection in terms of treatment efficacy. In three other CN injury-ED studies by two other research groups, SCs were injected periprostatically with [109,110] or without [111] concomitant IC injection. Direct comparison showed that periprostatic and IC injections produced similar therapeutic effects, but concomitant periprostatic and IC injections did not produce better outcomes than either injection alone [110].

Autologous nerve graft has been tested for the repair of damaged CN [178, 179]. However, the harvest of autologous nerves causes donor site morbidity. Thus, in a recently published study we tested whether acellular matrix seeded with SCs can be used as a nerve graft for CN repair [99]. Specifically, based on consideration that large quantities of adipose tissue are routinely removed from plastic surgery patients, we proposed that such "medical wastes" could be processed into acellular matrix for the seeding of ADSCs. Grafting of the seeded matrix to repair resected CNs resulted in improved erectile function that slightly missed statistical significance (, due to large variations). Thus, we believe that the approach is feasible but requires improvements in fabrication of the acellular matrix.

We have previously shown that both intraorgan (urinary bladder or urethra) and intravenous (IV) injections of ADSCs improved urinary function in rat models of stress urinary incontinence and detrusor overactivity [180, 181]. In a more recent study we showed that IV injection of ADSC also improved erectile function in post-RT ED rats [105]. Thus, IV injection appears to be a feasible option for SC transplantation. TA reconstruction with grafts is often performed on PD patients with large plaques. However, the procedure is associated with postoperation complications, such as ED. In a recent study, TA reconstruction with ADSC-seeded SIS was found to have a lower rate of ED complication than using unseeded SIS [78]. In another recent study, ADSC was injected into the TA that was undergoing fibrotic changes due to a prior TGF- injection [79]. This intratunical ADSC injection resulted in significantly less TA fibrosis and better erectile function when compared to intratunical saline injection.

FUNCTIONAL ASSESSMENT

Whether SC treatment improves erectile function is most commonly assessed at 4 weeks after treatment by measurement of intracavernous pressure (ICP) in response to electrostimulation of CN. Such stimulation mimics sexual stimulation and causes an increase of ICP that can approach systemic blood pressure. In fact, to account for variations in individual animal's systemic blood pressure, ICP is often normalized to mean arterial pressure (MAP). Thus, after the animal is anesthetized, a 25 G needle connected to a heparin-filled PE-50 tubing is inserted into the aortic bifurcation, the carotid artery, or the femoral artery for the measurement of MAP, and another similarly connected 25 G needle is inserted into the crura for the measurement of ICP. The MAP and ICP values are acquired via a pressure transducer connected to a data acquisition system. Electrostimulation is applied through a stainless steel bipolar hook placed on the CN approximately 5 mm distal to the MPG. Electricity is typically applied at a fixed frequency of 20 Hz, pulse width of 0.2 ms, and duration of 50 seconds. Three different amperage settings of 0.5, 1, and 1.5 mA are typically tested to obtain a range of erectile responses, and in between stimulations a rest period of 5–10 min is allowed for the CN to recover.

HISTOLOGICAL ASSESSMENT

The above-described functional assessment requires laparotomy followed by sacrificing the animal. The sacrificed animal is then subjected to the harvest of the penis, MPG, and any other tissues of interest. These tissues are then assessed histologically by IHC, IF, and/ or chemical staining. In the penis, IHC or IF staining is routinely used to assess the three key structures that regulate penile erection, namely, CEC, CSMC, and CN. The most commonly used markers for CEC are CD31, eNOS, RECA-1, and vWF. CN is mostly commonly evaluated by IHC or IF staining for the expression of nNOS in the dorsal nerves. For CSMC, the most commonly used method is IHC or IF staining for -smooth muscle actin. However, we have recently reported that staining with Alexa fluor-conjugated phalloidin was easier and quicker, and the resulting images were superior [18]. Masson's trichrome staining has also been commonly used to assess CSMC although the resulting red stains actually represent not only CSMC but also CEC, fibroblasts, and any other cells. For PD-related studies, the assessment of TA is usually done by trichrome staining or by IHC or IF staining for collagen-I and elastin. For studies using CN injury models, the examination of MPG is usually accomplished by IHC or IF staining for S100, neurofilaments, or other neural markers.

A few earlier SC-for-ED studies have attempted to identify transplanted SCs through histological examination of penile tissues. However, molecules or agents that were used to prelabel SCs all have inherent shortcomings [126]. In addition, we have shown that IC transplanted SCs quickly disappeared from penile tissues [101, 175]. As such, few recent studies have reported cell tracking data.

MAIN OUTCOMES

Up to November 2013 a total of 35 SC-for-ED studies have been published, and 29 of them are concerned with either CN injury (19 studies) or DM (10 studies). So, the discussion of SC-for-ED studies' main outcomes will be divided according to these two types of ED.

Diabetic ED

The first such studies were published in 2010, both dealing with T2DM, with one being clinical trial and the other preclinical. The clinical trial was carried out in Korea and involved treating each of seven T2DM patients (57 to 87 years of age) with IC injection of 15 million allogeneic UCBSCs [80]. At one month after treatment, three patients regained morning erection, and at 3 months, three additional patients regained morning erection. However, despite having increased penile rigidity, these patients were still unable to achieve vaginal penetration unless taking sildenafil before coitus. Nevertheless, at 11-month follow-up, one patient was able to maintain sufficient erection for coitus. Interestingly, all patients except the oldest had reduced levels of blood glucose and glycosylated hemoglobin, suggesting SC therapy might have antidiabetes effects, and supporting our observation that IC injection is a systemic application (see Stem Cell Transplantation).

The preclinical study was conducted by our group [85] and it utilized the ZDF rats, which were found to develop T2DM within the first 10 weeks of age and to develop ED at 22 weeks of age. These T2DM-ED rats were randomized for treatment with IC injection of autologous ADSC or with saline. Three weeks later, the ADSC-treated rats were found to have significantly higher ICP/MAP values than the saline-treated rats. Histological examination of erectile tissue also found that ADSC-treated rats had lower levels of apoptosis and higher numbers of endothelia cells and nNOS-positive nerves.

Apart from the two studies mentioned above, all SC-for-diabetic ED studies employed STZ-induced T1DM animal models. In one of two studies published in 2011, Gou et al. [86] reported using IC injection of VEGF-transfected allogeneic EPC to treat diabetic ED in rats. While the cell may actually be BMMNC (see Endothelial Progenitor Cell), ICP values obtained at 3 weeks after treatment were 56.22, 20.46, and 20.24 for rats treated with VEGF-transfected cell, blank vector-transfected cell, and untransfected cell, respectively. However, it should be noted that there were no normal or untreated controls; therefore, it cannot be determined whether the ICP value of 56.22 indicates treatment efficacy, or whether the ICP values of 20.46 and 20.24 indicate treatment inefficacy. It should also be pointed out that the SCs were transfected with a VEGF-expressing plasmid; therefore, they cannot be expected to maintain VEGF expression.

In the other 2011 study Qiu et al. [87] employed IC injection of allogeneic BMSC, and ICP/MAP values obtained four weeks later were 0.8, 0.6, and 0.4 for normal (nondiabetic), BMSC-treated, and untreated rats, respectively. In 2012, the same team of researchers published a similar study, this time adding a group of rats treated with VEGF-transduced BMSC [88]. The resulting ICP/MAP values were 0.82, 0.59,

0.48, and 0.36 for normal (nondiabetic), VEGF-BMSC-treated, BMSC-treated, and untreated rats, respectively. Therefore, the two studies had similar ICP/MAP values for both the positive (nondiabetic) and negative (untreated diabetic) controls. However, the ICP/MAP value for the BMSC-treated group changed from 0.6 in 2011 to 0.48 in 2012. Thus, this discrepancy needs to be resolved before a conclusion can be made on whether VEGF transduction indeed improved therapeutic efficacy.

Three additional studies were published in 2012. Nishimatsu et al. [90] demonstrated that the therapeutic effects of IC injected allogeneic ADSC's were mediated by adrenomedullin. The study by Sun et al. [89] is unusual in that an emphasis was placed on CN nerve regeneration (as opposed to endothelial preservation or restoration) as the therapeutic mechanism for IC injected BMSC in a diabetic ED animal model. The study by Ryu et al. [91] is unique in that the animal model was murine and the treatment cell was syngeneic SVF. More importantly, this study tested SVF cells at three different dosages. While 10,000 cells had no effects, 100,000 and 200,000 improved ICP to 82% of normal control. Such data is valuable in that they validated the importance of SC and identified a potential optimal dosage.

Two studies were published in 2013. He et al. [92] reported that BMSC transduced with KCNMA1 (a potassium channel) was better than untransfected BMSC. Liu et al. [93] showed that VEGF-transduced ADSC was better than untransfected ADSC.

CN-Injury ED

The first such study transplanted BDNF-transduced ESC into a CN crush injury rat model by either IC or intra-MPG injection [94]. Erectile function was assessed by ICP measurement at 3 months, and the resulting peak ICP values (in cmH_2O) were 96.9 for sham-treated group, 30.5 for untreated group, 55.1 for intra-MPG group, and 54.1 for IC group. While both treated groups were significantly better than the untreated group, there was no significant difference between the two treated groups. Histological analysis outcomes paralleled erectile functional outcomes.

The second study transplanted allogeneic SkMSC into a CN transection injury rat model by IC injection [95]. Functional analyses at 2 and 4 weeks both showed significantly better ICP values in treated versus untreated groups. The third study transplanted allogeneic BMMNC into a 5 mm CN resection injury rat model by IC injection [96]. Functional analyses at 3 and 5 weeks both showed significantly better ICP values in treated versus untreated groups.

Two CN crush injury studies were published in 2010. One emphasized on comparing between allogeneic BMSC and a specific population of allogeneic BMSC that was selected for cell surface expression of p75 low affinity nerve growth factor receptor (p75LNGFR) [98]. The other was interested in comparing between autologous ADSC and cell lysate that was prepared from autologous ADSC [97]. Functional and histological analyses at 4 weeks showed that p75LNGFR-selected BMSC was significantly better than unselected BMSC, and ADSC and ADSC lysates were equally effective in treating CN crush injury ED. Two additional studies were published in 2011. One is similar to the abovementioned 2006 study [95], as acknowledged in its discussion, in that the same animal model (CN transection), same SC type (SkMSC), and same injection route (IC) were employed, and similar functional outcome (ICP value) obtained [100]. The other is unique in that SC was employed as seeded cells on an acellular matrix, which was then grafted to repair a 5 mm gap in resected CNs [99]. The functional outcomes were favorable but slightly missed statistical significance.

Six CN injury studies were published in each of 2012 and 2013. Three of the 2012 studies are from our group. First, Fandel et al. [101] provided the first evidence that IC injected SCs (autologous ADSCs in this case) rapidly disappeared from the injection site and migrated to MPG in CN injury rats. Second, Qiu et al. [105] for the first time established a post-RT ED as target for SC therapy and also for the first time used IV injection for SC transplantation. Third, for the first time we showed that IC injection of SCs (autologous SVF cells in this case) was able to treat both acute (immediate) and chronic (4 weeks) CN injury-induced ED [106]. This study is also the first to examine functional and histological outcomes at 3 months post-SC injection, instead of the more commonly chosen one-month time point.

The remaining three 2012 studies all investigated combinatory SC therapy. Kovanecz et al. [103] showed that IC injection of SkMSC (xenogeneic mouse cells) alone or in combination with oral sildenafil was able to normalize erectile function in CN injury rats, but the combination of SkMSC with sildenafil was not superior to SkMSC or sildenafil alone. Kim et al. [102] employed intra-MPG injection of BDNF-transduced allogeneic BMSCs; the results showed that both BMSC and BDNF-BMSC were efficacious, but the latter was better. Piao et al. [104] employed BDNF-immobilized PLGA membrane with and without ADSC (xenogeneic human cells); the results showed that the combinatory treatment was better than single-agent treatments.

The same research group that conducted the above-mentioned BDNF-BMSC and BDNF-ADSC studies published two additional CN-injury studies in 2013. The one by Jeong et al. [107] is essentially the same as Piao et al. [104], except for adding a third treatment agent, udenafil, which is a newly developed PDE5I. The other by Kim et al. [108] used NGF instead of BDNF and hydrogel instead of PLGA. In any event, all four studies conducted by this research group (2 each in 2012 and 2013) indicated that any tested agent, whether BMSC, ADSC, BDNF, NGF, hydrogel, PLGA, or udenafil, was able to provide an additional level of therapeutic efficacy.

In two separate studies [109, 110], You et al. tested human BMSC and human ADSC (thus, both were xenogeneic), respectively, for treatment of CN-injury ED in rats. These studies' novelty was the hypothesis that a combination of IC and periprostatic injections might be better than IC or periprostatic injection alone. But, while the BMSC study obtained results that supported this hypothesis, the ADSC study did not.

Choi et al. [111] recently reported the isolation of MSCs from human testes. While such cells would seem suited for treating infertility, they were tested in a CN injury rat ED model. In any event, the results showed that these cells were as effective as BMSCs in preserving erectile function, and this led the authors to conclude that these cells might represent a promising new autologous cell source for clinical use. However, it should be pointed out that in this study the SC was xenogeneic, not autologous, and if indeed future clinical application of this SC will be done autologously, patients may have difficulty deciding whether excision of their testicle tissue for SC isolation is acceptable.

The last CN injury study [112] to be discussed here performed functional and histological assessments at 3 months after IC injection of ADSC. Thus, it reinforced our earlier observation [106] that a single-bolus IC injection of autologous ADSC could preserve erectile function for a prolonged period.

THERAPEUTIC MECHANISM

MSC's therapeutic capacity has been demonstrated across all medical disciplines, but how they exert such effects remains poorly understood. As mentioned earlier in the "Stem Cell Basics" section, two seemingly opposing mechanisms, cellular differentiation and paracrine action, have been considered. For cellular differentiation as a therapeutic mechanism, direct evidence has been scarce, and the difficulty in obtaining such evidence lies with the fact that cell-tracking labels are unreliable [126] and transplanted SCs rapidly disappear from the injection site [101, 175]. Thus, most SC-for-ED studies have come to the conclusion that paracrine action was responsible for their SC's therapeutic effects. However, direct evidence for paracrine action as a therapeutic mechanism is similarly scant, as summarized below.

Kendirci et al. [98] found that rat BMSC abundantly secreted basic fibroblast growth factor in culture. Albersen et al. [97] showed that lysate preparation from ADSC was just as good as intact ADSC in repairing CN injury. And, Zhang et al. [176, 177] found that rat ADSC abundantly secreted CXCL5 in culture, and this cytokine had potent angiogenic and neurotrophic activities. Thus, these four studies provided indirect or suggestive evidence for paracrine action as a therapeutic mechanism. On the other hand, the study by Nishimatsu et al. [90] provided direct evidence by using siRNA to knock down the expression of adrenomedullin in ADSC and demonstrating that such ADSC had reduced ability to preserve erectile function in diabetic ED rats. However, it must be pointed out that in this study, ADSCs with or without adrenomedullin knockdown were cultured in a medium specifically formulated for endothelial cells, and we have shown that ADSCs cultured in this medium spontaneously differentiated into endothelial cells [182]. Therefore, while providing direct evidence for paracrine action as a therapeutic mechanism, the study might have unintentionally employed endothelially induced ADSC rather than regular (uninduced) ADSC. In another study by Ryu et al. [91] VEGF neutralizing antibody was injected subcutaneously immediately before IC injection of SVF cells in STZ-induced diabetic ED mice. Such treatment effectively abolished SVF cell-induced angiogenesis in the CC and improvement of erectile function. Thus, apart from the fact that SVF cell preparation is a mixture of ADSCs and non-SCs, this study can be considered as providing solid direct evidence for paracrine action as a mechanism for SC's therapeutic effects.

CONCLUSIONS

SC therapy for ED has been investigated in 34 preclinical studies and one clinical trial. In responding to clinical needs, 19 of these studies targeted CN injury ED and 10 diabetic ED. ADSC is the most commonly employed SC, likely due to its ease of isolation from an abundant tissue source. However, deviating from expected clinical practices, allogeneic and xenogeneic SCs have increasingly been used in these studies. The reasons are (1) autologous SCs must be isolated from each tested animal, and this usually means more than 30 SC preparations in a typical preclinical study, (2) only one SC preparation is needed for allogeneic or xenogeneic transplantation, and it can even be obtained through purchase, and (3) the abundance of lipoaspirates produced from plastic surgeries has encouraged the use of human ADSC as a convenient SC source. Regardless of the reason, when allogeneic or xenogeneic SCs are used, their immunocompatibility issue should be properly addressed.

In more recent studies, SCs tend to be modified by transfection with angiogenic or neurotrophic genes, or their transplantation supplemented with such growth factors. While these modifications and supplementations were usually reported to increase therapeutic efficacy, the degree of improvement has always been small. So, it remains to be seen whether the benefit can outweigh the risk when it comes to clinical applications. Regardless, SC transplantation has mostly been done by IC injection, but more recent studies tend to try alternative routes, such as IV injection, periprostatic injection, and scaffolding. However, with few head-on comparisons with IC injection, it remains uncertain whether these alternatives are more advantageous.

All 35 studies reported improved erectile function with SC transplantation in ED patients or animal models. But the improvement as determined by ICP measurement is usually around 70% when compared to non-ED controls. Thus, it remains to be seen whether this level of improvement is sufficient for ED patients to successfully perform intercourse. In some preclinical studies SC transplantation also resulted in improved muscle, endothelium, and/or nerve in the erectile tissue, but few of these studies reported differentiation or engraftment of the transplanted SCs. Thus, authors of these studies often stated that paracrine action was likely responsible for SC's therapeutic effects. However, while convenient, such a hypothesis has received little support from actual investigations. Therefore, in terms of improving our understanding of how SCs exert their therapeutic effects, there needs to be a shift of research effort from the current preference for functional outcomes toward mechanism findings. For example, if indeed a particular growth factor is believed to be important, it should be investigated by means of specific inhibition or blockade of its action, or by using cell lines or animals that lack its expression. Such tasks are obviously technically challenging, but if successfully executed, they can truly advance the field of SC-for-ED research.

REFERENCES

1. N. C. Panel, "Impotence," NIH Consens Statement, vol. 10, pp. 1–33, 1992.
2. B. A. Inman, J. L. St. Sauver, D. J. Jacobson et al., "A population-based, longitudinal study of erectile dysfunction and future coronary artery disease," Mayo Clinic Proceedings, vol. 84, no. 2, pp. 109–113, 2009.
3. G. Jackson, N. Boon, I. Eardley et al., "Erectile dysfunction and coronary artery disease prediction: evidence-based guidance and consensus," International Journal of Clinical Practice, vol. 64, no. 7, pp. 848–857, 2010.
4. K. Chew, J. Finn, B. Stuckey et al., "Erectile dysfunction as a predictor for subsequent atherosclerotic cardiovascular events: findings from a linked-data study," The Journal of Sexual Medicine, vol. 7, no. 1, pp. 192–202, 2010.
5. J. Dong, Y. Zhang, and L. Qin, "Erectile dysfunction and risk of cardiovascular disease: meta-analysis of prospective cohort studies," Journal of the American College of Cardiology, vol. 58, no. 13, pp. 1378–1385, 2011.
6. G. Wagner, K. S. Fugl-Meyer, and A. R. Fugl-Meyer, "Impact of erectile dysfunction on quality of life: patient and partner perspectives," International Journal of Impotence Research, vol. 12, supplement 4, pp. S144–S146, 2000.

7. J. J. Sánchez-Cruz, A. Cabrera-León, A. Martín-Morales, A. Fernández, R. Burgos, and J. Rejas, "Male erectile dysfunction and health-related quality of life," European Urology, vol. 44, no. 2, pp. 245–253, 2003.
8. T. Kushiro, A. Takahashi, F. Saito et al., "Erectile dysfunction and its influence on quality of life in patients with essential hypertension," American Journal of Hypertension, vol. 18, no. 3, pp. 427–430, 2005.
9. M. S. Sand, W. Fisher, R. Rosen, J. Heiman, and I. Eardley, "Erectile dysfunction and constructs of masculinity and quality of life in the multinational Men's Attitudes to Life Events and Sexuality (MALES) study," The Journal of Sexual Medicine, vol. 5, no. 3, pp. 583–594, 2008.
10. G. V. Fernandes, R. R. dos Santos, W. Soares et al., "The impact of erectile dysfunction on the quality of life of men undergoing hemodialysis and its association with depression," The Journal of Sexual Medicine, vol. 7, no. 12, pp. 4003–4010, 2010.
11. A. Avasthi, S. Grover, A. Bhansali et al., "Erectile dysfunction in diabetes mellitus contributes to poor quality of life," International Review of Psychiatry, vol. 23, no. 1, pp. 93–99, 2011.
12. I. A. Aytaç, J. B. McKinlay, and R. J. Krane, "The likely worldwide increase in erectile dysfunction between 1995 and 2025 and some possible policy consequences," BJU International, vol. 84, no. 1, pp. 50–56, 1999.
13. A. Melman and K. Davies, "Gene therapy for erectile dysfunction: what is the future?" Current Urology Reports, vol. 11, no. 6, pp. 421–426, 2010.
14. A. R. McCullough, J. H. Barada, A. Fawzy, A. T. Guay, and D. Hatzichristou, "Achieving treatment optimization with sildenafil citrate (Viagra) in patients with erectile dysfunction," Urology, vol. 60, no. 2, pp. 28–38, 2002.
15. M. Kendirci and W. J. G. Hellstrom, "Current concepts in the management of erectile dysfunction in men with prostate cancer," Clinical Prostate Cancer, vol. 3, no. 2, pp. 87–92, 2004.
16. V. Phé and M. Rouprêt, "Erectile dysfunction and diabetes: a review of the current evidence-based medicine and a synthesis of the main available therapies," Diabetes and Metabolism, vol. 38, no. 1, pp. 1–13, 2012.

17. T. F. Lue, "Erectile dysfunction," The New England Journal of Medicine, vol. 342, no. 24, pp. 1802–1813, 2000.
18. G. Lin, X. Qiu, T. M. Fandel et al., "Improved penile histology by phalloidin stain: circular and longitudinal cavernous smooth muscles, dual-endothelium arteries, and erectile dysfunction-associated changes," Urology, vol. 78, no. 4, pp. 970.e1–970.e8, 2011.
19. X. Qiu, T. M. Fandel, G. Lin et al., "Cavernous smooth muscle hyperplasia in a rat model of hyperlipidaemia- associated erectile dysfunction," BJU International, vol. 108, no. 11, pp. 1866–1872, 2011.
20. A. Awad, B. Alsaid, T. Bessede, S. Droupy, and G. Benoît, "Evolution in the concept of erection anatomy," Surgical and Radiologic Anatomy, vol. 33, no. 4, pp. 301–312, 2011.
21. W. G. Dail, D. Trujillo, D. de la Rosa, and G. Walton, "Autonomic innervation of reproductive organs: analysis of the neurons whose axons project in the main penile nerve in the pelvic plexus of the rat," Anatomical Record, vol. 224, no. 1, pp. 94–101, 1989.
22. C. S. Lin, "Lue TF Cyclic nucleotide signaling in vascular and cavernous smooth muscle: aging-related changes," in Advances in Cell Aging and Gerontology, E. Bittar, Ed., vol. 16, pp. 57–106, Elsevier, 2004.
23. C. Lin, G. Lin, and T. F. Lue, "Cyclic nucleotide signaling in cavernous smooth muscle," The Journal of Sexual Medicine, vol. 2, no. 4, pp. 478–491, 2005.
24. C. Lin, Z. Xin, Z. Wang, G. Lin, and T. F. Lue, "Molecular Yin and Yang of erectile function and dysfunction," Asian Journal of Andrology, vol. 10, no. 3, pp. 433–440, 2008.
25. K. J. Hurt, B. Musicki, M. A. Palese et al., "Akt-dependent phosphorylation of endothelial nitric-oxide synthase mediates penile erection," Proceedings of the National Academy of Sciences of the United States of America, vol. 99, no. 6, pp. 4061–4066, 2002.
26. T. J. Bivalacqua, M. F. Usta, H. C. Champion, P. J. Kadowitz, and W. J. G. Hellstrom, "Endothelial dysfunction in erectile dysfunction: role of the endothelium in erectile physiology and disease,"Journal of Andrology, vol. 24, pp. S17–S37, 2003.

27. A. L. Burnett, "Novel nitric oxide signaling mechanisms regulate the erectile response," International Journal of Impotence Research, vol. 16, supplement 1, pp. S15–S19, 2004.
28. G. Corona, L. Petrone, E. Mannucci et al., "Difficulties in achieving vs maintaining erection: organic, psychogenic and relational determinants," International Journal of Impotence Research, vol. 17, no. 3, pp. 252–258, 2005.
29. H. Wessells, T. H. Teal, K. Engel et al., "Fluid shear stress-induced nitric oxide production in human cavernosal endothelial cells: inhibition by hyperglycaemia," BJU International, vol. 97, no. 5, pp. 1047–1052, 2006.
30. T. Michel and O. Feron, "Nitric oxide synthases: which, where, how, and why?" The Journal of Clinical Investigation, vol. 100, no. 9, pp. 2146–2152, 1997.
31. C. Lin, A. Lau, E. Bakircioglu et al., "Analysis of neuronal nitric oxide synthase isoform expression and identification of human nNOS-μ," Biochemical and Biophysical Research Communications, vol. 253, no. 2, pp. 388–394, 1998.
32. H. Ning, X. Qiu, L. Baine, et al., "Effects of high glucose on human cavernous endothelial cells,"Urology, vol. 80, pp. 1162. e7–1162. e11, 2012.
33. C. Lin, "Phosphodiesterase type 5 regulation in the penile corpora cavernosa," The Journal of Sexual Medicine, vol. 6, supplement 3, pp. 203–209, 2009.
34. C. Lin, G. Lin, Z. Xin, and T. F. Lue, "Expression, distribution and regulation of phosphodiesterase 5,"Current Pharmaceutical Design, vol. 12, no. 27, pp. 3439–3457, 2006.
35. R. Shamloul and H. Ghanem, "Erectile dysfunction," The Lancet, vol. 381, pp. 153–165, 2013.
36. A. A. Carvalheira, N. M. Pereira, J. Maroco, et al., "Dropout in the treatment of erectile dysfunction with PDE5: a study on predictors and a qualitative analysis of reasons for discontinuation," The Journal of Sexual Medicine, vol. 9, pp. 2361–2369, 2012.
37. National Diabetes Statistics, National Diabetes Information Clearinghouse, National Institute of Diabetes and Digestive and Kidney Diseases (NIDDK), National Institutes of Health, 2011,http://diabetes.niddk.nih.gov/dm/pubs/statistics/index.aspx.

38. G. Danaei, M. M. Finucane, Y. Lu et al., "National, regional, and global trends in fasting plasma glucose and diabetes prevalence since 1980: systematic analysis of health examination surveys and epidemiological studies with 370 country-years and 2·7 million participants," The Lancet, vol. 378, no. 9785, pp. 31–40, 2011.
39. IDF Diabetes Atlas, International Diabetes Federation, http://www.idf.org/diabetesatlas/5e/the-global-burden.
40. R. W. Lewis, K. S. Fugl-Meyer, G. Corona et al., "Definitions/epidemiology/risk factors for sexual dysfunction," The Journal of Sexual Medicine, vol. 7, no. 4, pp. 1598–1607, 2010.
41. H. A. Feldman, I. Goldstein, D. G. Hatzichristou, R. J. Krane, and J. B. McKinlay, "Impotence and its medical and psychosocial correlates: results of the Massachusetts Male Aging study," Journal of Urology, vol. 151, no. 1, pp. 54–61, 1994.
42. A. Ponholzer, C. Temml, K. Mock, M. Marszalek, R. Obermayr, and S. Madersbacher, "Prevalence and risk factors for erectile dysfunction in 2869 men using a validated questionnaire," European Urology, vol. 47, no. 1, pp. 80–85, 2005.
43. V. Fonseca, A. Seftel, J. Denne, and P. Fredlund, "Impact of diabetes mellitus on the severity of erectile dysfunction and response to treatment: analysis of data from tadalafil clinical trials,"Diabetologia, vol. 47, no. 11, pp. 1914–1923, 2004.
44. D. F. Penson, D. M. Latini, D. P. Lubeck, K. L. Wallace, J. M. Henning, and T. F. Lue, "Do impotent men with diabetes have more severe erectile dysfunction and worse quality of life than the general population of impotent patients? Results from the Exploratory Comprehensive Evaluation of Erectile Dysfunction (ExCEED) database," Diabetes Care, vol. 26, no. 4, pp. 1093–1099, 2003.
45. M. Albersen, G. Lin, T. M. Fandel et al., "Functional, metabolic, and morphologic characteristics of a novel rat model of type 2 diabetes-associated erectile dysfunction," Urology, vol. 78, no. 2, pp. 476.e1–476.e8, 2011.
46. M. R. Dashwood, A. Crump, X. Shi-Wen, and A. Loesch, "Identification of neuronal nitric oxide synthase (nNOS) in human penis: a potential role of reduced neuronally-derived nitric oxide

in erectile dysfunction," Current Pharmaceutical Biotechnology, vol. 12, no. 9, pp. 1316–1321, 2011.

47. F. Zhou, H. Xin, T. Liu, et al., "Effects of icariside II on improving erectile function in rats with streptozotocin-induced diabetes," Journal of Andrology, vol. 33, pp. 832–844, 2012.
48. S. Cellek, N. A. Foxwell, and S. Moncada, "Two phases of nitrergic neuropathy in streptozotocin-induced diabetic rats," Diabetes, vol. 52, no. 9, pp. 2353–2362, 2003.
49. X. Qiu, G. Lin, Z. Xin, et al., "Effects of low-energy shockwave therapy on the erectile function and tissue of a diabetic rat model," The Journal of Sexual Medicine, vol. 10, pp. 738–746, 2013.
50. C. Costa, R. Soares, Â. Castela et al., "Increased endothelial apoptotic cell density in human diabetic erectile tissue—comparison with clinical data," The Journal of Sexual Medicine, vol. 6, no. 3, pp. 826–835, 2009.
51. H. Ning, G. Lin, T. F. Lue, et al., "A coculture system of cavernous endothelial and smooth muscle cells," International Journal of Impotence Research, vol. 25, pp. 63–68, 2013.
52. K. Park, K. S. Ryu, W. J. Li, S. W. Kim, and J. Paick, "Chronic treatment with a type 5 phosphodiesterase inhibitor suppresses apoptosis of corporal smooth muscle by potentiating Akt signalling in a rat model of diabetic erectile dysfunction," European Urology, vol. 53, no. 6, pp. 1282–1288, 2008.
53. A. Jemal, R. Siegel, J. Xu, and E. Ward, "Cancer statistics," CA Cancer Journal for Clinicians, vol. 60, no. 5, pp. 277–300, 2010.
54. J. Brandeis, C. L. Pashos, J. M. Henning, et al., "A nationwide charge comparison of the principal treatments for early stage prostate carcinoma," Cancer, vol. 89, pp. 1792–1799, 2000.
55. R. C. Dean and T. F. Lue, "Neuroregenerative strategies after radical prostatectomy," Reviews in Urology, vol. 7, supplement 2, pp. S26–S32, 2005.
56. M. Kendirci, J. Bejma, and W. J. G. Hellstrom, "Update on erectile dysfunction in prostate cancer patients," Current Opinion in Urology, vol. 16, no. 3, pp. 186–195, 2006.
57. M. J. Resnick, T. Koyama, K. H. Fan, et al., "Long-term functional outcomes after treatment for localized prostate cancer," The New England Journal of Medicine, vol. 368, pp. 436–445, 2013.

58. V. Ficarra, G. Novara, T. E. Ahlering, et al., "Systematic review and meta-analysis of studies reporting potency rates after robot-assisted radical prostatectomy," European Urology, vol. 62, pp. 418–430, 2012.
59. Y. Pardo, F. Guedea, F. Aguilo, et al., "Quality-of-life impact of primary treatments for localized prostate cancer in patients without hormonal treatment," Journal of Clinical Oncology, vol. 28, pp. 4687–4696, 2010.
60. M. Fode, D. A. Ohl, D. Ralph, et al., "Penile rehabilitation after radical prostatectomy: what the evidence really says," BJU International, vol. 112, no. 7, pp. 998–1008, 2013.
61. M. Albersen, M. Kendirci, F. van der Aa, W. J. G. Hellstrom, T. F. Lue, and J. L. Spees, "Multipotent stromal cell therapy for cavernous nerve injury-induced erectile dysfunction," The Journal of Sexual Medicine, vol. 9, no. 2, pp. 385–403, 2012.
62. M. G. Ferrini, H. H. Davila, I. Kovanecz, S. P. Sanchez, N. F. Gonzalez-Cadavid, and J. Rajfer, "Vardenafil prevents fibrosis and loss of corporal smooth muscle that occurs after bilateral cavernosal nerve resection in the rat," Urology, vol. 68, no. 2, pp. 429–435, 2006.
63. L. T. Klein, M. I. Miller, R. Buttyan et al., "Apoptosis in the rat penis after penile denervation," Journal of Urology, vol. 158, no. 2, pp. 626–630, 1997.
64. J. J. Lysiak, S. Yang, A. P. Klausner, H. Son, J. B. Tuttle, and W. D. Steers, "Tadalafil increases Akt and extracellular signal-regulated kinase 1/2 activation, and prevents apoptotic cell death in the penis following denervation," Journal of Urology, vol. 179, no. 2, pp. 779–785, 2008.
65. S. Leungwattanakij, T. J. Bivalacqua, M. F. Usta et al., "Cavernous neurotomy causes hypoxia and fibrosis in rat corpus cavernosum," Journal of Andrology, vol. 24, no. 2, pp. 239–245, 2003.
66. W. Hu, L. Hu, J. Song et al., "Fibrosis of corpus cavernosum in animals following cavernous nerve ablation," Asian Journal of Andrology, vol. 6, no. 2, pp. 111–116, 2004.
67. F. Iacono, R. Giannella, P. Somma, G. Manno, F. Fusco, and V. Mirone, "Histological alterations in cavernous tissue after radical prostatectomy," Journal of Urology, vol. 173, no. 5, pp. 1673–1676, 2005.

68. S. Carrier, H. Hricak, S.-S. Lee et al., "Radiation-induced decrease in nitric oxide synthase—containing nerves in the rat penis," Radiology, vol. 195, no. 1, pp. 95–99, 1995.

69. M. Kimura, H. Yan, Z. Rabbani et al., "Radiation-induced erectile dysfunction using prostate-confined modern radiotherapy in a rat model," The Journal of Sexual Medicine, vol. 8, no. 8, pp. 2215–2226, 2011.

70. G. Garaffa, L. W. Trost, E. C. Serefoglu, et al., "Understanding the course of Peyronie›s disease,"International Journal of Clinical Practice, vol. 67, pp. 781–788, 2013.

71. T. J. Walsh, J. M. Hotaling, T. F. Lue, et al., "How curved is too curved? The severity of penile deformity may predict sexual disability among men with Peyronie›s disease," International Journal of Impotence Research, vol. 25, pp. 109–112, 2013.

72. J. A. Lopez and J. P. Jarow, "Penile vascular evaluation of men with Peyronie›s disease," Journal of Urology, vol. 149, no. 1, pp. 53–55, 1993.

73. M. Çulha, B. Alici, O. Acar, N. Mutlu, and A. Gökalp, "The relationship between diabetes mellitus, impotence and veno-occlusive dysfunction in Peyronie›s disease patients," Urologia Internationalis, vol. 60, no. 2, pp. 101–104, 1998.

74. J. F. Stecker Jr. and C. J. Devine Jr., "Evaluation of erectile dysfunction in patients with Peyronie›s disease," Journal of Urology, vol. 132, no. 4, pp. 680–681, 1984.

75. T. J. Bivalacqua, E. K. Diner, T. E. Novak et al., "A rat model of Peyronie›s disease associated with a decrease in erectile activity and an increase in inducible nitric oxide synthase protein expression,"Journal of Urology, vol. 163, no. 6, pp. 1992–1998, 2000.

76. D. Martinez, C. E. Ercole, T. S. Hakky, et al., "Peyronie›s disease: still a surgical disease," Advances in Urology, vol. 2012, Article ID 206284, 5 pages, 2012.

77. A. Kadioglu, O. Sanli, T. Akman, et al., "Graft materials in Peyronie›s disease surgery: a comprehensive review," The Journal of Sexual Medicine, vol. 4, pp. 581–595, 2007.

78. L. Ma, Y. Yang, S. C. Sikka et al., "Adipose tissue-derived stem cell-seeded small intestinal submucosa for tunica albuginea grafting

and reconstruction," Proceedings of the National Academy of Sciences of the United States of America, vol. 109, no. 6, pp. 2090–2095, 2012.

79. F. Castiglione, P. Hedlund, F. van der Aa, et al., "Intratunical injection of human adipose tissue-derived stem cells prevents fibrosis and is associated with improved erectile function in a rat model of Peyronie›s disease," European Urology, vol. 63, pp. 551–560, 2013.

80. J. Y. Bahk, J. H. Jung, H. Han, S. K. Min, and Y. S. Lee, "Treatment of diabetic impotence with umbilical cord blood stem cell intracavernosal transplant: preliminary report of 7 cases,"Experimental and Clinical Transplantation, vol. 8, no. 2, pp. 150–160, 2010.

81. T. J. Bivalacqua, W. Deng, M. Kendirci et al., "Mesenchymal stem cells alone or ex vivo gene modified with endothelial nitric oxide synthase reverse age-associated erectile dysfunction," American Journal of Physiology—Heart and Circulatory Physiology, vol. 292, no. 3, pp. H1278–H1290, 2007.

82. G. Nolazco, I. Kovanecz, D. Vernet et al., "Effect of muscle-derived stem cells on the restoration of corpora cavernosa smooth muscle and erectile function in the aged rat," BJU International, vol. 101, no. 9, pp. 1156–1164, 2008.

83. M. T. Abdel Aziz, S. El-Haggar, T. Mostafa et al., "Effect of mesenchymal stem cell penile transplantation on erectile signaling of aged rats," Andrologia, vol. 42, no. 3, pp. 187–192, 2010.

84. Y. Huang, H. Ning, A. W. Shindel et al., "The effect of intracavernous injection of adipose tissue-derived stem cells on hyperlipidemia-associated erectile dysfunction in a rat model," The Journal of Sexual Medicine, vol. 7, no. 4, pp. 1391–1400, 2010.

85. M. M. Garcia, T. M. Fandel, G. Lin et al., "Treatment of erectile dysfunction in the obese Type 2 diabetic ZDF rat with adipose tissue-derived stem cells," The Journal of Sexual Medicine, vol. 7, no. 1, pp. 89–98, 2010.

86. X. Gou, W. He, M. Xiao et al., "Transplantation of endothelial progenitor cells transfected with VEGF165 to restore erectile

function in diabetic rats," Asian Journal of Andrology, vol. 13, no. 2, pp. 332–338, 2011.

87. X. Qiu, H. Lin, Y. Wang et al., "Intracavernous transplantation of bone marrow-derived mesenchymal stem cells restores erectile function of streptozocin-induced diabetic rats," The Journal of Sexual Medicine, vol. 8, no. 2, pp. 427–436, 2011.

88. X. Qiu, C. Sun, W. Yu et al., "Combined strategy of mesenchymal stem cell injection with vascular endothelial growth factor gene therapy for the treatment of diabetes-associated erectile dysfunction," Journal of Andrology, vol. 33, no. 1, pp. 37–44, 2012.

89. C. Sun, H. Lin, W. Yu et al., "Neurotrophic effect of bone marrow mesenchymal stem cells for erectile dysfunction in diabetic rats," International Journal of Andrology, vol. 35, pp. 601–607, 2012.

90. H. Nishimatsu, E. Suzuki, S. Kumano et al., "Adrenomedullin mediates adipose tissue-derived stem cell-induced restoration of erectile function in diabetic rats," The Journal of Sexual Medicine, vol. 9, no. 2, pp. 482–493, 2012.

91. J. K. Ryu, M. Tumurbaatar, H. R. Jin, et al., "Intracavernous delivery of freshly isolated stromal vascular fraction rescues erectile function by enhancing endothelial regeneration in the streptozotocin-induced diabetic mouse," The Journal of Sexual Medicine, vol. 9, pp. 3051–3065, 2012.

92. Y. He, W. He, G. Qin, et al., "Transplantation KCNMA1 modified bone marrow-mesenchymal stem cell therapy for diabetes mellitus-induced erectile dysfunction," Andrologia, 2013.

93. G. Liu, X. Sun, J. Bian, et al., "Correction of diabetic erectile dysfunction with adipose derived stem cells modified with the vascular endothelial growth factor gene in a rodent diabetic model," PLoS ONE, vol. 8, Article ID e72790, 2013.

94. D. Bochinski, G. T. Lin, L. Nunes et al., "The effect of neural embryonic stem cell therapy in a rat model of cavernosal nerve injury," BJU International, vol. 94, no. 6, pp. 904–909, 2004.

95. Y. Kim, F. de Miguel, I. Usiene et al., "Injection of skeletal muscle-derived cells into the penis improves erectile function," International Journal of Impotence Research, vol. 18, no. 4, pp. 329–334, 2006.

96. P. A. Fall, M. Izikki, L. Tu, et al., "Apoptosis and effects of intracavernous bone marrow cell injection in a rat model of postprostatectomy erectile dysfunction," European Urology, vol. 56, pp. 716–725, 2009.
97. M. Albersen, T. M. Fandel, G. Lin et al., "Injections of adipose tissue-derived stem cells and stem cell lysate improve recovery of erectile function in a rat model of cavernous nerve injury," The Journal of Sexual Medicine, vol. 7, no. 10, pp. 3331–3340, 2010.
98. M. Kendirci, L. Trost, B. Bakondi, M. J. Whitney, W. J. G. Hellstrom, and J. L. Spees, "Transplantation of nonhematopoietic adult bone marrow stem/progenitor cells isolated by p75 nerve growth factor receptor into the penis rescues erectile function in a rat model of cavernous nerve injury," Journal of Urology, vol. 184, no. 4, pp. 1560–1566, 2010.
99. G. Lin, M. Albersen, A. M. Harraz et al., "Cavernous nerve repair with allogenic adipose matrix and autologous adipose-derived stem cells," Urology, vol. 77, no. 6, pp. 1509.e1–1509.e8, 2011.
100. J. C. Woo, W. J. Bae, S. J. Kim et al., "Transplantation of muscle-derived stem cells into the corpus avernosum restores erectile function in a rat model of cavernous nerve injury," Korean Journal of Urology, vol. 52, no. 5, pp. 359–363, 2011.
101. T. M. Fandel, M. Albersen, G. Lin et al., "Recruitment of intracavernously injected adipose-derived stem cells to the major pelvic ganglion improves erectile function in a rat model of cavernous nerve injury," European Urology, vol. 61, no. 1, pp. 201–210, 2012.
102. S. J. Kim, S. W. Choi, K. J. Hur, et al., "Synergistic effect of mesenchymal stem cells infected with recombinant adenovirus expressing human BDNF on erectile function in a rat model of cavernous nerve injury," Korean Journal of Urology, vol. 53, pp. 726–732, 2012.
103. I. Kovanecz, S. Rivera, G. Nolazco, et al., "Separate or combined treatments with daily sildenafil, molsidomine, or muscle-derived stem cells prevent erectile dysfunction in a rat model of cavernosal nerve damage," The Journal of Sexual Medicine, vol. 9, pp. 2814–2826, 2012.
104. S. Piao, I. G. Kim, J. Y. Lee, et al., "Therapeutic effect of adipose-derived stem cells and BDNF-immobilized PLGA membrane in

a rat model of cavernous nerve injury," The Journal of Sexual Medicine, vol. 9, pp. 1968–1979, 2012.

105. X. Qiu, J. Villalta, L. Ferretti et al., "Effects of intravenous injection of adipose-derived stem cells in a rat model of radiation therapy-induced erectile dysfunction," The Journal of Sexual Medicine, vol. 9, pp. 1834–1841, 2012.
106. X. Qiu, T. M. Fandel, L. Ferretti, et al., "Both immediate and delayed intracavernous injection of autologous adipose-derived stromal vascular fraction enhances recovery of erectile function in a rat model of cavernous nerve injury," European Urology, vol. 62, pp. 720–727, 2012.
107. H. H. Jeong, S. Piao, J. N. Ha, et al., "Combined therapeutic effect of udenafil and adipose-derived stem cell (ADSC)/brain-derived neurotrophic factor (BDNF)-membrane system in a rat model of cavernous nerve injury," Urology, vol. 81, pp. 1108. E7–1108. e14, 2013.
108. I. G. Kim, S. Piao, J. Y. Lee, et al., "Effect of an adipose-derived stem cell and nerve growth factor-incorporated hydrogel on recovery of erectile function in a rat model of cavernous nerve injury,"Tissue Engineering A, vol. 19, pp. 14–23, 2013.
109. D. You, M. J. Jang, J. Lee, et al., "Periprostatic implantation of human bone marrow-derived mesenchymal stem cells potentiates recovery of erectile function by intracavernosal injection in a rat model of cavernous nerve injury," Urology, vol. 81, pp. 104–110, 2013.
110. D. You, M. J. Jang, J. Lee, et al., "Comparative analysis of periprostatic implantation and intracavernosal injection of human adipose tissue-derived stem cells for erectile function recovery in a rat model of cavernous nerve injury," Prostate, vol. 73, pp. 278–286, 2013.
111. W. Y. Choi, H. G. Jeon, Y. Chung, et al., "Isolation and characterization of novel, highly proliferative human CD34/CD73-double-positive testis-derived stem cells for cell therapy," Stem Cells and Development, vol. 22, pp. 2158–2173, 2013.
112. C.Ying, M.Yang, X.Zheng, et al., "Effects of intracavernous injection of adipose-derived stem cells on cavernous nerve regeneration in a rat model," Cellular and Molecular Neurobiology, vol. 33, pp. 233–240, 2013.

113. B. F. Koontz, H. Yan, M. Kimura, Z. Vujaskovic, C. Donatucci, and F. Yin, "Feasibility study of an intensity-modulated radiation model for the study of erectile dysfunction," The Journal of Sexual Medicine, vol. 8, no. 2, pp. 411–418, 2011.
114. G. J. van der Wielen, M. Vermeij, B. W. D. de Jong et al., "Changes in the penile arteries of the rat after fractionated irradiation of the prostate: a pilot study," The Journal of Sexual Medicine, vol. 6, no. 7, pp. 1908–1913, 2009.
115. L. da Silva Meirelles, P. C. Chagastelles, and N. B. Nardi, "Mesenchymal stem cells reside in virtually all post-natal organs and tissues," Journal of Cell Science, vol. 119, no. 11, pp. 2204–2213, 2006.
116. M. Crisan, S. Yap, L. Casteilla et al., "A perivascular origin for mesenchymal stem cells in multiple human organs," Cell Stem Cell, vol. 3, no. 3, pp. 301–313, 2008.
117. G. Lin, M. Garcia, H. Ning et al., "Defining stem and progenitor cells within adipose tissue," Stem Cells and Development, vol. 17, no. 6, pp. 1053–1063, 2008.
118. J. Braun, A. Kurtz, N. Barutcu, et al., "Concerted regulation of CD34 and CD105 accompanies mesenchymal stromal cell derivation from human adventitial stromal cell," Stem Cells and Development, vol. 22, pp. 815–827, 2013.
119. M. Corselli, C. W. Chen, B. Sun, et al., "The tunica adventitia of human arteries and veins as a source of mesenchymal stem cells," Stem Cells and Development, vol. 21, pp. 1299–1308, 2012.
120. G. Lin, Z. Xin, H. Zhang et al., "Identification of active and quiescent adipose vascular stromal cells,"Cytotherapy, vol. 14, no. 2, pp. 240–246, 2012.
121. M. Maumus, J.-A. Peyrafitte, R. D›Angelo et al., "Native human adipose stromal cells: localization, morphology and phenotype," International Journal of Obesity, vol. 35, no. 9, pp. 1141–1153, 2011.
122. L. Zimmerlin, V. S. Donnenberg, M. E. Pfeifer et al., "Stromal vascular progenitors in adult human adipose tissue," Cytometry A, vol. 77, no. 1, pp. 22–30, 2010.

123. C. S. Lin and T. F. Lue, "Defining vascular stem cells," Stem Cells and Development, vol. 22, pp. 1018–1026, 2013.
124. M. Dominici, K. Le Blanc, I. Mueller et al., "Minimal criteria for defining multipotent mesenchymal stromal cells. The International Society for Cellular Therapy position statement," Cytotherapy, vol. 8, no. 4, pp. 315–317, 2006.
125. C. S. Lin and T. F. Lue, "Adipose-derived stem cells: therapy through paracrine actions," in Stem Cells and Cancer Stem Cells, M. A. Hayat, Ed., vol. 4, pp. 203–216, Springer, New York, NY, USA, 2012.
126. C. S. Lin, Z. C. Xin, J. Dai, et al., "Commonly used mesenchymal stem cell markers and tracking labels: limitations and challenges," Histology and Histopathology, vol. 28, pp. 1109–1116, 2013.
127. C. S. Lin, H. Ning, G. Lin, et al., "Is CD34 truly a negative marker for mesenchymal stromal cells?"Cytotherapy, vol. 14, pp. 1159–1163, 2012.
128. P. J. Simmons and B. Torok-Storb, "Identification of stromal cell precursors in human bone marrow by a novel monoclonal antibody, STRO-1," Blood, vol. 78, no. 1, pp. 55–62, 1991.
129. P. J. Simmons and B. Torok-Storb, "CD34 expression by stromal precursors in normal human adult bone marrow," Blood, vol. 78, no. 11, pp. 2848–2853, 1991.
130. C. M. Kolf, E. Cho, and R. S. Tuan, "Mesenchymal stromal cells. Biology of adult mesenchymal stem cells: regulation of niche, self-renewal and differentiation," Arthritis Research and Therapy, vol. 9, no. 1, pp. 204–213, 2007.
131. G. Lin, G. Liu, L. Banie et al., "Tissue distribution of mesenchymal stem cell marker stro-1," Stem Cells and Development, vol. 20, no. 10, pp. 1747–1752, 2011.
132. A. I. Caplan and D. Correa, "The MSC: an injury drugstore," Cell Stem Cell, vol. 9, no. 1, pp. 11–15, 2011.
133. D. J. Prockop and J. Y. Oh, "Medical therapies with adult stem/progenitor cells (MSCs): a backward journey from dramatic results in vivo to the cellular and molecular explanations," Journal of Cellular Biochemistry, vol. 113, no. 5, pp. 1460–1469, 2012.
134. M. B. Murphy, K. Moncivais, and A. I. Caplan, "Mesenchymal stem cells: environmentally responsive therapeutics for regenerative

medicine," Experimental & Molecular Medicine, vol. 45, article e54, 2013.

135. D. Brenin, J. Look, M. Bader, N. Hübner, G. Levan, and P. Iannaccone, "Rat embryonic stem cells: a progress report," Transplantation Proceedings, vol. 29, no. 3, pp. 1761–1765, 1997.

136. M. Kawamata and T. Ochiya, "Establishment of embryonic stem cells from rat blastocysts," Methods in Molecular Biology, vol. 597, pp. 169–177, 2010.

137. M. Schulze, H. Ungefroren, M. Bader, and F. Fändrich, "Derivation, maintenance, and characterization of rat embryonic stem cells in vitro," Methods in Molecular Biology, vol. 329, pp. 45–58, 2006.

138. H. Ning, G. Lin, T. F. Lue, and C. Lin, "Neuron-like differentiation of adipose tissue-derived stromal cells and vascular smooth muscle cells," Differentiation, vol. 74, no. 9-10, pp. 510–518, 2006.

139. A. B. Mathiasen, E. Jorgensen, A. A. Qayyum, et al., "Rationale and design of the first randomized, double-blind, placebo-controlled trial of intramyocardial injection of autologous bone-marrow derived Mesenchymal Stromal Cells in chronic ischemic Heart Failure (MSC-HF Trial)," American Heart Journal, vol. 164, pp. 285–291, 2012.

140. T. Asahara and J. M. Isner, "Endothelial progenitor cells for vascular regeneration," Journal of Hematotherapy and Stem Cell Research, vol. 11, no. 2, pp. 171–178, 2002.

141. C. Foresta, N. Caretta, A. Lana, A. Cabrelle, G. Palù, and A. Ferlin, "Circulating endothelial progenitor cells in subjects with erectile dysfunction," International Journal of Impotence Research, vol. 17, no. 3, pp. 288–290, 2005.

142. C. Foresta, N. Caretta, A. Lana et al., "Relationship between vascular damage degrees and endothelial progenitor cells in patients with erectile dysfunction: effect of vardenafil administration and PDE5 expression in the bone marrow," European Urology, vol. 51, no. 5, pp. 1411–1419, 2007.

143. C. Foresta, A. Ferlin, L. de Toni et al., "Circulating endothelial progenitor cells and endothelial function after chronic Tadalafil treatment in subjects with erectile dysfunction," International

Journal of Impotence Research, vol. 18, no. 5, pp. 484–488, 2006.

144. M. Baumhäkel, N. Werner, M. Böhm, and G. Nickenig, "Circulating endothelial progenitor cells correlate with erectile function in patients with coronary heart disease," European Heart Journal, vol. 27, no. 18, pp. 2184–2188, 2006.

145. K. Esposito, M. Ciotola, M. I. Maiorino et al., "Circulating CD34+KDR– endothelial progenitor cells correlate with erectile function and endothelial function in overweight men," The Journal of Sexual Medicine, vol. 6, no. 1, pp. 107–114, 2009.

146. T. E. Ichim Z. Zhong, N. A. Mikirova et al., "Circulating endothelial progenitor cells and erectile dysfunction: possibility of nutritional intervention?" Panminerva Medica, vol. 52, no. 2, pp. 75–80, 2010.

147. S. la Vignera, R. Condorelli, E. Vicari, R. D›Agata, and A. E. Calogero, "Circulating endothelial progenitor cells and endothelial microparticles in patients with arterial erectile dysfunction and metabolic syndrome," Journal of Andrology, vol. 33, no. 2, pp. 202–209, 2012.

148. S. la Vignera, R. Condorelli, E. Vicari, R. D›Agata, and A. Calogero, "Original immunophenotype of blood endothelial progenitor cells and microparticles in patients with isolated arterial erectile dysfunction and late onset hypogonadism: effects of androgen replacement therapy," Aging Male, vol. 14, no. 3, pp. 183–189, 2011.

149. S. la Vignera, R. A. Condorelli, E. Vicari, R. D›Agata, and A. E. Calogero, "New immunophenotype of blood endothelial progenitor cells and endothelial microparticles in patients with arterial erectile dysfunction and late-onset hypogonadism," Journal of Andrology, vol. 32, no. 5, pp. 509–517, 2011.

150. M. C. Yoder and D. A. Ingram, "Endothelial progenitor cell: ongoing controversy for defining these cells and their role in neoangiogenesis in the murine system," Current Opinion in Hematology, vol. 16, no. 4, pp. 269–273, 2009.

151. A. Mohammad and A. Shuaib, "Endothelial progenitor cells and vascular disease: are they for real?"Neurology, vol. 75, no. 23, pp. 2050–2051, 2010.

152. M. Prokopi, G. Pula, U. Mayr et al., "Proteomic analysis reveals presence of platelet microparticles in endothelial progenitor cell cultures," Blood, vol. 114, no. 3, pp. 723–732, 2009.

153. M. C. Yoder, "Is endothelium the origin of endothelial progenitor cells?" Arteriosclerosis, Thrombosis, and Vascular Biology, vol. 30, pp. 1094–1103, 2010.

154. M. R. Richardson and M. C. Yoder, "Endothelial progenitor cells: quo vadis?" Journal of Molecular and Cellular Cardiology, vol. 50, no. 2, pp. 266–272, 2011.

155. M. C. Yoder, "Endothelial progenitor cell: a blood cell by many other names may serve similar functions," Journal of Molecular Medicine, vol. 91, pp. 285–295, 2013.

156. F. Timmermans, J. Plum, M. C. Yöder, D. A. Ingram, B. Vandekerckhove, and J. Case, "Endothelial progenitor cells: identity defined?" Journal of Cellular and Molecular Medicine, vol. 13, no. 1, pp. 87–102, 2009.

157. J. Z. Shi, H. Zhang, M. Hou et al., "Is it possible to obtain "true endothelial progenitor cells" by in vitro culture of bone marrow mononuclear cells?" Stem Cells and Development, vol. 16, no. 4, pp. 683–690, 2007.

158. J. L. Goldberg, M. J. Laughlin, and V. J. Pompili, "Umbilical cord blood stem cells: implications for cardiovascular regenerative medicine," Journal of Molecular and Cellular Cardiology, vol. 42, no. 5, pp. 912–920, 2007.

159. J. H. Park, I. Hwang, S. H. Hwang, et al., "Human umbilical cord blood-derived mesenchymal stem cells prevent diabetic renal injury through paracrine action," Diabetes Research and Clinical Practice, vol. 98, pp. 465–473, 2012.

160. T. Yokoyama, R. Pruchnic, J. Y. Lee et al., "Autologous primary muscle-derived cells transfer into the lower urinary tract," Tissue Engineering, vol. 7, no. 4, pp. 395–404, 2001.

161. T. Yokoyama, N. Yoshimura, R. Dhir et al., "Persistence and survival of autologous muscle derived cells versus bovine collagen as potential treatment of stress urinary incontinence," Journal of Urology, vol. 165, no. 1, pp. 271–276, 2001.

162. A. Furuta, L. K. Carr, N. Yoshimura, et al., "Advances in the understanding of sress urinary incontinence and the promise

of stem-cell therapy," Reviews in Urology, vol. 9, pp. 106–112, 2007.

163. P. A. Zuk, M. Zhu, H. Mizuno et al., "Multilineage cells from human adipose tissue: implications for cell-based therapies," Tissue Engineering, vol. 7, no. 2, pp. 211–228, 2001.
164. Y. C. Halvorsen, W. O. Wilkison, and J. M. Gimble, "Adipose-derived stromal cells—their utility and petential in bone formation," International Journal of Obesity, vol. 24, supplement 4, pp. S41–S44, 2000.
165. S. Gronthos, D. M. Franklin, H. A. Leddy, et al., "Surface protein characterization of human adipose tissue-derived stromal cells," Journal of Cellular Physiology, vol. 189, pp. 54–63, 2001.
166. Y. C. Halvorsen, A. Bond, A. Sen et al., "Thiazolidinediones and glucocorticoids synergistically induce differentiation of human adipose tissue stromal cells: biochemical, cellular, and molecular analysis,"Metabolism, vol. 50, no. 4, pp. 407–413, 2001.
167. Y.-D. C. Halvorsen, D. Franklin, A. L. Bond et al., "Extracellular matrix mineralization and osteoblast gene expression by human adipose tissue-derived stromal cells," Tissue Engineering, vol. 7, no. 6, pp. 729–741, 2001.
168. A. Sen, Y. R. Lea-Currie, D. Sujkowska, et al., "Adipogenic potential of human adipose derived stromal cells from multiple donors is heterogeneous," Journal of Cellular Biochemistry, vol. 81, pp. 312–319, 2001.
169. P. Wu, K. Sato, S. Yukawa, Y. Hikasa, and K. Kagota, "Differentiation of stromal-vascular cells isolated from canine adipose tissues in primary culture," Journal of Veterinary Medical Science, vol. 63, no. 1, pp. 17–23, 2001.
170. P. Pettersson, M. Cigolini, and L. Sjostrom, "Cells in human adipose tissue developing into adipocytes," Acta Medica Scandinavica, vol. 215, no. 5, pp. 447–451, 1984.
171. B. M. Strem, K. C. Hicok, M. Zhu et al., "Multipotential differentiation of adipose tissue-derived stem cells," Keio Journal of Medicine, vol. 54, no. 3, pp. 132–141, 2005.
172. T. K. Kim and J. H. Eberwine, "Mammalian cell transfection: the present and the future," Analytical and Bioanalytical Chemistry, vol. 397, no. 8, pp. 3173–3178, 2010.

173. C. S. Lin, G. Lin, and T. F. Lue, "Allogeneic and xenogeneic transplantation of adipose-derived stem cells in immunocompetent recipients without immunosuppressants," Stem Cells and Development, vol. 21, pp. 2770–2778, 2012.
174. J. M. Hare, J. E. Fishman, G. Gerstenblith, et al., "Comparison of allogeneic vs autologous bone marrow-derived mesenchymal stem cells delivered by transendocardial injection in patients with ischemic cardiomyopathy: the POSEIDON randomized trial," Journal of the American Medical Association, vol. 308, pp. 2369–2379, 2012.
175. G. Lin, X. Qiu, T. Fandel et al., "Tracking intracavernously injected adipose-derived stem cells to bone marrow," International Journal of Impotence Research, vol. 23, no. 6, pp. 268–275, 2011.
176. H. Zhang, H. Ning, L. Banie et al., "Adipose tissue-derived stem cells secrete CXCL5 cytokine with chemoattractant and angiogenic properties," Biochemical and Biophysical Research Communications, vol. 402, no. 3, pp. 560–564, 2010.
177. H. Zhang, R. Yang, Z. Wang, G. Lin, T. F. Lue, and C. Lin, "Adipose tissue-derived stem cells secrete CXCL5 cytokine with neurotrophic effects on cavernous nerve regeneration," The Journal of Sexual Medicine, vol. 8, no. 2, pp. 437–446, 2011.
178. E. D. Kim, R. Nath, K. M. Slawin, D. Kadmon, B. J. Miles, and P. T. Scardino, "Bilateral nerve grafting during radical retropubic prostatectomy: extended follow-up," Urology, vol. 58, no. 6, pp. 983–987, 2001.
179. B. A. Nelson, S. S. Chang, M. S. Cookson, and J. A. Smith Jr., "Morbidity and efficacy of genitofemoral nerve grafts with radical retropubic prostatectomy," Urology, vol. 67, no. 4, pp. 789–792, 2006.
180. G. Lin, G. Wang, L. Banie et al., "Treatment of stress urinary incontinence with adipose tissue-derived stem cells," Cytotherapy, vol. 12, no. 1, pp. 88–95, 2010.
181. Y. Huang, A. W. Shindel, H. Ning et al., "Adipose derived stem cells ameliorate hyperlipidemia associated detrusor overactivity in a rat model," Journal of Urology, vol. 183, no. 3, pp. 1232–1240, 2010.

182. H. Ning, G. Liu, G. Lin, R. Yang, T. F. Lue, and C. Lin, "Fibroblast growth factor 2 promotes endothelial differentiation of adipose tissue-derived stem cell," The Journal of Sexual Medicine, vol. 6, no. 4, pp. 967–979, 2009.

Chapter 2

Biochemical Alterations in Semen of Varicocele Patients: A Review of the Literature

Antonio Mancini[1], Roberto Festa[2], Sebastiano Raimondo[1], Andrea Silvestrini[3], Elena Giacchi[4], Gian Paolo Littarru[5], Alfredo Pontecorvi[1], andElisabetta Meucci[3]

[1]Division of Endocrinology, Department of Internal Medicine, Catholic University of the Sacred Heart, Rome 00168, Italy

[2]Department of Molecular Pathology, University of Marche, Ancona 60020, Italy

[3]Institute of Biochemistry and Clinical Biochemistry, Catholic University of the Sacred Heart, Rome 00168, Italy

[4]Centre for Study and Research on Natural Fertility Regulation, Catholic University of the Sacred Heart, Rome 00168, Italy

[5]Department of Biology, Biochemistry and Genetics, University of Marche, Ancona 60020, Italy

ABSTRACT

Oxidative stress is a mechanism underlying different kinds of infertility in human males. However, different results can be observed in relation to the method used for its evaluation. Varicocele patients show a number of biochemical abnormalities, including an altered distribution of coenzyme Q between seminal plasma and sperm cells and also an apparent defect in the utilization of antioxidants. Moreover, an influence of systemic hormones on seminal antioxidant system was observed too. Finally, the effects of surgical treatment on oxidativestress indexes and the possible usefulness of some medical therapies, like coenzyme Q supplementation, are discussed. In conclusion, published data show a role of oxidative stress in varicocele-related male infertility, but at present we do not know the precise molecular mechanisms underlying these phenomena.

OXIDATIVE STRESS IN MALE INFERTILITY

An excess of reactive oxygen species (ROS) and other oxidant radicals, in the body but in particular at genital level, has been associated with male infertility [1–5]. The high content of polyunsaturated fatty acids within the spermatozoa plasma membrane and the low concentration of cytoplasmic scavenging enzymes make these cells highly susceptible to peroxidation in the presence of high levels of ROS in seminal fluid [6–8]. It has been shown that the time of permanence of spermatozoa in the epididymis is longer in oligozoospermic patients, resulting in a higher exposure to ROS [9–11]. The source of ROS in seminal fluid is due to both sperm cells and infiltrating leukocytes [12]. There is also a correlation between leukocyte concentrations, ROS levels, lipid peroxidation, and functional damage [13].

To counteract the potentially damaging effects of oxidative stress (OS), sperm cells and seminal plasma are endowed with some protective antioxidant systems. Spermatozoa have a rather low level of enzymatic antioxidant defence, including catalase, superoxide dismutase (SOD), and glutathione peroxidise. On the contrary, seminal plasma is well endowed with antioxidant buffer capacity [14]. The role of ascorbic acid and uric acid, among the low-molecular-weight antioxidants in seminal plasma, has also been highlighted [14].

Studies in infertile men have shown an impaired seminal plasma nonenzymatic antioxidant capacity [15]. The total oxyradical scavenging capacity (TOSC) is a recently developed assay measuring the overall capability of biological fluids or cellular antioxidants to neutralize the toxicity of various oxyradicals [16, 17]. The TOSC assay can discriminate between different forms of ROS, allowing to identify the role of specific antioxidants in the onset of pathological processes. An early application of the TOSC assay in andrology showed a reduced antioxidant efficiency in seminal fluid of infertile men with a significant correlation between the scavenging capacity of hydroxyl radicals and the parameters of sperm cell motility [18]. Another simpler method to measure the total antioxidant system (TAOS), also called total antioxidant capacity (TAC), was conceived by Rice-Evans and Miller [19]. In this method, the system metmyoglobin-H_2O_2 is used as source of radicals, which interaction with the chromogenic 2,2^{I} -azinobis-3-ethylbenzothiazoline-6-sulphonate (ABTS) generates a radical cation which is spectroscopically detectable. Antioxidants contrast this reaction, so that the lag time in the formation of $ABTS^{+0}$ is proportional to the antioxidant content. In a 2003 study, for the first time we applied this method, with minor modifications, to seminal plasma from varicocele infertile patients [20].

STUDIES WITH VARICOCELE PATIENTS

Varicocele (VAR) is a model of male infertility particularly interesting, from the andrological point of view, not only for its prevalence (19–41% of infertile men) [21] but also in relation to an open debate on the real need of surgical or sclerotherapic treatment and on its role in causing infertility. Furthermore, different studies suggest that OS is a common mechanism underlying VAR, as well as X-irradiation, exposure to environmental toxicants, or other physical conditions such as cryptorchidism. All these stress conditions can cause changes in testicular microvascular blood flow and endocrine signalling, eventually leading to germ cell apoptosis and hypospermatogenesis

[22]. Other studies suggest that VAR patients have high OS also in the case of normozoospermia. DNA fragmentation index (the percentage of sperm cells with denatured DNA), determined by flow cytometry, and the percentage of TUNEL-positive cells, another estimate of sperm DNA damage, have been found significantly greater in VAR, either with normal or abnormal semen profile, than in control fertile subjects. Likewise, ROS levels were significantly higher in both sub-groups of VAR patients [23]. Sakamoto and colleagues showed a significantly higher hexanoyl-l-lysine (HEL) concentration and SOD activity in seminal plasma in azoospermic and oligozoospermic patients; those with VAR had a significantly higher NO, HEL, and SOD activity in plasma. Oligozoospermic patients with VAR presented significantly higher IL-6 in seminal plasma. After varicocelectomy, a significant increase in sperm concentration was found together with a reduction in NO, HEL, 8-Hydroxydeoxyguanosine (8-OHdG) levels, and SOD activity, a reduction in IL-6, and a decrease in the percentage of apoptosis-positive sperm, evaluated by sperm DNA fragmentation [24].

A prospective study, before and after varicocelectomy, was also performed in subfertile patients. The parameters for evaluating OS changes were (a) 4977 bp deletion of mitochondrial DNA in sperm, as detected by PCR, (b) 8-OHdG content in spermatozoa DNA, measured by HPLC electrochemical method, (c) seminal plasma protein thiols and ascorbic acid. Varicocelectomy had a positive effect on seminal parameters in 22/30 patients, with a decrease in 4977 bp deletion of mitochondrial DNA and 8-OHdG levels, and an increase in plasma thiols and ascorbic acid. Interestingly, also in eight patients in whom semen quality did not improve after surgery, a significant decrease in 8-OHdG in sperm DNA and an increase in thiols and ascorbic acid were observed [25].

A standardized semen quality score, proposed by Pasqualotto and colleagues, applying principal component analysis to nine semen characteristics, did not show differences between infertile and fertile subjects with VAR; however, the mean quality score was lower than that in healthy controls. Moreover, the authors showed significant lower ROS-TAC scores in infertile males compared with control subjects, but the scores of non-VAR fertile subjects were not significantly different from those of fertile men with VAR [26]. Therefore, it can be reasonably hypothesized that the fertility potential in VAR can decline due to OS.

A meta-analysis has been published, collecting 23 human studies on the topic of OS in VAR-associated infertility [27], Four studies of these were selected for the similar methods of measuring ROS. The overall estimate showed higher concentrations of ROS and lower total antioxidant capacity in VAR than in controls. In the mentioned paper by Meucci et al. [20], we showed a Lag value (TAC) significantly greater in VAR patients than in non-VAR. But it should be remembered that measuring TAC is different from measuring ROS. Oligospermic VAR patients showed the greatest values of TAC. Lag and sperm motility significantly correlated in VAR normospermic patients. Follicle-stimulating hormone (FSH) showed significant inverse association with Lag in the same group. This partially unexpected results was interpreted as an ineffective utilization of antioxidants in oligospermic VAR, while in normozoospermic VAR the direct correlation between TAC and motility suggested a protective role toward sperm motility. Finally, in the same subgroup, the inverse correlation with FSH suggested a better utilization of antioxidants thanks to the increasing FSH levels, with a compensation with still unknown mechanisms. However, in the light of the last studies, sperm density could be seen as a factor of antioxidant consumption.

Another important antioxidant is the lipophilic molecule Coenzyme Q_{10} (CoQ), also known as ubiquinone, for its ubiquitous presence in animals and different tissues. It is a component of the mitochondrial respiratory chain, therefore potentially involved in spermatozoa function both for energetic and antioxidant properties. We assayed for the first time CoQ levels both in total seminal fluid and in seminal plasma (obtained by centrifugation) [28]. In this original study, conducted on 77 subjects with normal or pathological findings at a standard semen analysis (according to WHO criteria [29]), CoQ levels, measured by HPLC, showed a significant correlation with sperm count and sperm motility. However VAR patients represented an interesting exception; in fact in these patients the correlation with sperm concentration was preserved, whereas the correlation with sperm motility was lacking. Moreover, they showed an increased plasma to total seminal CoQ ratio in comparison with the other subjects. We suggested a possible molecular defect in VAR; a relative deficiency or a defective utilization of CoQ in sperm cells could contribute to the respiratory chain defect reported in spermatozoa of these subjects, where a reduction in O_2 consumption had been showed [30].

In a following study, we also determined CoQ in the cell pellet of spermatozoa, obtained after centrifugation of semen [31]. We found, once again, a differential pattern in VAR and non-VAR subjects. In non-VAR, a higher concentration of CoQ (expressed as ng per million of cells) was present in the spermatozoa of oligo- and asthenozoospermic patients. This relationship was not observed in VAR, who also showed slightly lower intracellular absolute values of CoQ. Since CoQ is involved in the cell defence against free radical damage, a higher intracellular concentration may represent a mechanism of protection for spermatozoa. In VAR patients, this mechanism seems to be defective, leading to higher sensitivity to oxidative damage. The results were confirmed in extended groups of patients, compared to controls, matched with VAR according to seminal parameters (idiopathic oligozoospermia, isolated asthenozoospermia, normal fertile men) [32]. We remarked the significantly higher proportion of CoQ in seminal plasma; as it reflects an interchange between intra- and extracellular compartments, the different distribution in VAR patients could represent a greater sensitivity to peroxidative damage and could suggest its reduced utilization for energy and therefore a defective motility even in patients with normal sperm count.

More recently, we studied a group of unselected infertile patients (n = 100; divided into 3 subgroups: VAR, infections, other etiologies) and 31 fertile men, also correlating Lag values (TAC) with circulating hormones: gonadotropins, testosterone, estradiol, fT3, fT4, TSH, and prolactin (PRL) [33]. We confirmed the finding of a higher TAC in VAR than controls, while lower values were in patients with inflammation. The regression analysis between hormones and seminal parameters showed an inverse correlation between PRL and sperm motility and a direct correlation of TAC with PRL or fT4, but not with gonadotropins or gonadal steroids. Interesting was the suggestion that systemic hormones may play a role in regulating seminal TAC, even hormones, such as thyroid ones and prolactin, which are not usually tested in the first-level evaluation of male patients with fertility problems. Figure 1 shows the main results found in that study, with respect to TAC differences in the various groups.

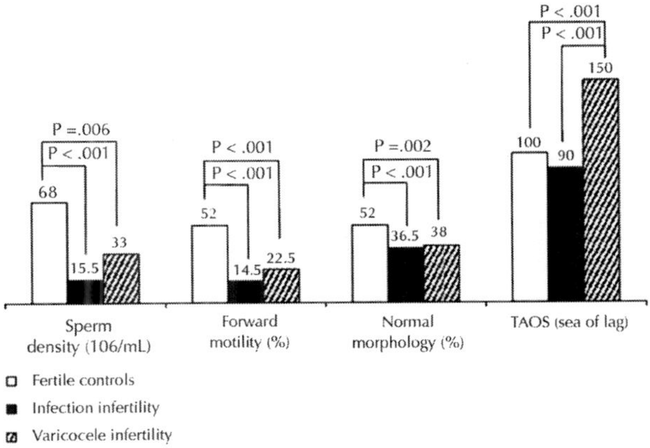

Figure 1: Standard sperm analysis and total antioxidant status (values are medians; data from [33]).

In another study, a multivariate analysis, including FSH, Lag, percentage of forward-progressive spermatozoa, oligozoospermia, and VAR, had showed a strong inverse correlation between FSH and motility ($r^2 = 0.31$, $P > F = 0.0007$), not modified by Lag ($r^2 = 0.31$, $P > F = 0.002$) suggesting that the link between FSH levels and sperm motility is probably represented by the length of Lag phase, suggesting a compensatory role of FSH in modulating antioxidant systems [34].

EFFECTS OF SURGICAL TREATMENT

The effect of varicocelectomy on OS, similarly, is not so univocally clear. Vitamin E has been demonstrated to be positively affected by surgical VAR repair [35]. The relationship between varicocelectomy and plasma OS has been studied also in children (10–16 years) with left-sided VAR and ipsilateral testicular hypoplasia, by evaluating basal (presurgery) thiobarbituric acid reactive substances and plasma peroxidation susceptibility (lag time and slope) both in peripheral blood samples and in samples from the pampinous plexus. Peripheral blood samples were re-evaluated 1 year after surgery. Both parameters were comparable in peripheral and pampinous blood and higher compared with controls. After surgery they significantly decreased, again suggesting that surgical varicocelectomy with a venous shunt construction reduces OS. The study highlights that OS is present in children and adolescents with VAR [36].

Our group also studied VAR patients in an attempt to verify whether varicocelectomy had an effect on CoQ distribution in seminal fluid [37]. Only a partial reversion was observed, since the seminal plasma CoQ/total CoQ ratio (higher in VAR vs controls) decreased, but the correlation between total CoQ and motility was not restored; instead, a peculiar correlation between cellular CoQ and motility (an inverse correlation, observed at variance with normal subjects, before surgery) was no longer detectable in postoperative VAR patients.

EFFECTS OF EXOGENOUS COQ TREATMENT

The findings mentioned in the previous paragraphs constitute the rationale for treating infertile subjects, particularly VAR, with exogenous CoQ.

Lewin and Lavon [38] originally reported the effect of CoQ on sperm motility in vitro: a significant increase in motility had been observed in sperm obtained from asthenozoospermic men, incubated with exogenous CoQ, whereas no significant variation was reported in the motility of sperm cells from normal subjects. The same study also reported the effect of exogenous CoQ in vivo, in a group of patients with low fertilization rates, after in vitro fertilization with intracytoplasmatic sperm injection for male factor infertility. No significant changes were reported in most sperm parameters, but a significant improvement was noticed in the fertilization rate after a treatment with CoQ at the dosage of 60 mg/day for a mean period of 103 days.

To investigate a potential therapeutic role, Balercia et colleagues administered CoQ to a group of 22 idiopathic asthenozoospermic infertile patients [39], classified according to WHO-1999 criteria [29]. Patients were given CoQ, 200 mg/day divided into two doses per os, for 6 months. Semen analysis, including computer-assisted sperm analysis and motility (C.A.S.A.), CoQ, and phosphatidylcholine assays, were performed at baseline and after 6 months of therapy. A semen analysis was further performed after 6 months from interruption of therapy (wash-out). After treatment, an increase in CoQ and phosphatidylcholine concentrations were found both in seminal plasma and in sperm cells. Regarding semen, a significant difference was found in forward motility of sperm cells after 6 months of CoQ oral supplementation. But the main result was the improvement of sperm motility, also confirmed by means of computer-assisted determination of kinetic parameters (significant increase of VCL and VSL). A positive dependence (using the Cramer's index of association) was evident among the relative variations of seminal plasma or intracellular CoQ content and of C.A.S.A. kinetic parameters (Cramer's V 1/4 0.4637; 0.3818; 0.3467; 0.5148, resp.). A significant reduction in sperm forward motility was reported after 6 months of washout, whereas no significant differences were found in sperm cells concentration and morphology. These results constitute the first demonstration that exogenous administration of CoQ increases its levels in seminal plasma and in spermatozoa. The increment was important, especially in seminal plasma where posttreatment levels were three times higher than basal ones. Similar increases of CoQ concentration (two-threefold higher than baseline value) are commonly found in blood plasma after chronic administration of the quinone [40].

As CoQ is a highly lipophylic molecule, we could reasonably hypothesize its diffusion through the phospholipid bilayer of cellular membranes, but we presently do not know whether transport from blood plasma to testicular and accessory male genital glands is passive or involves an active mechanism. Nevertheless, the good degree of association among these variables, according to Cramer's V index of association, supports the hypothesis of a pathogenetic role of CoQ in asthenozoospermia, according to previously reported data [32]. Apparent improvement of the spontaneous pregnancy rate, even though this was not a primary endpoint of the study, also suggests that this therapeutic approach may be beneficial.

These results were confirmed by a double-blind placebo-controlled clinical trial, realized by the same group [41], using CoQ dosage similar to that used in the previous open trial on male infertility. The study design was: 1 month run in, 6 months of therapy (30 patients) or placebo (30 patients), and a further 3-month followup. The study confirmed the increase in CoQ levels both in seminal plasma and sperm cells; also CoQH (the reduced form of CoQ, with a higher antioxidant efficacy) showed a similar increase. A significant improvement of sperm cell total motility and forward motility was observed in the treated group after 6 months of CoQ administration. The improvement of sperm cell kinetic parameters was also confirmed after computer-assisted analysis, with a significant increase both in VCL and VSL after treatment. Moreover, patients with lower baseline value of motility and lower levels of CoQ had a statistically significant higher probability to be responders to the treatment. Wash-out data confirmed the expected treatment-related results. Nine spontaneous pregnancies were achieved during the observation period. After opening the randomisation list, it was found that six of the patients who had impregnated their female partner had undergone CoQ therapy (three after 4 months, one after 5 months and one after 6 months of treatment). Three pregnancies occurred in partners of patients undergoing placebo treatment: one after 2 months of treatment and the other 2 after 3 months of washout.

A positive effect of CoQ treatment on sperm features was also confirmed in a study by Safarinejad [42], in which 212 infertile men with idiopathic oligoastenospermia were treated either with CoQ (300 mg/day) or placebo. Treatment lasted 26 weeks and was followed by a 30-week washout. Significant improvement in sperm concentration and motility was found with CoQ therapy for both parameters. The Kruger classification sperm morphology revealed an increase in the percent of normal forms in the CoQ group. The CoQ group also showed a significant decrease in serum FSH and LH at 26-week treatment phase. By the end of treatment phase, percentage of acrosome reaction increased in the CoQ group whereas it remained unchanged in the placebo group. Monitoring pregnancy rate was not among the aims of this study.

Taken together, these studies show an improved sperm motility upon exogenous CoQ administration, which could be explained on the basis of the well known involvement of CoQ in mitochondrial bioenergetics and of its widely recognized antioxidant properties. The increased concentration of CoQ in seminal plasma and sperm cells, the improvement of semen kinetic features after treatment, and the evidence of a direct correlation between CoQ concentrations and sperm motility strongly support a direct cause/effect relationship.

CONCLUSIONS

Even if it is clear that Oxidative Stress is present in varicocele as a pathogenic mechanism, however the interpretation of analytical data is not so simple. In fact, antioxidants values can be influenced by different modulatory factors, and anyway they always represent the balance between synthesis and utilization.

A deeper insight into these molecular mechanisms could lead to a greater knowledge of the so-called unexplained infertility. However, different aspects of varicocele physiopathology need to be still investigated, including the age-related effect of oxidative stress, the biochemical composition of seminal plasma.

These data are waiting for being integrated with the novel approaches to infertility studies including genetic and proteomic investigation, which can further clarify to what extent varicocele can affect sperm function and which predictive values we can dispose to better give an indication to surgical or medical therapy in such a condition.

REFERENCES

1. R. J. Aitken, J. S. Clarkson, and S. Fishel, "Generation of reactive oxygen species, lipid peroxidation, and human sperm function," Biology of Reproduction, vol. 40, no. 1, pp. 183–197, 1989.
2. R. J. Aitken, M. A. Baker, G. N. de Iuiliis, and B. Nixon, "New insights into sperm physiology and pathology," Handbook of Experimental Pharmacology, vol. 198, pp. 99–115, 2010.
3. N. Desai, E. Sabanegh Jr., T. Kim, and A. Agarwal, "Free radical theory of aging: implications in male infertility," Urology, vol. 75, no. 1, pp. 14–19, 2010.
4. F. Deepinder, M. Cocuzza, and A. Agarwal, "Should seminal oxidative stress measurement be offered routinely to men presenting for infertility evaluation," Endocrine Practice, vol. 14, no. 4, pp. 484–491, 2008.
5. G. Balercia, S. Moretti, A. Vignini et al., "Role of nitric oxide concentrations on human sperm motility,"Journal of Andrology, vol. 25, no. 2, pp. 245–249, 2004.
6. R. Jones, T. Mann, and R. Sherins, "Peroxidative breakdown of phospholipids in human spermatozoa, spermicidal properties of fatty acid peroxides, and protective action of seminal plasma," Fertility and Sterility, vol. 31, no. 5, pp. 531–537, 1979.

7. R. J. Aitken and J. S. Clarkson, "Cellular basis of defective sperm function and its association with the genesis of reactive oxygen species by human spermatozoa," Journal of Reproduction and Fertility, vol. 81, no. 2, pp. 459–469, 1987.
8. R. K. Sharma and A. Agarwal, "Role of reactive oxygen species in male infertility," Urology, vol. 48, no. 6, pp. 835–850, 1996.
9. H. Wolff, J. A. Politch, A. Martinez, F. Haimovici, J. A. Hill, and D. J. Anderson, "Leukocytospermia is associated with poor semen quality," Fertility and Sterility, vol. 53, no. 3, pp. 528–536, 1990.
10. L. Johnson and D. D. Varner, "Effect of daily spermatozoan production but not age on transit time of spermatozoa through the human epididymis," Biology of Reproduction, vol. 39, no. 4, pp. 812–817, 1988.
11. W. C. L. Ford and K. Whittington, "Antioxidant treatment for male subfertility: a promise that remains unfulfilled," Human Reproduction, vol. 13, no. 6, pp. 1416–1419, 1998.
12. R. J. Aitken, D. W. Buckingham, J. Brindle, E. Gomez, H. W. Baker, and D. S. Irvine, "Analysis of sperm movement in relation to the oxidative stress created by leukocytes in washed sperm preparations and seminal plasma," Human Reproduction, vol. 10, no. 8, pp. 2061–2071, 1995.
13. R. J. Aitken, K. West, and D. Buckingham, "Leukocytic infiltration into the human ejaculate and its association with semen quality, oxidative stress, and sperm function," Journal of Andrology, vol. 15, no. 4, pp. 343–352, 1994.
14. R. Smith, D. Vantman, J. Ponce, J. Escobar, and E. Lissi, "Total antioxidant capacity of human seminal plasma," Human Reproduction, vol. 11, no. 8, pp. 1655–1660, 1996.
15. S. E. Lewis, P. M. Boyle, K. A. McKinney, I. S. Young, and W. Thompson, "Total antioxidant capacity of seminal plasma is different in fertile and infertile men," Fertility and Sterility, vol. 64, no. 4, pp. 868–870, 1995.
16. G. W. Winston, F. Regoli, A. J. Dugas Jr., J. H. Fong, and K. A. Blanchard, "A rapid gas chromatographic assay for determining oxyradical scavenging capacity of antioxidants and biological fluids," Free Radical Biology and Medicine, vol. 24, no. 3, pp. 480–493, 1998.

17. F. Regoli and G. W. Winston, "Quantification of total oxidant scavenging capacity (TOSC) of antioxidants for peroxynitrite, peroxyl radicals, and hydroxyl radicals," Toxicology and Applied Pharmacology, vol. 156, no. 2, pp. 96–105, 1999.
18. G. Balercia, F. Mantero, T. Armeni, G. Principato, and F. Regoli, "Oxyradical scavenging capacity toward different reactive species in seminal plasma and sperm cells. A possible influence on kinetic parameters," Clinical Chemistry and Laboratory Medicine, vol. 41, no. 1, pp. 13–19, 2003.
19. C. Rice-Evans and N. J. Miller, "Total antioxidant status in plasma and body fluids," Methods in Enzymology, vol. 234, pp. 279–293, 1994.
20. E. Meucci, D. Milardi, A. Mordente et al., "Total antioxidant capacity in patients with varicoceles,"Fertility and Sterility, vol. 79, no. 3, pp. 1577–1583, 2003.
21. C. K. Naughton, A. K. Nangia, and A. Agarwal, "Pathophysiology of varicoceles in male infertility,"Human Reproduction Update, vol. 7, no. 5, pp. 473–481, 2001.
22. T. T. Turner and J. J. Lysiak, "Oxidative stress: a common factor in testicular dysfunction," Journal of Andrology, vol. 29, no. 5, pp. 488–498, 2008.
23. R. Smith, H. Kaune, D. Parodi et al., "Increased sperm DNA damage in patients with varicocele: relationship with seminal oxidative stress," Human Reproduction, vol. 21, no. 4, pp. 986–993, 2006.
24. Y. Sakamoto, T. Ishikawa, Y. Kondo, K. Yamaguchi, and M. Fujisawa, "The assessment of oxidative stress in infertile patients with varicocele," British Journal of Urology International, vol. 101, no. 12, pp. 1547–1552, 2008.
25. S. S. Chen, W. J. Huang, L. S. Chang, and Y. H. Wei, "Attenuation of oxidative stress after varicocelectomy in subfertile patients with varicocele," Journal of Urology, vol. 179, no. 2, pp. 639–642, 2008.
26. F. F. Pasqualotto, A. Sundaram, R. K. Sharma, E. Borges Jr., E. B. Pasqualotto, and A. Agarwal, "Semen quality and oxidative stress scores in fertile and infertile patients with varicocele," Fertility and Sterility, vol. 89, no. 3, pp. 602–607, 2008.

27. A. Agarwal, S. Prabakaran, and S. S. Allamaneni, "Relationship between oxidative stress, varicocele and infertility: a meta-analysis," Reproductive BioMedicine Online, vol. 12, no. 5, 2200, pp. 630–633, 2006.
28. A. Mancini, L. de Marinis, A. Oradei et al., "Coenzyme Q10 concentrations in normal and pathological human seminal fluid," Journal of Andrology, vol. 15, no. 6, pp. 591–594, 1994.
29. World Health Organization (WHO), Laboratory Manual for the Examination of Human Semen and Semen-Cervical Mucus Interaction, Cambridge University Press, Cambridge, UK, 4th edition, 1999.
30. E. de Carlo, P. Arisan, R. Mioni, and C. Foresta, "La determinazione del consumo di ossigeno nello studio del metabolismo dello spermatozoo umano," in Il Laboratorio in Andrologia, C. Foresta and C. Scandellari, Eds., pp. 55–72, Panda Edizioni, Padova, Italy, 1990.
31. A. Mancini, G. Conte, D. Milardi, L. De Marinis, and G. P. Littarru, "Relationship between sperm cell ubiquinone and seminal parameters in subjects with and without varicocele," Andrologia, vol. 30, no. 1, pp. 1–4, 1998.
32. A. Mancini, D. Milardi, G. Conte et al., "Coenzyme Q10: another biochemical alteration linked to infertility in varicocele patients?" Metabolism, vol. 52, no. 4, pp. 402–406, 2003
33. A. Mancini, R. Festa, A. Silvestrini et al., "Hormonal regulation of total antioxidant capacity in seminal plasma," Journal of Andrology, vol. 30, no. 5, pp. 534–540, 2009.
34. A. Mancini, D. Milardi, A. Bianchi et al., "Increased total antioxidant capacity in seminal plasma of varicocele patients: a multivariate analysis," Archives of Andrology, vol. 53, no. 1, pp. 37–42, 2007.
35. T. Mostafa, T. H. Anis, A. El-Nashar, H. Imam, and I. A. Othman, "Varicocelectomy reduces reactive oxygen species levels and increases antioxidant activity of seminal plasma from infertile men with varicocele," International Journal of Andrology, vol. 24, no. 5, pp. 261–265, 2001.

36. R. M. Cervellione, G. Cervato, N. Zampieri et al., "Effect of varicocelectomy on the plasma oxidative stress parameters," Journal of Pediatric Surgery, vol. 41, no. 2, pp. 403–406, 2006.
37. A. Mancini, D. Milardi, G. Conte, R. Festa, L. de Marinis, and G. P. Littarru, "Seminal antioxidants in humans: preoperative and postoperative evaluation of coenzyme Q10 in varicocele patients," Hormone and Metabolic Research, vol. 37, no. 7, pp. 428–432, 2005.
38. A. Lewin and H. Lavon, "The effect of coenzyme Q10 on sperm motility and function," Molecular Aspects of Medicine, vol. 18, supplement 1, pp. s213–s219, 1997.
39. G. Balercia, F. Mosca, F. Mantero et al., "Coenzyme Q10 supplementation in infertile men with idiopathic asthenozoospermia: an open, uncontrolled pilot study," Fertility and Sterility, vol. 81, no. 1, pp. 93–98, 2004.
40. P. Langsjoen, A. Langsjoen, R. Willis, and K. Folkers, "Treatment of hypertrophic cardiomyopathy with coenzyme Q10," Molecular Aspects of Medicine, vol. 18, supplement 1, pp. 145s–151s, 1997.
41. G. Balercia, E. Buldreghini, A. Vignini et al., "Coenzyme Q10 treatment in infertile men with idiopathic asthenozoospermia: a placebo-controlled, double-blind randomized trial," Fertility and Sterility, vol. 91, no. 5, pp. 1785–1792, 2009.
42. M. R. Safarinejad, "Efficacy of coenzyme Q10 on semen parameters, sperm function and reproductive hormones in infertile men," Journal of Urology, vol. 182, no. 1, pp. 237–248, 2009.

Chapter 3

Recent Advances in Reproductive Biotechnologies in Sheep and Goat

Basil Alexander[1, 2], Gabriela Mastromonaco[1, 3], and W. Allan King[1]

[1]Department of Biomedical Sciences, Ontario Veterinary College (OVC), University of Guelph, Ontario, Canada

[2]Department of Farm Animal Production and Health, Faculty of Veterinary Medicine and Animal Science, University of Peradeniya, Sri Lanka

[03]Reproductive Physiology, Toronto Zoo, 361A Old Finch Avenue, Scarborough, ON, M1B 5K7

ABSTRACT

This review focuses on the platform of recent advances in reproductive biotechnologies in sheep and goat. Here, we discuss some aspects of veterinary and biomedical importance in artificial insemination using sexed semen, in vitro/in vivo fertilization, interspecies in vitro fertilization, multiple ovulation and embryo transfer (MOET), somatic cell nuclear transfer and transgenic animal production in sheep and goat. Some of these technologies are already widely used in the cattle industry, and some are new to the goat and sheep industry.

INTRODUCTION

The world sheep and goat populations in 2006 were recorded as 416 and 489 million, respectively [1]. Reproductive biotechnologies are playing an increasingly important role in the production and management of these species. Animal biotechnology encompasses the application of science and engineering principles to the processing or production of materials to provide services or goods for human use [2]. Examples of current animal biotechnologies include artificial insemination using fresh, frozen or sexed semen, embryo transfer using fresh or frozen in vivo or in vitro produced embryos, cloning using somatic cell nuclear transfer procedures and production of transgenic animals. Recent advances in reproductive biotechnologies have shown important developments in the technologies and their delivery that promise to yield significant benefits for their application within the livestock industry as well as in biomedical sciences. This review focuses on the recent advances of biotechnologies in sheep and goats.

METHODS

Artificial Insemination (Ai)

Artificial insemination is the procedure involving the mechanical deposition of pre-collected semen into the uterus of an estrous female by a technician. The widespread commercial application of AI, a robust tool in livestock breeding, began in earnest in the 1950's after researchers developed methods to successfully freeze cattle semen [3]. This technology, which is the most extensively applied reproductive biotechnology in the world, has many valuable advantages such as reducing venereal diseases, rapidly increasing genetic merits of the production animals through selective breeding and eliminating lethal alleles. The potential to pass high genetic merits of a selected male to thousands of females makes this a far more efficient technology for producing large numbers (1.5 x 108) of offspring per year compared to female based technologies, such as embryo transfer (ET), which can only produce a few progeny from a selected female. More recently, the advent of separation of sperm into X- and Y-chromosome fractions using flow cytometry has added a new dimension to livestock production [4].

Since the first report of live rabbit pups of predetermined sex using X and Y-enriched sorted semen over 20 years ago [5], there have been more than 40,000 births of live animals resulting from the so- called Beltsville sperm sexing technology [4]. This sperm sexing technology has proven to be a reliable and more efficient method of obtaining predetermined sex in animals compared to other relatively wasteful methods of embryo sexing and pre-implantation genetic diagnosis [6 - 8]. Live offspring born from fresh sex- sorted semen have been reported in many species including cattle [9], pigs [10, 11], horses [12, 13] and sheep [14, 15]. As the sorting procedure can separate sperm only at a speed of approximately 10 million per hour, inseminations have to be carried out using limited numbers of sperm in each insemination dose compared to the conventional standards for AI. To obtain high success rates with sorted semen AI, most trials have been carried out using fresh sorted semen, nevertheless, use of frozen sorted semen is ultimately more beneficial to the livestock industry as it can be stored for long duration and easy to transport anywhere in the world.

Semen Sexing Technology

Semen sexing is the process of separating spermatozoa into two subpopulations containing X-chromosome and Y-chromosome bearing spermatozoa. In theory, use of the X-bearing spermatozoa fraction for insemination will result in female progeny, while the Y-bearing spermatozoa fraction will give male progeny. Considerable efforts have been made in this area over the past 30-40 years, but only recently has there been considerable progress, particularly in cattle [16]. The most commonly applied technique for the separation of a fresh semen sample into X and Y-chromosome bearing fractions is fluorescence activated cell sorting (FACS). The concept behind this technique is described below:

Fluorescence Activated Cell Sorting (FACS)

This technique involves the separation of X- and Y- bearing spermatozoa in small quantities based on the DNA content of the spermatozoa so that they can then be used in in vitro fertilization and AI programs [17]. The procedure is relatively slow and requires expensive infrastructure at least for mass scale commercial application. The technique is based on the biological principle that the DNA content of the X and Y chromosomes as X-chromosome has 3.8% more DNA than Y-chromosome [9]. This difference can, nonetheless, be detected with FACS technique. Before the spermatozoa are passed through the cell sorter, the sample is exposed to a nontoxic DNA dye that specifically binds to DNA to allow measurement of the DNA content of each spermatozoa. The cell suspension is then passed through an extremely fine nozzle that vibrates at high frequency causing the fluid stream to disperse into micro-drops which, optimally holds only one spermatozoa after the conditions are calibrated. When the stream of micro-droplets is passing through a UV laser beam, the already stained DNA will start to glow or emit fluorescence. The strength (intensity) of the florescence is measured by a detector, and if the florescence is in the range designated for the Y-bearing spermatozoa, that micro-drop is given an electric charge. Furthermore, if the intensity is within the range for X-bearing spermatozoa, the micro-drop is given an opposite electric charge. The charged micro-drops fall between two charged plates, resulting in two groups of droplets to be separated into different pools (Figure 1). Droplets that fall outside of the fluorescence range for X or Y are collected into a third group where the sex cannot be determined. The disadvantages of the technique are its relatively slow process and increased wastage of unsorted spermatozoa. The advantage is it can give up to 95% purity sexed semen samples.

Application of Sexed Semen in Goat and Sheep Production

Although the sexed semen technology is gaining in popularity in commercial cattle industries, its use has yet to be developed in the sheep and goat industries. Nevertheless recent attempts to separate the X- and Y-chromosomal fractions using flow cytometers on ram semen has been attempted and yielded fraction purity greater than 90% [18]. In flow cytometers, the sperm extending medium plays a critical role in the efficiency of separation and the viability of the sperm after sorting [17, 19, and 20]. Ram sperm have to be diluted 20- fold before sorting and a further 200-fold dilution takes place when it passes through the cell sorter resulting in capacitation-like changes that lead to reduced fertility of sexed sheep semen [17, 20]. It has also been shown that suspension of ram semen in Tries-based medium without egg- yolk, improves the staining of the DNA and efficiency of separation of sperm without reducing its viability [8, 18, 21].

When working with frozen sex- sorted semen in sheep, it is believed that the semen should be deposited in the oviduct or deep within the uterus to obtain high success rates, although it appears to be not as critical in cattle [16]. In sheep, frozen semen is usually deposited laparoscopic ally into the uterus and these same methods have been used effectively to produce offspring from frozen sexsorted semen [15]. Oviductal deposition of frozen semen in sheep is not practical if large numbers of sheep are to be inseminated. To our knowledge, there have been no reports of attempts to inseminate sheep or goat using sex- sorted semen in the cervix or transcervically.

The minimum number of sperm in an intrauterine AI dose in sheep varies between 5 x 106 and 25 x 106, but in Australia it has been suggested as 25 x 106 motile spermatozoa. Although it is not known exactly the minimum number of frozen sex-sorted sperm for intrauterine insemination of sheep, it is expected that it should be in the range of standard commercial intrauterine AI semen dose [20]. However, it is acceptable that the number of sperm in frozen sex sorted semen should be increased in line with the negative effects of the sorting process to obtain high efficiency.

The timing of AI also plays a significant role in AI success in sheep but recent findings have suggested that the best results can be achieved with sex–sorted frozen sperm when inseminated just before the expected ovulation time in ovulation- synchronized progesterone treated ewes. Using sex sorted frozen semen (40 million sperm per AI dose), optimal results can be expected when ewes are inseminated at 58 h after sponge removal or 36 h after GnRH injection [20].

Embryo Production and Transfer

Multiple ovulation and embryo transfer (MOET): This breeding model has been extensively used to multiply genetically superior goats and sheep and many protocols have been developed to optimize its application in research as well as in commercial practice [22-25]. In most domestic farm animals, especially in cattle, the genetic gain is limited on the female side due to low reproductive rate with only one calf being produced per year and also relatively long intervals between generations. To overcome these limitations MOET has been developed. Using this method, a female is hormonally stimulated to have multiple ovulations (superovulation). Most MOET programs in sheep and goat consist of a 14 to 17 day progesterone exposure, with FSH injections beginning 2 days before the removal of the progesterone releasing device. Following six or eight FSH injections given twice daily, the animals are allowed to breed naturally or by artificial insemination. The ovulated ova are allowed to fertilize in vivo following artificial insemination or natural mating. After fertilization and initiation of embryo development, 6-7 day old embryos (morula/ blastocyst stage) are recovered from within the uterus using embryo flushing techniques. In sheep, this is done surgically [26]. These embryos are then transferred to non-pregnant estrus-synchronized recipients 6-7 days post estrus or frozen in liquid nitrogen (-196i° C) for future use.

It is well-known that the superovulation protocols in small ruminants do not guarantee the recovery of quality transferable embryos due to various factors that affect the success of the program [25]. These factors can be listed as extrinsic and intrinsic factors. The extrinsic factors include: a) source and purity of the gonadotrophins, b) protocol of gonadotrophin injection, and c) the type of progesterone treatment protocol [25]. Intrinsic factors include: age, breed, nutrition and reproductive status of the animals [25]. However, despite all the achievements in the MOET programs in small ruminants so far, the success of obtaining high quality transferable embryos still remains

Figure 1: Schematic representation of the concept behind the Florescent Activated Cell Sorting technique used in separation of X- and Y-bearing chromosomes in a fresh semen sample. Low and more studies are needed to investigate the optimization of these programs.

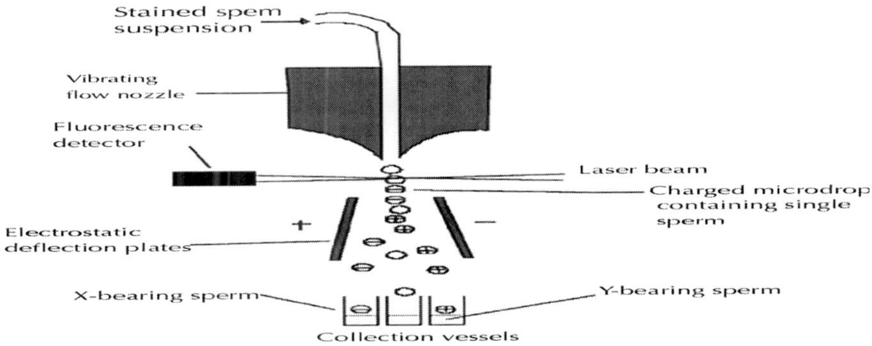

Figure 1: Schematic representation of the concept behind the Florescent Activated Cell Sorting technique used in separation of X- and Y-bearing chromosomes in a fresh semen sample.

Embryo Transfer (ET)

According to the available data from the International Embryo Transfer Society (IETS), the number of embryo transfers carried out in small ruminants is shown in Table 1. In sheep and goat, ET is usually carried out by laparoscopic surgery 6-7 days post estrus [27], (Figure 2). Estrus is generally synchronized in sheep as follows. On day-1 of the program, progesterone releasing intravaginal sponges (Veramix®, 60mg medroxyprogesterone acetate, Pharmacia & Upjohn, Orangeville, Canada) are inserted in to the vagina. On day- 14, the sponges are removed and 300 IU PMSG (Folligon®, Intervet) are injected intramuscularly to each ewe at the time of sponge withdrawal. Vasectomised rams are introduced on day-15 and ewes in estrus are identified between 12-36 h post PMSG injections. Surgical embryo transfer is then performed on day-22 of the program [27].

The embryos are usually evaluated for morphology according to the IETS criteria [28] and only the excellent quality blastocysts/ morulae are transferred into recipient ewes. Ewes are anesthetized using xylazine (0.2mg/kg) injection intravenously, and are secured on a laparoscopic cradle. An incision of approximately 1 cm is made in the skin approximately 3 cm to the left of the mid line and approximately 5 cm from the udder, using a scalpel blade (Figure 2B-D). A trochar and cannula are inserted into the abdominal cavity through the incision made in the skin (Figure 2E-F). The uterine horns and the ovaries with corpora lutea are visualized using a laparoscope (Figure 2G). The uterine horn is punctured close to the utero-tubular junction using a blunt 18-gauge needle and the embryos are loaded into an embryo transfer catheter and transferred into the lumen of the uterine horn (Figure 2H). The ewes are then monitored postoperatively for a few hours and released to the paddocks.

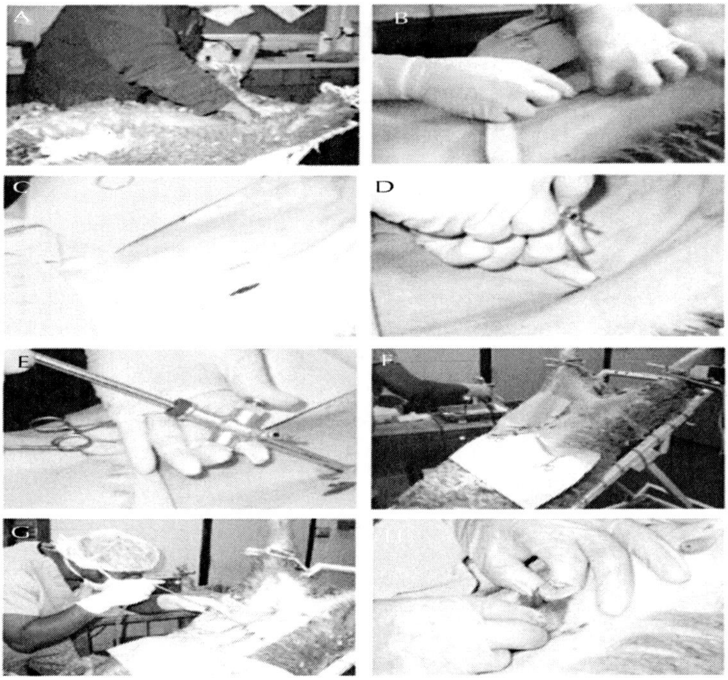

Figure 2: Embryo Transfer in sheep and goat. Embryo Transfer in sheep and goats (A–H): (A), preparation of anesthetized ewe on a cradle; (B) and (C), two skin incisions (each 1cm) are made on either side of the mid ventral line, 5 cm away from the udder; (D, E and F), insertion of trocar and cannula, cannula is left on the abdomen through which endoscope is inserted into the abdomen; (G), insertion of the endoscope through the cannula to visualize

the ovaries, corpora lutea and reproductive tract; (H), a uterine horn is punctured close to the utero-tubular junction using a blunt-end 18 Gauge needle, embryos are loaded into an ET catheter and transferred into the lumen.

Table 1: World embryo transfer activity in small ruminants in 2008

Species	**Trans-ferable embryos**	**Transferred embryos**		
		Fresh	Frozen	Total
Sheep	18828	4793	433	5226
Goat	3141	824	278	1102
Cervids	980	840	0	840

Source: Embryo transfer Newsletter, IETS, September 2009

Recently, a goat ET group in Sri Lanka reported that they have produced ET born goat kids (Figure 2B) from fresh embryos in a field embryo transfer program without using sophisticated equipment [22], thus validating the field application of the technique in veterinary practice to multiply genetically valuable goats to establish an elite goat herd under local production conditions. Moreover, ET in small ruminants is still carried out using the conventional ET techniques employing laparoscopic techniques with an average pregnancy rate of 60% with fresh embryo transfers. The pregnancy rates can vary due to many factors such as donor, recipient, embryo and operator. The transcervical ET procedure seems to be not practical in these species due to the problems associated with handling of the cervix and its anatomy. Recently, a research group [29] reported that anestrus sheep cervix can be dilated using prostaglandin 12 h prior to the insertion of AI gun into the uterus suggesting possibility of trans cervical ET in sheep. However, more studies are needed to optimize this technique in small ruminants to obtain high success rates.

In Vitro Embryo Production in Sheep and Goat

In vitro embryo production in sheep and goat provides an alternate source of low cost embryos for transfer in breeding programs such as

MOET. The process consists of 3 main steps: 1) oocyte collection and In vitro maturation (IVM) of cumulus-oocyte complexes (COCs), 2) In vitro fertilization (IVF) and 3) in vitro culture of embryos. These steps have been reviewed in detail by others [30 - 33]. Here we will highlight the important differences between species.

Oocyte Collection and In Vitro Maturation

Prior to in vitro fertilization, COCs are collected either by minimally invasive laparoscopic ovum pick up (LOPC) or postmortem from slaughtered females [32, 34]. Cumulus-oocyte complexes are collected from live sheep by a laparotomy followed by aspiration of oocytes from ovaries using an aspiration pump. This method is often called as laparoscopic ovum pick-up (LOPU) and seems to be very efficient for the recovery and quality of the COCs obtained in sheep and goats. Usually, in sheep, a short repeated gonadotrophin treatment is followed by LOPU [35-38]. In contrast, goats can be stimulated with a 'one shot' regime of gonadotropins (one shot of follicular stimulating hormone (FSH) plus equine chorionic gonadotropin (eCG), compared to the traditional multi-dose gonadotrophin regimes. The results revealed no differences in the efficiency of COCs recovered and their quality [36, 39]. It has also been shown that 'one shot' regime can be performed as a 4-day treatment regime followed by LOPU in sheep and goats without reducing the efficiency in oocyte recovery and quality [40]. The most common method of oocyte collection is from abattoir derived ovaries from sheep or goat. Ovaries are transported to the laboratory at 37°C in phosphate buffered saline (PBS) after which they are finely sliced with a scalpel blade and rinsed in oocyte collection medium consisting of 2% steer serum in Ham's F10 medium [34].

In vitro maturation of abattoir derived oocytes from sheep and goats (for comprehensive reviews see 32, 31) rely on methods based on bi-carbonate buffered TCM 199 medium supplemented with L-glutamine, ovine FSH (10 μg/ml), ovine LH (10 μg/ml, estrogen (1 μg/ml) and 10% fetal bovine serum [34]. Some researchers have used mature follicular fluid supplementation in the IVM medium to enhance the maturation of sheep oocytes [31]. Under these conditions, goat and sheep oocytes tend to extrude first polar body between 16-24 h of in vitro maturation [41]. In contrast, it is accepted that supplementation of the glutathione precursor cysteamine (100 μM) in IVM medium enhances the in vitro maturation process of goat oocytes [41]. In addition, a recent study [42] showed that cysteamine and BSA added to IVM medium for sheep, resulted in high blastocyst rates (42% blastocyst rate from total cultured oocytes) and high survival rate of blastocysts after embryo transfer. It is obvious that artificial oocyte maturation and culture systems have detrimental effects on embryo development compared to their in vivo counterparts. Recent fluorescent in situ hybridization cytogenetic studies from our laboratory using whole chromosome painting probes have revealed that high incidence of chromosomal abnormalities in sheep blastocysts derived from IVP systems, compared to in vivo derived blastoctsts [43] emphasizing the inherent differences in the two production methods.

In Vitro Fertilization

In vitro fertilization of the oocytes is usually carried out following 24 h maturation in the IVM medium. Surrounding cumulus cells are removed by gentle pippetting and washing in fertilization medium and groups of 40-50 oocytes are placed in 4-well dishes in 500 μl of synthetic oviductal fluid (SOF) covered by 200 μl of mineral oil [31,43]. Motile sperm are obtained by centrifugation of frozen-thawed semen in Percoll gradient (45%/90%) at 500 g for 10 min in room temperature. Percoll gradient separation of spermatozoa seems to be an effective means of yielding motile sperm from frozen-thawed semen [44]. Motile sperm are collected from the bottom of the 90% fraction and diluted to a concentration of 107 spermatozoa/ml in media. Recent studies have shown that incubation of spermatozoa for a further 1 h period in media supplemented with heat-inactivated estrus serum enhances the capacitation process of spermatozoa (sheep and goat : [41]; deer : [45,46]). In our laboratory we routinely add heat – inactivated sheep serum (2%) to the IVF medium and incubate oocytes with motile spermatozoa for 17 hours resulting acceptable levels of blastocyst development [43]. Although 17 h co-incubation is practiced in IVF, it has been shown that even 4 h co-incubation was enough to obtain acceptable cleavage and blastocyst rates in sheep [41]. Further application of in vitro fertilization in obtaining sex pre-determined offspring will be an advantage for the livestock industry [20, 47]. In vitro fertilization of prepubertal oocytes and oocytes recovered from LOPU [37] are also important areas to be developed further.

In Vitro Culture

Following in vitro fertilization, embryos are washed several times and then placed in in vitro culture (IVC) media for further development. There are 3 methods available for embryo culture after fertilization, such as co-culture with somatic cells, culture in semi-defined media and culture of embryos in in vivo systems (oviducts) of the same or different species [41]. Co-culture systems in sheep and goat are usually based on including oviductal cells in TCM-199 medium. Semi-defined medium is also used often in small ruminant IVC based on the components of the sheep oviductal fluid (SOF), a medium containing essential and non-essential amino acids supplemented with BSA [43,48]. In our laboratory, sheep embryos cultured in SOF medium supplemented with amino acids and BSA at 38°C in 5% O2, 5% CO2, 90% N2 humidified atmosphere resulted in 19.2% blastocyst rates from total oocytes cultured [43]. This rate is confirmed by [38], who showed that SOF culture systems supplemented with BSA and amino acids produce high quality blastocysts in sheep. Addition of fetal bovine serum (FBS) on day 2 or 3 of culture does result in high embryo survival post-embryo transfer and normal viable offspring [41]. However, some studies have reported that sheep embryos reduce their viability by 15%–25% when produced in SOF systems supplemented with serum compared to co-culture [48] or in in vivo systems of culturing the embryos in oviducts [49]. It has been noted that adding steer serum or human serum to sheep and goat IVC media may attribute to many abnormalities in the offspring [50, 51].

Interspecies in Vitro Fertilization

Investigating interspecies fertilization provides valuable insights into the role of cytoplasmic and nuclear events that regulate full term development. Due to species specific molecular, morphological and chronological markers these embryo models are unique for examining the paternal and maternal interactions and their vital role in development. Interesting findings from our laboratory revealed that ram spermatozoa is not able to fertilize bovine oocytes in vivo, however, in vitro fertilization occurs and the resulting hybrid embryos, confirmed by cytogenetic analysis (Figure 3), arrested at 4-8 cell stage [52] even when zygotes were transferred to sheep oviducts for early development. Similar developmental arrest occurs with the reverse cross. Hybridization between sheep and goats through cross or chance breeding like many species, appears to be polar with the success or efficiency dependent of the parent of origin [53]. Goats bred to rams conceive and pregnancies will progress to second trimester while in the case of the reverse cross, sheep oocytes exposed to buck sperm in vivo do not fertilize [52]. However, a few cases of sheep X goat hybrids born to goats have been documented [54]. In vitro sheep and goat oocytes, could be fertilized by buck or ram sperm and embryos developed to the blastocyst stage, hatched and, following transfer into the uteri of sheep or goats, they established pregnancies. However, retarded fetal growth, defects in placentae formation and pregnancy failure during the second month of gestation were observed [52]. The in vitro production of hybrid embryos is particularly amenable to facilitate further study of the reproductive barriers and species differences in imprinted and epigenetic, regulation of early embryo development that are key to embryo survival and development.

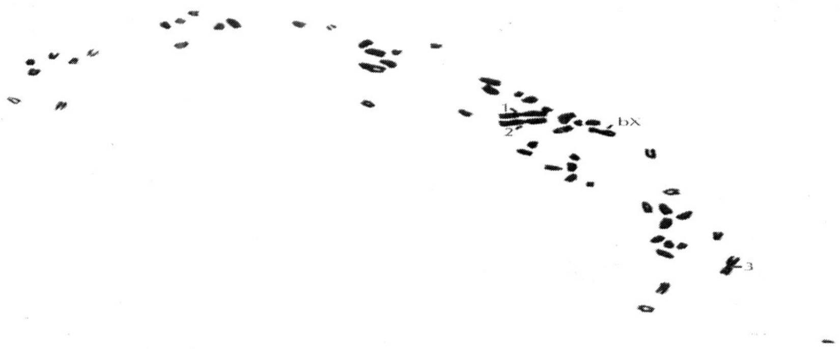

Figure 3: Metaphase spread from a 4-cell sheep-cattle hybrid embryo showing 57 chromosomes (30 cattle and 27 sheep). Note the 3 metacentric sheep chromosomes labeled 1, 2 and 3 and the cattle X chromosome labeled bX. (King and Kelk, unpublished data).

Somatic Cell Nuclear Transfer (Cloning)

A new era in reproductive biotechnology began when Wilmut and colleagues produced the first somatic cell nuclear transfer (SCNT) derived viable sheep, "Dolly", from transplanting an adult somatic cell into an enucleated sheep oocyte [55]. Following this breakthrough, theoretically, it seems to be a promising technology to produce unlimited numbers of genetic copies from an adult animal or a fetus; and so far many species including farm, pet and endangered animals have been cloned using this technology [56]. Obtaining a viable offspring through this technology still imposes a great challenge for researchers due to its relatively low success rate and in some instances compromised health status of offspring [57, 58]. At present, cloning is carried out for biomedical and research purposes, and agriculture production. Although extensive reviews are available on animal cloning, here we emphasize some recent findings that are important in small ruminant cloning.

The standard SCNT technique in sheep/goat in most of the laboratories follows some common steps such as oocyte maturation, removal of cumulus cells from oocytes, enucleation, transplantation of the somatic cell into the perivitelline space of the oocyte, electrofusion of the cell couplet, activation of the embryo and in vitro embryo culture. When the embryos develop to blastocyst, they are transplanted into the uteri of estrus-synchronized surrogate animals 6-7 day post estrus [27]. In most cases, the oocytes are collected from abattoir ovaries using the slicing method and undergo IVM for 17h (goat: [59-61], Sheep: [27, 34]). Some laboratories that conduct goat SCNT programs preferred in vivo derived oocytes either following ovulation [62, 63] or LOPU [64, 65]. This may be due to the decreased availability of goat abattoirs in different countries or the higher success rates from in vivo matured oocytes. Following maturation, the cumulus cells are removed by vortexing in 3% Sodium citrate medium [27] for 1-2 minute or in 0.01% hyaluronidase. Cumulus –free oocytes with first polar body extrusion are selected and after a short exposure to cytochalasin B and Hoechst stain, enucleation is carried out in a micromanipulator equipped with UV light [27,61,64,65]. Following oocyte enucleation, cell cycle-synchronized donor cells are transplanted into the perivitelline space of the oocytes in a manner that both cell membranes attach firmly to each other. The cellcouplets are then electrofused in a 0.3

M mannitol fusion medium. One hour following fusion, cell-couplets are activated by culturing for 5 min in ionomycin containing medium followed by culturing them in 6-DMAP or cycloheximide containing medium [27,34,61]. Recent studies in our laboratory revealed that a greater incidence of chromosomal abnormalities occur when SCNT-sheep embryos are cultured in 6-DMAP containing medium compared to cycloheximide [27, 34]. After activation, embryos are cultured in IVC medium and are surgically transferred into uteri of estrus –synchronized ewes [27] or into the oviducts of the does [61]. Pregnancy confirmation is done by ultrasound scanning beginning on day 35 of pregnancy. Pregnancy loss in sheep following SCNT-derived embryo transfer can be monitored by ultrasound imaging combined with serum progesterone levels [27].

Recently, there has been some controversy on the biological age of the SCNT-derived offspring, and whether they may susceptible for pre-mature death compared to their age-matched control counterparts [56]. A good example of this was the premature death of "Dolly". The hypothesis behind this is that donor somatic cells from adults may correlate with offspring carrying shortened telomere lengths compared to normal controls. Telomeres are located at the end of the chromosomes and become shorter in each cell cycle when somatic cells replicate. When the telomere length reaches a critical length the cell either enters senescence or enters a 'crisis' state associated with the development of cancer cells. This phenomenon does not happen in the germ line and in embryonic cells as these cells possess telomerase, an enzyme that adds telomere sequences to chromosomes during cell replication thus preventing telomere shortening from occurring. In most somatic cells, the telomerase enzyme is not present, leading to continuous telomere shortening when cells replicate [66].

Recent findings in telomere lengths in animal clones revealed cases of shorter [67, 68] not different [69-71] and surprisingly even longer lengths compared to those measured in their age matched control counterparts [72]. These findings have triggered much speculation on the fate of clones. However, this makes animal clones derived from adult somatic cells appropriate models for studying cellular rejuvenation and aging in vivo since they are generated from aged and culture propagated somatic cells known to contain shorten telomeres. Following SCNT, the differentiated donor nucleus undergoes extensive remodeling and reprogramming by the recipient oocyte cytoplasm

[73], which has been shown to cause altered gene expression profiles [74] and chromatin modifications [75] that likely contribute to the high incidence of abnormalities, prenatal and post natal losses found in clones [73]. Altered expression of telomerase activity [71] and donor cell type-dependent telomere length differences [76] further support inappropriate genome reprogramming, however, the precise etiology of altered telomere lengths in vivo are not clear for clones. Recent studies from our laboratory on SCNT-derived small ruminants showed that shortened telomere lengths in sheep cloned using adult donor cells compared to controls [67] and a similar phenomenon was observed in SCNTderived goats [77]. Interestingly, the offspring derived from natural breeding between cloned parents, did not show any discrepancies in telomere length [67] suggesting that telomere length was reset in the germ line of the cloned offspring. To date we do not possess enough data on telomere length of clones and "Dolly" cannot be considered the only incidence in this nature, thus more research is needed to investigate the lifespan of cloned offspring; at this stage the data available is inconclusive.

Production of Transgenic Sheep and Goats

Transgenic animals are produced either to carry an exogenous gene or to have a "knock out" gene from their own genome. Many transgenic animals have been produced for biomedical research interests as well as to test their application in livestock production [78]. There are many techniques available for the production of transgenic animals, such as pronuclear microinjection [37, 79, and 80], sperm-mediated transgenesis [81] and somatic cell nuclear transfer [65, 82, and 83]. During the last decade, research has focused on producing transgenic animals which secrete recombinant proteins in their milk. These animals produce relatively high quantities of recombinant proteins compared to other conventional methods due to the physiological nature of the mammary gland for its unique ability to synthesize proteins [78,84,85,86,87,88]. A few examples of transgenic small ruminants producing recombinant proteins in milk for pharmaceutical and biomedical interest are sheep producing human clotting factor VIII [89] and factor IX [82] and goats synthesizing human antithrombin III [90], human alpha-fetoprotein [91], human monoclonal antibodies [92, 93], malaria antigens [94] spider silks [95], human granulocyte colony stimulating factor (96) and human butyryl-cholinesterase [97,98]. Although these animals have shown high expression of the transgene product in the milk, a recent report suggests that the transgene may have some negative effects on the physiology of mammary gland function, leading to a compromised situation [87]. However, the first protein produced by transgenic animals, ATryn, a recombinant human anti-thrombin produced in transgenic goats' milk, received approval for use in humans in 2009.

CONCLUSIONS

In this review, we have focused on some aspects of reproductive biotechnology that are of veterinary and biomedical importance in sheep and goat that have been reported in the recent past. It is well known that most biotechnologies take many years to come into full practice after enormous amounts of laboratory and field research. Therefore, more focus should be carried out in emerging areas like artificial insemination of sheep and goat using sexed semen, in vitro and in vivo embryo production systems, transgenic animal production and cloning using stem cells.

ACKNOWLEDGEMENTS

The authors gratefully acknowledge the assistance provided by Ed R Reyes, Elizabeth St. John, Pamela Hasson in the University of Guelph, the MITACS Accelerate internship program, Canada, the Canadian Commonwealth Scholarship Plan and the University of Peradeniya in preparation of this manuscript.

REFERENCES

1. Zygoyiannis D (2006) Sheep production in the world and in Greece. Small Rumin Res 62: 143-147.
2. Ghadar F, Spindler H (2005) the growth of biotechnology. Industrial Management 47: 19-26.

3. Polge C (1968) Frozen semen and the A.I. Programme in Proc. 2nd Tech. Conf. Artif. Insem. Reprod. NAAB, Columbia, MO: 46-51.

4. Johnson LA, Rath D, Vazquez JM, Maxwell WMC, Dobrinsky JR (2005) Preselection of sex of offspring in swine for production: current status of the process and its application. Theriogenology 63: 615-624.

5. Johnson LA, Flook JP, Hawk HW (1989) Sex preselection in rabbits: live births from X and Y sperm separated by DNA and cell sorting. Biol Reprod 41: 199-203.

6. Garner DL (2001) Sex-sorting mammalian sperm: concept to application in mammals. J Androl 22: 519-526.

7. Seidel GE Jr, Garner DL (2002) Current status of sexing mammalian spermatozoa. Reproduction 124: 733-743.

8. Evans G, Hollinshead FK, Maxwell WMC (2004) Preservation and artificial insemination of sexed semen in sheep. Reprod Fertil Dev 16: 455-464.

9. Seidel GE, Schenk JL, Herickhoff LA, Doyle SP, Brink Z, et al. (1999) Insemination of heifers with sexed sperm. Theriogenology 52: 1407-1420.

10. Vazquez JM, Martinez EA, Parrilla I, Roca J, Gill MA, et al. (2003) Birth of piglets after deep intrauterine insemination with flow cytometrically sorted boar spermatozoa. Theriogenology 59: 1605-1614.

11. Rath D, Ruiz S, Sieg B (2003) Birth of female piglets following intrauterine insemination of a sow using flow cytometrically sexed boar semen. Vet Rec 152: 400-401.

12. Buchanan BR, Seidel GE, McCue PM, Schenk JL, Heickhoff LA, et al. (2000) Insemination of mares with low numbers of either unsexed or sexed spermatozoa. Theriogenology 53: 1333-1344.

13. Lindsey AC, Schenk JL, Graham JK, Bruemmer JE, Squires EL (2002) Hysteroscopic insemination of low numbers of flow sorted fresh and frozen thawed stallion spermatozoa. Equine Vet J 34: 121-127.

14. Catt SL, Catt JW, Gomez MC, Maxwell WMC, Evans G (1996) The birth of a male lamb derived from an in vitro matured oocyte

fertilized by intra-cytoplasmic injection of a single presumptive male sperm. Vet Rec 139: 494-495.

15. Hollinshead FK, O'Brien JK, Maxwell WMC, Evans G (2002) Production of lambs of pre-determined sex after the insemination of ewes with low numbers of X- or Y-chromosome bearing spermatozoa. Reprod Fertil Dev 14: 503-508.
16. Garner DL, Seidel GE Jr (2003) past, present and future perspectives on sexing sperm. Can J Anim Sci 83: 375-384.
17. Maxwell WMC, Johnson LA (1997) Chlortetracycline analysis of boar spermatozoa after incubation, flow cytometric sorting, cooling or cryopreservation. Mol Reprod Dev 46: 408-418.
18. Hollinshead FK, O' Brien JK, Gillan L, Mayers M, Maxwell WMC, et al. (2004) Liquid storage of flow cytometrically sorted ram spermatozoa. Theriogenology 62: 587-605.
19. Catt SL, O'Brian JK, Maxwell WMC, Evans G (1997) Assessment of ram and boar spermatozoa during cell-sorting by flow cytometry. Reprod Domestic Anim 32: 251- 258.
20. Hollinshead FK, Gillan L, O'Brian JK, Evans G, Maxwell WMC (2003) In vitro and in vivo assessment of functional capacity of flow cytometrically sorted ram spermatozoa after freezing and thawing. Reprod Fertil Dev 15: 351-359.
21. De Graaf SP, Gillan L, Evans G, Maxwell WMC, O'Brian JK (2004). The effect of the sheath fluid on the quality of sex-sorted ram spermatozoa. Reprod Fertil Dev 16: 284-285.
22. Perera GDRK, Pushpakumara PGA, De Silva LNA, Alexander B (2008) Production of genetically superior goats through embryo transfer technology in Sri Lanka. Tropi Agri Res 20: 177-184.
23. Bartlewski PM, Alexander BD, Rawlings NC, Barrett DMW, King WA (2008) Ovarian responses, hormonal profiles and embryo yields in anoestrus ewes superovulated with Folltropin-V after pretreatment with medroxyprogesterone acetate (MAP)- releasing vaginal sponges and a single dose of estradiol-17ß (E2-17ß). Reprod Domest Anim 43: 299 – 307.
24. Bartlewski PM, Alexander BD, King WA (2008a) Ovarian and endocrine determinants of superovulatory responses in anestrous ewes. Small Rumin Res 75: 210-216.

25. Gonzalez-Bulnes A, Baird DT, Campbell BK, Cocero MJ, Garcia-Garcia RM, et al. (2004) Multiple factors affecting the efficiency of multiple ovulation and embryo transfer in sheep and goats. Reprod Fertil Dev 16: 421-435.

26. Menchaca A, Vilarino M, Pinczak A, Kmaid S, Saldana JM (2009) Progesterone treatment, FSH plus eCG, GnRH administration, and Day 0 Protocol for MOET programs in sheep. Theriogenology 72: 477-483.

27. Alexander B, Coppola G, Mastromonaco GF, John ES, Reyes ER, et al. (2008) Early Pregnancy Diagnosis by Serum Progesterone and Ultrasound in Sheep Carrying Somatic Cell Nuclear Transfer - Derived Pregnancies. Repro Domest Anim 43: 207-211.

28. String fellow and Seidel (1998) Manual of the International Embryo Transfer Society.

29. Candappa IBR, Bainbridge HC, Price NT, Hourigan KR, Bartlewski PM (2009) A preliminary study on the suitability of Cervidil to induce cervical dilation for artifi cial insemination in ewes. Res Vet Sci 87: 204-206.

30. Garcia-Garcia R, Ward F, Fair S, O'Meara C, Wade M, et al. (2007) Development and quality of sheep embryos cultured in commercial G1.3/G2. 3 sequential media. Anim Reprod Sci 98: 233-240.

31. Cognie Y, Poulin N, Locatelli Y, Mermillod P (2004) State-of-the-art production, conservation and transfer of in-vitro-produced embryos in small ruminants. Reprod Fertil Dev 16: 437-445.

32. Wani NA (2002) In vitro maturation and in vitro fertilization of sheep oocytes. Small Rumin Res 44: 89-95.

33. Wang S, Liu Y, Holyoak GR, Evans RC, Bunch TD (1998) A protocol for in vitro maturation and fertilization of sheep oocytes. Small Rum Res 29: 83-88.

34. Alexander B, Coppola G, Di Berardino D, Rho GJ, St John E, et al. (2006) The effect of 6-dimethylaminopurine (6-DMAP) and cycloheximide (CHX) on the development and chromosomal complement of sheep parthenogenetic and nuclear transfer embryos. Mol Reprod Dev 73: 20-30.

35. Alberio R, Olivera J, Roche A, Alabart J, Folch J (2002) Performance of a modified ovum pick-up system using three different FSH stimulation protocols in ewes. Small Rumin Res 46: 81-87.

36. Baldassarre H, Wang B, Kafi di N, Keefer C, Lazaris A, et al. (2002) Advances in the production and propagation of transgenic goats using laparoscopic ovum pickup and in vitro embryo production technologies. Theriogenology 57: 275-284.

37. Baldassarre H, Wang B, Kafi di N, Gauthier M, Neveu N, et al. (2003) Production of transgenic goats by pronuclear microinjection of in vitro produced zygotes derived from oocytes recovered by laparoscopy. Theriogenology 56: 83-839.

38. Wan PC, Haoa ZD, Zhoub P, Wua Y, Yanga L (2009) Effects of SOF and CR1 media on developmental competence and cell apoptosis of ovine in vitro fertilization embryos. Anim Reprod Sci 114: 279-288.

39. Baldassarre H, Furnus CC, De Matos DG, Pessi H (1996) In vitro production of sheep embryos using laparoscopic folliculocentesis: Alternative gonadotrophin treatments

40. Gibbons A, Bonnet FP, Cueto MI, Catala M, Salamone DF, et al. (2007) Procedure for maximizing oocyte harvest for in vitro embryo production in small ruminants. Reprod Dom Anim 42: 423-440.

41. Cognie Y, Baril G, Poulin N, Mermillod P (2003) Current status of embryo technologies in sheep and goat. Theriogenology 59: 171-188.

42. Accardo C, Dattena M, Pilichi S, Mara L, Chessa B, et al. (2004) Effects of recombinant human FSH and LH on in vitro maturation of sheep oocytes: embryo development and viability. Anim Reprod Sci 81: 77-86.

43. Coppola G, Alexander B, Di Berardino D, St John E, Basrur PK, et al. (2007) Use of cross-species in-situ hybridization (ZOO-FISH) to assess chromosome abnormalities in day-6 in vivo- or in vitro-produced sheep embryos. Chromosome Res 15: 399-408.

44. Rho GJ, Hahnel AC, Betteridge KJ (2001) Comparison of oocyte maturation times and of three methods of sperm preparation for their effects on the production of goat embryos in vitro. Theriogenology 56: 503-516.

45. Comizzoli P, Mermillod P, Cognie Y, Chal N, Legendre X, et al. (2001) Successful in vitro production of embryos in red deer (Cervus elaphus) and the sika deer (Cervus nippon). Theriogenology 55: 649-659.
46. Berg DK, Thompson JG, Asher GW (2002) Development of In Vitro Embryo Production Systems for Red Deer (Cervus Elaphus). Part 3. In Vitro Fertilisation Using Sheep Serum as a Capacitating Agent and the Subsequent Birth of Calves. Anim Reprod Sci 70: 85-98.
47. O' Brien JK, Hollinshead FK, Maxwell WMC (2004) In vivo development capacity of in vitro produced embryos derived from sex-sorted and re-cryopreserved frozen-thawed ram-sperm. Reprod Fertil Dev 16: 286.
48. Hoshi H (2003) In vitro production of bovine embryos and their application for embryo transfer. Theriogenology 59: 675-685.
49. Holm P, Walker SK, Seamark RF (1996) Embryo viability, duration of gestation and birth weight in sheep after transfer of in vitro matured and in vitro fertilized zygotes cultured in vitro or in vivo. J Reprod Fertil 107: 175-181.
50. Sinclair KD, McEvoy TG, Maxfi eld EK, Maltin CA, Young LE, et al. (1999) Aberrant fetal growth and development after in vitro culture of sheep zygotes. J Reprod Fertil 116: 177-186.
51. Walker S, Hill J, Kleeman D, Nancarrow C (1996) Development of ovine embryos in synthetic oviductal fluid containing amino acids at oviductal fluid concentrations. Biol Reprod 55: 703-708.
52. Kelk DA (1997) Development characteristics of interspecific hybrid embryos. PhD Thesis. University of Guelph, Ontario, Canada.
53. Anderson GB (1988) interspecific pregnancy: barriers and prospects. Biol Reprod 38: 1-15.
54. Pinheiro LEL, Guimaraes SEF, Almeida IL, Mikich AB (1989) the natural occurrence of sheep X goat hybrids. Theriogenology 32: 987 – 994.
55. Wilmut I, Schnieke AE, McWhir J, Kind AJ, Campbell KH (1997) Viable offspring derived from fetal and adult mammalian cells. Nature 385: 810-813.

56. Vajta G, Gjerris M (2006) Science and technology of farm animal cloning: state of the art. Anim Reprod Sci 92: 211-230.

57. Hill JR, Roussel AJ, Cibelli JB, Edwards JF, Hooper NL, et al. (1999) Clinical and pathological features of cloned transgenic calves and fetuses (13 case studies). Theriogenology 51: 1451-1465.

58. Rho GJ, Coppola G, Sosnowski J, Kasimanickam R, Johnson WH, et al. (2007) Use of somatic cell nuclear transfer to study meiosis in female cattle carrying a sex-dependent fertility-impairing X-chromosome abnormality. Cloning Stem Cells 9: 118-29.

59. Ma S, Lan G, Miao Y, Wang Z, Chang Z, et al. (2003) Hypoxanthine (HX) inhibition of in vitro meiotic resumption in goat oocytes. Mol Reprod Dev 66: 306-313.

60. Lan GC, Han D, Wu YG, Han ZB, Ma SF, et al. (2005) Effects of duration, concentration and timing of ionomycin and 6-dimethylaminopurine (6-DMAP) treatment on activation of goat oocytes. Mol Reprod Dev 71: 380-388

61. Lan GC, Chang ZL, Luo MJ, Jiang YL, Han D, et al. (2006) Production of Cloned Goats by Nuclear Transfer of Cumulus Cells and Long-Term Cultured Fetal Fibroblast Cells Into Abattoir-Derived Oocytes. Mol Reprod Dev 73: 834-840.

62. Zou X, Wang Y, Cheng Y, Yang Y, Ju H, et al. (2002) Generation of cloned goats (Capra hircus) from transfected foetal fibroblast cells, the effect of donor cell cycle. Mol Reprod Dev 61: 164-172.

63. Behboodi E, Memili E, Melican DT, Destrempes MM, Overton SA, et al. (2004) Viable transgenic goats derived from skin cells. Transgenic Res 13: 215-224.

64. Keefer CL, Stone RK, Bhatia B, Lazaris A, Begin I, et al.(2000) Efficient production of viable goat offspring following nuclear transfer using adult somatic cells. Biol Reprod 62: 192.

65. Keefer CL, Baldassarre H, Keyston R, Wang B, Bhatia B, et al. (2001) Generation of dwarf goat (Capra hircus) clones following nuclear transfer with transfected and nontransfected fetal fibroblasts and in vitro-matured oocytes. Biol Reprod 64: 849-856.

66. Xu J, Yang X (2003) Will cloned animals suffer premature aging - the story at the end of clone's chromosomes. Reprod Biol Endocrinol 1: 105-110.

67. Alexander B, Coppola G, Perrault SD, Peura TT, Betts DH, et al. (2007) Telomere length of sheep clones and their offspring. Mol Reprod Dev 74: 1525-1537.

68. Shiels PG, Jardine AG (2003) Dolly, no longer the exception: Telomeres and implications for transplantation. Cloning stem cells 5: 157-160.

69. Jiang L, Carter DB, Xu J, Yang X, Prather RS, et al. (2004) Telomere lengths in cloned transgenic pigs. Biol Reprod 70: 1589-1593. Betts DH, Bordingnon V, Hill JR, Winger Q, Westhusing ME, et al. (2001) Reprogramming of telomerase activity and rebuilding of telomere length in cloned cattle. Proc Natl Acad Sci USA 98: 1077-1082.

70. Betts DH, Bordingnon V, Hill JR, Winger Q, Westhusing ME, et al. (2001) Reprogramming of telomerase activity and rebuilding of telomere length in cloned cattle. Proc Natl Acad Sci USA 98: 1077-1082.

71. Tian XC, Xu J, Yang X (2000) Normal telomere lengths found in cloned cattle. Nat Genet 26: 272-273.

72. Lanza R, Cibelli JB, Blackwell C, Cristofalo VJ, Francis MK, et al. (2000) Extension of cell life- span and telomere length in animals cloned from senescent somatic cells. Science 288: 665-669.

73. Reik W, Dean W (2002) Epigenetic reprogramming: back to the beginning. Nature 420: 127.

74. Humpherys D, Eggan K, Akatsu H, Friedman A, Hoechedlinger K, et al. (2002) Abnormal gene expression in cloned mice derived from embryonic stem cell and cumulus cell nuclei. Proc Natl Acad Sci USA 99: 12889-12894.

75. Dean W, Santos F, Stojkovic M, Zakhartchenko V, Walter J, et al. (2001) Conservation of methylation reprogramming in mammalian development: aberrant reprogramming in cloned embryos. Proc Natl Acad Sci USA 98: 13734- 13738.

76. Miyashita N, Shiga K, Yonai M, Keneyama K, Kobayashi S, et al. (2002) Remarkable differences in telomere lengths among

cloned calves derived from different cell types. Biol Repro 66: 1649-1655.

77. Betts DH, Perrault SD, Petrik J, Lin L, Favetta LA, et al. (2005) Telomere length analysis in goat clones and their offspring. Mol Reprod Dev 72: 461-470.
78. Wheeler MB, Walters EM, Clark SG (2003) transgenic animals in biomedicine and agriculture: outlook for the future. Anim Reprod Sci 79: 265-289.
79. Ebert KM, Selgrath JP, DiTullio P, Denman J, Smith TE, et al. (1991) Transgenic production of a variant of human tissue-type plasminogen activator in goat milk: generation of transgenic goats and analysis of expression. Biotechnology 9: 835- 838.
80. Baldassarre H, Wang B, Gauthier M (1999) Embryo transfer in a commercial transgenic production program using BELE® goat embryos. Theriogenology 51: 415.
81. Celebi C, Guillaudeux T, Auvray P, Vallet-Erdtmann V, Jegou B (2003) The making of "transgenic spermatozoa". Biol Reprod 68: 1477-1483.
82. Schnieke AE, Kind AJ, Ritchie WA, Mycock K, Scott AR, et al. (1997) Human Factor IX transgenic sheep produced by nuclear transfer of nuclei form transfected fetal fibroblasts. Science 278: 2130-2133.
83. Keefer CL, Lazaris A, Keyston R (2002) Cloning using somatic cells for the production and propagation of transgenic Nigerian dwarf and dwarf-crossed goats. Theriogenology 57: 422.
84. Houdebine LM (2000) transgenic animal bioreactors Transgenic Res 9: 305-320.
85. Keefer CL (2004) Production of bioproducts through the use of transgenic animal models. Anim Reprod Sci 82: 5-12.
86. Baldassarre H, Wang B, Pierson J, Neveu N, Sneek L, et al. (2004) Prepubertal Propagation of Transgenic Cloned Goats by Laparoscopic Ovum Pick-Up and in Vitro Embryo Production. Cloning Stem Cells 6: 25-29.
87. Baldassarre H, Hockley DK, Dore M, Brochu E, Hakier B, et al. (2008a) Lactation performance of transgenic goats expressing recombinant human butyrylcholinesterase in the milk. Transgenic Res 17: 73-84.

88. Baldassarre H, Hockley DK, Olaniyan B, Brochu E, Zhao X, et al. (2008b) Milk composition studies in transgenic goats expressing recombinant human butyrylcholinesterase in the mammary gland. Transgenic Res 17: 863-872.

89. Niemann H, Halter R, Carnwath JW, Herrmann D, Lemme E, et al. (1999) Expression of blood clotting factor VIII in the mammary gland of transgenic sheep. Transgenic Res 8: 237-247.

90. Zhou Q, Kyazike J, Echelard Y, Meade HM, Higgins E, et al. (2005) Effect of genetic background on glycosylation heterogeneity in human antithrombin produced in the mammary gland of transgenic goats. J Biotechnol 117: 57-72.

91. Parker MH, Birck-Wilson E, Allard G, Masiello N, Day M, et al. (2004) Purification and characterization of a recombinant version of human alpha-fetoprotein expressed in the milk of transgenic goats. Protein Expr Purif 38: 177-183.

92. Young MW, Meade H, Curling JM, Ziomek CA, Harvey M (1998) Production of recombinant antibodies in the milk of transgenic animals. Res Immunol 149: 609- 610.

93. Pollock DP, Kutzko JP, Birck-Wilson E, Williams JL, Echerlard Y, et al. (1999) Transgenic milk as a method for the production of recombinant antibodies. J Immunol Methods 231: 147-157.

94. Behboodi E, Ayres SL, Memili E, O'Coin M, Chen LH, et al. (2005) Health and reproductive profi les of malaria antigen-producing transgenic goats derived by somatic cell nuclear transfer. Cloning Stem Cells 7: 107-118.

95. Karatzas CN, Zhou FJ, Huang Y, Duguay F, Chretien N, et al. (1999) Production of recombinant spider silk (BioSteel®) in the milk of transgenic animals. Transgenic Res 8: 476-477.

96. Ko JH, Lee CS, Kim KH, Pang MG, Koo JS, et al. (2000) Production of biologically active human granulocyte colony stimulating factor in the milk of transgenic goat. Transgenic Res 9: 215-222.

97. Cerasoli DM, Griffi ths EM, Doctor BP, Saxena A, Fedorko JM, et al. (2005) In vitro and in vivo characterization of recombinant human butyrylcholinesterase (Protexia) as a potential nerve agent bioscavenger. Chem Biol Interact 158: 363- 365.

98. Huang YJ, Huang Y, Baldassarre H, Wang B, Lazaris A, et al. (2007) Recombinant human butyrylcholinesterase from milk of transgenic animals to protect against organophosphate poisoning. Proc Natl Acad Sci USA 104: 13603-13608.

chapter 4

Male Reproductive Traits of Full-Sibs of Different Age Classes in Three-Spined Sticklebacks (Gasterosteus Aculeatus)

Marion Mehlis* and Theo CM Bakker

ABSTRACT

The process of ageing is associated with negative effects of mutations acting late in life, which range from those affecting cells to those affecting the whole organism. In many animal taxa, the deterioration of the phenotype with age also affects traits such as males' primary and secondary sexual characteristics. In three-spined sticklebacks (*Gasterosteus aculeatus*), males usually reproduce at one or two years of age. To see whether sexual selection has the potential to differ between young and old males, full-sib brothers of different age classes were compared, which were bred and raised under standardised laboratory conditions. During two simulated, successive breeding seasons males were allowed to build their nest in single tanks either in the first ("young males") or in the second ("old males") breeding season. A comparison of reproductively active brothers of the first and second breeding season showed that older males produce more but smaller sperm, which might be of lower quality. The fact that older males stored more sperm is size dependent as the results show that larger males possess a greater absolute testis mass, which is inextricably linked to sperm number. However, independent of body size, old males had a lower intensity of red/orange and UV breeding coloration as well as a reduced testis melanisation, which might have consequences in female mate choice and sperm competition.

BACKGROUND

More than 300 different theories on the proximate and ultimate causes of ageing (Medvedev 1990) have been proposed over the past six decades (for reviews see Hughes and Reynolds 2005; Rose et al. 2008 ; Milewski 2010 ; Johnson and Gemmel 2012). Ultimate causes investigate the tension between longevity and reproduction. For example, Medawar ("mutation accumulation theory": Medawar 1952) postulates that due to natural selection (e.g. predation) individuals within a population do not live long enough to accumulate deleterious mutations that would reduce fitness late in life. Furthermore, Williams ("antagonistic pleiotropy": Williams 1957) reveals that some genes, which are responsible for an increased reproductive investment when being young, contribute to a lower rate of investment in maintenance and reproduction later in life. Researchers interested in proximate causes focus on mechanisms such as the accumulation of damage to cells and cell function over time caused by free radicals produced during cellular metabolism ("oxidative stress": Harman 1956). To date there is no universal theory of ageing, possibly because the process itself is multicausal (see Holliday 2006).

Theoretical considerations aside, there has recently been considerable interest in the effects of ageing on sexually selected traits. For example, two indicators of male sexual attractiveness, tail length in barn swallows () (Balbontín et al. *Hirundo rustica*2011) and foot colour in blue-footed boobies () (Velando et al. *Sula nebouxii*2011) were shown to decrease with age. In many animal taxa, ageing has effects on reproductive success, which may be negative (e.g. Dean et al. 2010) as well as positive (e.g. DuVal 2012). In some cases, males of intermediate age were most successful (e.g. Raveh et al. 2010). Also in humans (*Homo sapiens*), testicular volume was significantly different among age classes, with men between 30–60 years showing the greatest testicular volume (Yang et al. 2011). If old males are of lower quality, females will discriminate against them (Beck and Promislow 2007). This exactly happened in the house mouse (*Mus musculus domesticus*); old males and their scent were less attractive to females (Garratt et al.2011). Similarly, in the field cricket (*Gryllus bimaculatus*), females had a strong preference for the songs of young males (Verburgt et al. 2011). On the other hand, in *Drosophila bipectinata* females preferred to mate with older males, presumably due to the fact that old males mated faster, copulated longer and inseminated more (Somashekar and Krishna 2011). In guppies (*Poecilia reticulata*) old males produced longer but slower sperm and they had larger reserves of strippable sperm when compared to young males (Gasparini et al. 2010). However, artificial insemination did not reveal any effect of age on sperm competition success (Gasparini et al. 2010). Overall, a number of studies investigated the influence of ageing on reproductive traits resulting in contradictory findings, which might partly be explained by the different breeding systems of the study animals (see Johnson and Gemmel 2012 for an overview).

The three-spined stickleback (*Gasterosteus aculeatus*) is a good model system to study the influences of male age on reproductive traits for several reasons. Depending upon location, sticklebacks breed from April to August. Individuals normally reach reproductive age in their second (one-year-old) or third summer (two-year-old) and die after one or two breeding seasons (but see Gambling and Reimchen 2012 for a report of some populations in which individuals live for six years or more). During the breeding season males establish territories in the shallow shore region and build a nest composed of filamentous algae. Furthermore, males usually develop a conspicuous red/orange coloration in the cheek region, court many females and provide all of the parental care (Wootton 1976). The intensity of male breeding coloration is one of the key determinants of female mate-choice decisions (e.g. McLennan and McPhail 1990 ; Bakker and Milinski 1993). Once a female has made her choice, she pushes her way into the male's nest, deposits her eggs and then leaves as the territorial male enters the nest behind her to fertilise the clutch. Female choice can be circumvented to an extent by sneaking behaviour, in which an intruding male dashes through the nest to deposit sperm immediately before or after the territory holder. This is a common behavioural tactic of territorial males in many populations (e.g. Largiadèr et al. 2001), indicating that sperm competition is an important part of the stickleback breeding system. A recent study revealed that competitive males, which had succeeded in establishing a territory and attracting ripe females, performed most of the sneak attempts (Candolin and Vlieger2013).

In the three-spined stickleback spermatogenesis only occurs during the short photoperiods preceding the breeding season (Borg 1982), resulting in a larger number of sperm stored in testes of virgin males (e.g. early spring) compared to those of multiply mated males (e.g. late summer) (Zbinden et al. 2001). As stickleback males are sperm limited over the course of one breeding season, careful sperm allocation is a critical fitness component (Zbinden et al. 2003 , 2004). Overall then, both the intensity of males' breeding coloration (Bakker and Milinski 1993) and gonadal investment (Cubillos and Guderley 2000) have a positive influence on reproductive success. Hence, on the basis of stickleback males' breeding behaviour and the different theories of ageing it was investigated whether age has a negative influence on sexually selected reproductive traits (breeding coloration, testis and sperm traits) by using full-sib brothers of different age classes.

RESULTS

Statistical Analyses

The R 2.9.1 statistical package was used for analyses. All given p-values are based on two-tailed tests. For analyses different linear mixed effect models ("lme") were constructed using males' reproductive traits (breeding coloration, testis and sperm traits) as dependent variables and male age (young or old) as explanatory variable (Table 1). Furthermore, young and old males originated from the same family (see Methods) implying that they are not independent from each other on a genetic basis. Thus, in all models family identity was included as random factor and never removed to control for possible ancestral influences. Tests of significance were based on likelihood-ratio tests ("LRT"). The use of "lme" requires that the dependent variable is normally distributed. To achieve normal distributions of the residuals of the best explaining models according to Kolmogorov-Smirnov tests, some data were logarithmically transformed (body mass, absolute and relative testis mass, sperm number, total brightness (dorsal region) and sperm tail length), square-root transformed (relative red area of the breeding coloration in the cheek region), exponentially transformed (red/orange hue, testis melanisation (L^*_{total})) or reciprocally transformed (total brightness (cheek region)). For a detailed description of all measured reproductive traits see Methods.

Table 1: Listing of all conducted linear mixed effect models "lme"

Dependent variables	Explanatory variable male age		Explanatory variable body size		AIC male age	AIC body size	Sample size (N)	
	χ2	p-value	χ2	p-value			Young	Old
Body size [cm]	47.842	<0.001	/	/	61.707	/	60	101
Body mass [g]	39.942	<0.001	/	/	−90.424	/	60	101
Body condition	0.448	0.503	/	/	−315.952	/	60	101
Red area [%]	0.192	0.662	5.245	0.022	607.296	602.243	59	101
Carotenoid chroma (A)	5.312	0.021	4.447	0.035	−59.083	-58.218	59	99
UV chroma (A)	11.091	<0.001	0.855	0.355	−538.148	−527.912	59	99
Red/orange hue (A) [nm]	3.985	0.046	1.269	0.260	43316.630	43319.350	59	99
Total brightness (A)	8.210	0.004	6.903	0.009	−1240.811	−1239.504	59	99
Total brightness (R)	16.374	<0.001	1.595	0.207	262.555	277.334	59	101
Absolute testis mass [g]	54.517	<0.001	76.359	<0.001	−452.293	−474.135	60	96
Relative testis mass (GSI)	20.887	<0.001	3.304	0.069	45.989	63.572	60	96
Testis melanisation (L^*_{total})	64.591	<0.001	19.391	<0.001	1955.718	2008.869	60	96

Sperm number	4.256	0.039	11.441	<0.001	223.120	207.984	59	99
Head length [μm]	73.952	<0.001	15.977	<0.001	−277.861	−219.886	60	22
Tail length [μm]	11.816	<0.001	6.773	0.009	−163.597	−158.555	60	22
Head width [μm]	53.729	<0.001	9.646	0.002	−303.683	−259.599	60	22
Mid-piece width [μm]	4.268	0.039	0.676	0.411	−271.444	−267.852	60	22
Mid-piece volume [μm³]	9.003	0.003	3.934	0.047	−298.985	−293.916	60	22
Mid-piece length [μm]	2.537	0.111	2.369	0.124	−225.356	−225.187	60	22
Head to tail length ratio	0.052	0.819	0.036	0.849	−540.046	-540.030	60	22

(A) colour measurements were made directly below the eye (breeding coloration).

(R) measurements were taken at the dorsum below the first dorsal spine.

(GSI) gonadosomatic index after de Vlaming et al. (1982).

(L^*_{total}) testis brightness (see Mehlis et al. 2012 for details).

In all models family identity was included as random factor and never removed to control for possible ancestral influences. The model with the lowest AIC (Akaike's information criterion) value represents the best approximating model.

Mehlis and Bakker

Body Traits

Young (N_{young} = 60) and old males (N_{old} = 101) differed significantly in body size ("lme", ^{2} = 47.842, $P < 0.001$) and mass ("lme", ^{2} = 39.942, $P < 0.001$), showing that older males were on average larger and heavier than younger ones (Table 2). Hence, whether age or size affected the observed results (see below) is hard to distinguish due to the fact that age and body size are not statistically independent from each other. Accordingly, one has to mention that body size of the used individuals was determined by age as fish grow throughout their life time. It should be valid to use the base of differences (age) in the statistical analyses in order to find differences in reproductive traits and discuss them in an evolutionary context. Nevertheless, all models (Table 1) were run again but instead of using male age body size was included as explanatory variable. The results of these models are also listed in Table 1. Akaike's information criterion (AIC) was used for model comparison (male age or body size as explanatory variable); the model with the lowest AIC value represents the best approximating model (Symonds and Moussalli 2011). The results showed that, apart from the relative red area of males' breeding coloration, absolute testis mass and sperm number, male age is more appropriate in explaining the observed results than body size (Table 1). Thus, only the statistically relevant results concerning male body size are described in detail and discussed later on. Moreover, young and old males did not differ significantly in physical conditions ("lme", $\chi^2 = 0.448$, $P = 0.503$), indicating that they had the same pre-condition during life time (Table 2).]

Table 2: Descriptive statistics (median, first and third quartile) of body traits, breeding coloration variables and testis and sperm traits of young and old males used in the analyses

	Young			Old		
	Median	**1. Quartile**	**3. Quartile**	**Median**	**1. Quartile**	**3. Quartile**
Body size [cm]	4.90	4.70	5.10	5.20	4.95	5.40
Body mass [g]	1.562	1.372	1.712	1.812	1.617	2.031
Body condition	1.30	1.25	1.36	1.29	1.24	1.35
Red area [%]	14.84	6.22	27.21	13.74	6.29	21.94
Carotenoid chroma (A)	0.450	0.287	0.538	0.392	0.189	0.501
UV chroma (A)	0.271	0.244	0.291	0.245	0.209	0.273
Red/orange hue (A) [nm]	506.0	502.0	509.5	505.0	501.0	508.5
Total brightness (A)	2701.70	2072.17	3719.65	3267.38	2489.20	4939.09
Total brightness (R)	3075.86	2374.82	4326.12	1963.18	1402.66	3114.35
Absolute testis mass [g]	0.0107	0.0084	0.0140	0.0165	0.0135	0.0202
Relative testis mass (GSI)	0.697	0.585	0.862	0.951	0.731	1.103
Testis melanisation (L^*_{total})	39.00	26.88	47.13	60.50	49.38	67.50

Sperm number	$9.3_{*}10^{6}$	$6.0_{*}10^{6}$	$12.2_{*}10^{6}$	$10.7_{*}10^{6}$	$7.9_{*}10^{6}$	$14.4_{*}10^{6}$
Head length [μm]	1.106	1.067	1.128	0.991	0.958	1.011
Tail length [μm]	18.033	16.946	19.280	17.017	16.036	17.600
Head width [μm]	1.076	1.048	1.104	0.999	0.979	1.018
Mid-piece width [μm]	0.782	0.761	0.813	0.766	0.731	0.792
Mid-piece volume [$μm^3$]	0.284	0.268	0.311	0.256	0.239	0.281
Mid-piece length [μm]	0.587	0.548	0.614	0.583	0.515	0.621
Head to tail length ratio	0.094	0.089	0.099	0.091	0.087	0.098

(A) colour measurements were made directly below the eye (breeding coloration).

(R) measurements were taken at the dorsum below the first dorsal spine.

(GSI) gonadosomatic index after de Vlaming et al. (1982).

(L^{*}_{total}) testis brightness (see Mehlis et al. 2012 for details).

Mehlis and Bakker

Breeding Coloration

The relative area of red breeding coloration in the cheek region did not differ significantly between young and old males (N_{young} = 59, N_{old} = 101; "lme", ^{2} = 0.192, P = 0.662; Table 2) but it was significantly explained by body size ("lme", ^{2} = 5.245, P = 0.022), with larger males showing a significantly greater relative area of the red breeding coloration. However, young and old males differed significantly in carotenoid chroma (N_{young} = 59, N_{old} = 99; "lme", χ^2 = 5.312, P = 0.021) as well as in UV chroma (N_{young} = 59, N_{old} = 99; "lme", ^{2} = 11.091, $P < 0.001$), with larger chroma values for young males in both cases (Figure 1; Table 2). Thus, young males had a significantly more saturated coloration in the red/orange spectral region. In addition, the red/orange hue was significantly lower in old males (N_{young} = 59, N_{old} = 99; "lme", χ^2 = 3.985, P = 0.046), indicating a more red-shifted hue of the breeding coloration in young males compared to old males (Figure 1; Table 2). Moreover, younger males showed a significantly lower total brightness in the cheek region (N_{young} = 59, N_{old} = 99; "lme", χ^2 = 8.210, P = 0.004; Table 2) and a significantly higher total brightness in the dorsal region (N_{young} = 59, N_{old} = 101; "lme", χ^2 = 16.374, $P <$ 0.001; Figure 1; Table 2).

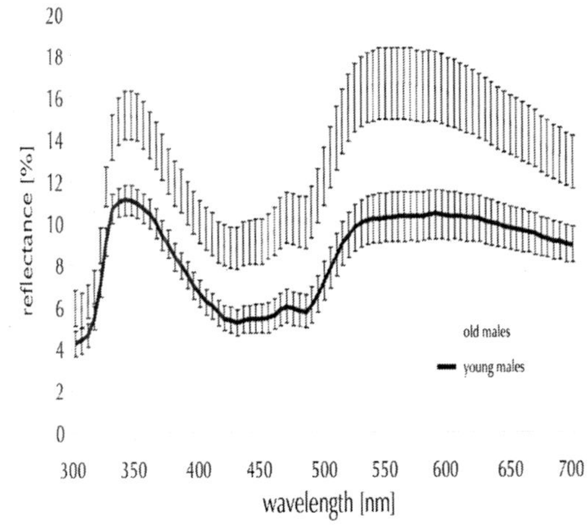

Figure 1: Representative reflectance spectrum of the carotenoid-based breeding coloration of three-spined stickleback males. Mean reflectance ± stan-

dard error (%) between 300 and 700 nm of the red/orange breeding coloration in the cheek region of reproductively active young (black line) and old (grey line) males. Reflectance was measured relative to a 98% Spectralon white standard.

Testis Traits

Young (N_{young} = 60) and old males (N_{old} = 96) differed significantly in absolute ("lme", $\chi^2 = 54.517$, $P < 0.001$) and relative testis mass ("lme", $^2 = 20.887$, $P < 0.001$) as well as in total testis brightness ("lme", $\chi^2 = 64.591$, $P < 0.001$), which is a measure of testicular melanisation (see Mehlis et al. 2012). While absolute and relative testis mass were both significantly higher in older males, the results show that testis melanisation was significantly lower in young males meaning that the testes of old males were less pigmented (Figure 2a-b; Table 2). However, it has to be mentioned that differences in absolute testis mass were better explained by differences in body size (lower AIC) than by male age alone, with larger males having significantly heavier testes ("lme", $^2 = 76.359$, $P < 0.001$).

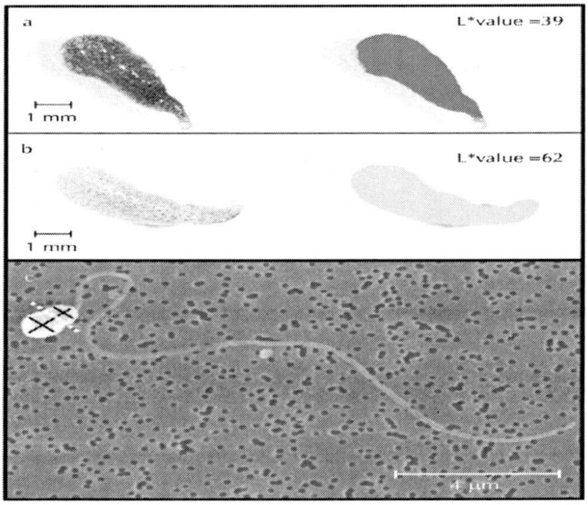

Figure 2: Representative testes and sperm of three-spined stickleback males. Testis of a young (a) and an old (b) male and on the right side the corresponding L*value for testis brightness as a measure of testis melanisation (see Mehlis et al. 2012). (c) Sperm head, mid-piece, and tail can be distinguished

on the SEM image. The black lines indicate head length and width as well as mid-piece length and width, the dotted white line indicates the boundary between head and mid-piece.

Sperm Traits

Stored sperm number differed significantly between young and old males (N_{young} = 59, N_{old} = 99; "lme", χ^2 = 4.256, P = 0.039), with older males having significantly more sperm (Table 2). However, the statistical analysis revealed that sperm number was explained in a more appropriate way by male body size (lower AIC) than by male age, with larger males having significantly more sperm ("lme", χ^2 = 11.441, P < 0.001). Young (N_{young} = 60) and old males (N_{old} = 22) differed significantly in sperm morphology traits (see Figure 2c), such as head length ("lme", χ^2 = 73.952, P < 0.001), tail length ("lme", χ^2 = 11.816, P < 0.001), head width ("lme", χ^2 = 53.729, P < 0.001), mid-piece width ("lme", χ^2 = 4.268, P = 0.039) and mid-piece volume ("lme", χ^2 = 9.003, P = 0.003), with young males showing higher values in all of these measures (Table 2). However, sperm of young and old males did not differ significantly in mid-piece length ("lme", χ^2 = 2.537, P = 0.111; Table 2) and head to tail length ratio ("lme", χ^2 = 0.052, P = 0.819; Table 2).

DISCUSSION

By comparing reproductive traits of lab-reared full-sib brothers of different ages in their first reproductive season (i.e. first nest building), the present study revealed that an advanced age can have considerable consequences on the expression of reproductive traits in three-spined sticklebacks, which might have an influence in inter- as well as intra-sexual contexts.

In three-spined sticklebacks sperm competition occurs in many populations (e.g. Goldschmidt et al. 1992 ; Jamieson and Colgan 1992 ; Rico et al. 1992 ; Largiadèr et al. 2001 ; Vlieger and Candolin 2009). Furthermore, it is generally accepted that sperm competition is a widespread and powerful selective force affecting sperm quantity and/or sperm quality in such a way to maximise competitive fertilisation success (e.g. Rowe and Pruett-Jones 2011). In a situation in which the risk of sperm competition is high, males should have larger testes and/ or a higher number of sperm per ejaculation (Harcourt et al. 1981 ; Stockley et al. 1997) assuming that fertilisation success follows a raffle-principle, so that males with more sperm will have an advantage (see Parker1990). In the American horseshoe crab (*Limulus polyphemus*) young males ejaculated more total sperm and had a significantly higher sperm concentration than old males (Sasson et al. 2012). In contrast, in the guppy (*Poecilia reticulata*) and in zebrafish (*Danio rerio*), the number of extractable sperm was higher in old males (Gasparini et al. 2010 ; Kanuga et al. 2011). In the zebrafish study the authors argued that this might be a consequence of fewer successful breeding attempts of old zebrafish males. In three-spined sticklebacks, the number of stored sperm is significantly positively correlated with testis mass (Zbinden et al. 2001), and gonad mass is related to reproductive success (Cubillos and Guderley 2000) as is body size (Kraak et al. 1999), showing the adaptive importance of these variables. In the present study, larger (older) stickleback males also had significantly more stored sperm as well as a higher absolute testis mass. It is hard to distinguish whether size or age affected the observed results, due to the fact that age and body size are not statistically independent from each other and especially in fish they are inextricably linked. However, all stickleback males used here were virgin as they had no opportunity to release sperm during their entire life span under laboratory conditions. In the rainbow trout (*Oncorhynchus mykiss*) it is known that unused sperm are reabsorbed during the post-spawning period, just before the next cycle of spermatogenesis begins (Billard and Takashima 1983), which could also be assumed for sticklebacks as in this species sperm production undergoes an annual cycle (Borg1982). Furthermore, in a previous study it was stated that at the end of the breeding season sticklebacks testes were drastically reorganised (Schneider 1969), which is supported by the fact that testis mass declines after the breeding season (e.g. Hoffmann et al. 2012). Hence, it is likely that the sperm, which were found in the two-year-old males, were solely produced during the second winter period, leading to the interpretation that larger old males produced both absolutely and relatively more sperm.

If a male produces more gametes, these sperm will be proportionally smaller, assuming that a fixed "resource budget" is available (Parker 1982) and in the present study sperm dimensions were indeed larger in young males. Sperm morphology traits, such as sperm size, are known to be good proxies of reproductive performance in several animal species (Gomendio and Roldan 1991). For example, some studies have shown that sperm swimming ability was positively correlated with either head length, tail length or the sum of both (Pitcher et al. 2007 ; Gomendio and Roldan 2008; Fitzpatrick et al. 2010). However, this topic is controversial (see Snook 2005 for an overview) and many studies found no relationship between sperm morphology traits and sperm swimming performance (e.g. Gage et al. 2002 ; Locatello et al. 2007). Nevertheless, there is evidence that sperm motility is associated with mid-piece volume (Anderson and Dixson 2002) and the evolution of sperm mid-piece volume has been affected by selection pressures resulting from sperm competition (Anderson et al. 2005); the higher the mid-piece volume the higher the mitochondrial loading and thus flagellum beating frequency (Cardullo and Baltz 1991). The results of the present study show that sperm size and mid-piece volume were significantly larger in young males, suggesting higher quality sperm, as in sticklebacks fertilisation success is predicted by longer tail length, greater mid-piece volume and smaller head to tail length ratio (TCMB et al. unpublished data). Young and old males did however not differ significantly in head to flagellum length ratio, another proxy for sperm motility (Humphries et al. 2008), leaving this issue open for further investigations.

Sperm are known to be highly prone to oxidative stress (e.g. Aitken and Baker 2006). Helfenstein et al. (2010) reported the first experimental evidence that development of carotenoid-based ornaments and sperm quality may be linked through oxidative stress. Carotenoid-based conspicuous yellow, orange and red colour patterns are widespread in many vertebrate species (e.g. Hill et al. 2002). The colour variables for the stickleback cheek region that were measured in the present study indicate a stronger deposition of carotenoids in terms of a more chromatic and darker breeding coloration in younger males (Gomez et al. 2011) as an indicator of higher individual quality compared to older males. In sticklebacks, the intensity of the red/orange breeding coloration is one of the key determinants of female mate-choice decisions (e.g. McLennan and McPhail 1990 ; Bakker and Milinski 1993). If carotenoid availability is limited, these pigments will be traded off between fitness components such as sexual ornamentation and immunoresponsive capacities (Lozano 1994), thereby maintaining the honesty of carotenoid-based signals (e.g. Blount et al. 2003 ; but see

Navara and Hill 2003 spec. larvae that contain a.o. lutein (Czeczuga). In the laboratory, both young and old males were fed *Chironomus*1970), a major carotenoid for the development of males' breeding coloration (Wedekind et al. 1998 . Since animals cannot synthesise carotenoids *de novo*(Goodwin 1984), the given food supply was the only carotenoid source for the males. The less developed breeding coloration of older males might imply that old males' ability to cope with oxidative stress may be reduced, thus supporting the oxidative stress ageing theory as suggested by Harman (1956).

Testis melanisation occurs in many animal taxa, for example in fish (Louiz et al. 2009), amphibians (Zieri et al. 2007), reptiles (Guillette et al. 1983), birds (Galván et al. 2011), and mammals (Poole and Lawton 2009). In birds, for example, testicular melanisation has been evolved in species with high rates of accumulated mitochondrial mutations and has been supposed to be an adaptive response related to the protective capacity of melanin against oxidative stress (Galván et al.2011). The current study showed that the testes of older stickleback males were less pigmented, indicating that younger males might be able to handle oxidative stress better than their older brothers (but see Andziak et al. 2006). At the same time younger males were less pigmented in the dorsal region. This may indicate a trade-off between the deposition of melanin pigments in skin and testis tissue. Such a correlation between the proportion of plumage coloured by melanin and occurrence of testicular melanisation has not been found in birds (Galván et al. 2011). However, the precise function and relevance of testis melanisation in sticklebacks is unknown and requires further investigation.

Older males were significantly larger and heavier than their younger brothers. This is not surprising due to the fact that fish have indeterminate growth and also in sticklebacks age is largely confounded with body size (Allen and Wootton 1982). Furthermore, in three-spined sticklebacks, larger males are more aggressive (Mehlis et al. 2010), have an advantage in dominance fights (Rowland 1989), and females find larger males more attractive possibly due to their higher paternal quality and/or territorial quality (Kraak et al. 1999). However, females also prefer more intensely red-coloured stickleback males (Bakker and Milinski 1993 ; Kraak et al.1999 ; Künzler and Bakker 2001) and the results of the present study show that the relative area of red breeding coloration was greater in large males. It remains unclear how the attractiveness in terms of breeding coloration (higher saturated coloration and hue in the red/orange spectral region in young males but greater area of red breeding coloration in large old males) is traded off against body size, and thus whether younger males have the edge over their older brothers.

CONCLUSIONS

To conclude, the results revealed that advanced age can have beneficial as well as detrimental effects on an individual male stickleback's reproductive traits. Older males were larger (dominance advantage) and had more sperm than their younger brothers. They might be, however, at a disadvantage in terms of mate acquisition (less intense nuptial signal) and fertilisation ability (lower quality sperm). The less developed nuptial colour, testis melanisation and sperm quality could be the result of oxidative stress to cells and tissues accumulating over time (Harman 1956). However, one has to mention that further investigations are needed to confirm that the results of this explanatory study are really important under natural conditions, especially when stickleback males are confronted with sperm competition and whether this influences males' fertilisation abilities and reproductive success. Furthermore, given the damaging effects of progressive ageing, it is interesting to note that most males from the study population do not live long enough to reach a second reproductive phase in the field. Taken together, these observations support ultimate ageing theories suggesting that an age-related decrease in fitness might select for an increased reproductive investment early in life (Medawar 1952 ; Williams 1957).

METHODS

Experimental Subjects

About 500 three-spined sticklebacks from an anadromous, genetically heterogeneous population (Heckel et al. 2002) were caught during their spring migration in April 2008 on the island of Texel, the Netherlands.

Sticklebacks were purchased from a commercial fisherman, who has the permission to catch the fish. Within 5–6 hours fish were transported in large boxes (half filled with sea- and tap-water) to the Institute for Evolutionary Biology and Ecology in Bonn, Germany, where they were kept together in a large outside-tank (750 l), with air ventilation and a constant supply of tap-water at a flow rate of 3l min^{-1} and fed with red mosquito larvae (*Chironomus* spec.). The probability that individuals from the used study population die after their first breeding season seems to be high due to two reasons. First, the frequency distribution of standard lengths of the sampled fish during spring migration was single-peaked (MM personal observation). Second, a previous study did not find any large individuals during autumn migration from the breeding sites to the sea (van Mullem and van der Vlugt 1964). Nevertheless, under laboratory conditions it is common that these fish live 30 months or even longer and still reproduce (e.g. Mehlis et al. 2008 ; Mehlis et al. 2012).

To achieve different family groups, a randomly chosen male was allowed to spawn with a randomly chosen female, which were transferred to the laboratory with simulated summer conditions (day length 16L:8D, temperature 17 ± 1°C) for reproduction; thereby 40 clutches were produced in June 2008. Parents were only used once to avoid pseudoreplication. Thus, males used in this study originated from the F1 generation of randomly crossed wild-caught sticklebacks. To exclude paternal effects clutches were removed from the males' tanks 2 h after fertilisation and split into two full-sib groups. Hatched fry were fed daily with *Artemia* nauplii during the first month of age and juveniles/adults were fed with red mosquito larvae (*Chironomus* spec.) *in excess* later on. At an age of three weeks group size was reduced to 50 individuals, which were kept in holding tanks measuring 30 cm × 20 cm × 20 cm (length × width × height). Twenty weeks later, fish were transferred to holding tanks measuring 50 cm × 30 cm × 30 cm. Groups that consisted of more than 20 individuals were split again (eleven groups originating from eight families) and families that consisted of fewer than 20 individuals were fused again (15 families). At this time point all holding tanks were placed in an air-conditioned room under standardised winter light-regime (8L:16D, 17 ± 1°C). In sticklebacks, sexual maturation is stimulated by long photoperiods (Borg et al. 2004). Hence, to start the breeding season the light regime was changed to summer conditions in May 2009 (16L:8D, 17 ± 1°C), which lasted five months and followed by a second simulated winter period. At an age of 20 months fish were put under summer conditions again.

During both simulated breeding seasons randomly chosen males that showed signs of nuptial coloration in their holding tanks were individually isolated in separate tanks (30 cm × 20 cm × 20 cm) for nest building. It was ensured that all males used were virgin, because they had no possibility to build a nest in their holding tank and they were not paired to any female in their nesting tank. Collecting data such as total testis mass and sperm count (see below) is invasive; hence it was not possible to measure these traits for one male through time. In addition, only males that had built a nest were used, which ensures that they were reproductively active. In total, 161 males originating from 32 families built a nest. This included 60 males from 32 families, which were allowed to build nests in their first summer ("young males") and 101 males from 22 families, which were not allowed to build nests until the following summer ("old males"). During both simulated breeding seasons data collection for young and old males followed the same pattern, which is subsequently explained in detail.

Measurement of Body Traits

Males' body size (S) and mass (M) were determined and afterwards their body condition (BC) was calculated following Bolger and Connolly (1989; $BC = 100 * M / S^3$). Body measures were taken before isolating the males and shortly before euthanising them (see below). Hence, for each male both values were averaged for further analyses.

Measurement of Breeding Coloration

To determine the red area of male breeding coloration standardised digital still photographs were taken inside a black photo box using a camera (Nikon D70s with a Nikkor micro lens) connected to two flashes (Metz 20 BC6). This is a method frequently used in sticklebacks (e.g. Bakker and Mundwiler 1994 ; Frommen et al. 2008). A black curtain was tightened around the photo box to prevent any stray light from entering the box.

Males that had a nest for two days were stimulated with a receptive female (swollen abdomen filled with eggs) for 15 min. Afterwards, the male was put into a transparent plastic box (9.5 cm × 7 cm × 7 cm) containing some water and the left lateral side, visible through high quality glass (Hoya HMC UV filter), was photographed with an exposure time of 1/125 s and focal aperture of 16. Images were processed using Adobe Photoshop CS4. A white Munsell card (N10) visible on each picture served as white balance. The shape of the fish head (from snout to gills) was marked using the magnetic-lasso-tool and subsequently saved on a white background (1400 × 1000 pixel). To finish the quantification of the red area, images of the fish head were uploaded in Sigma Scan Pro 5.0 and the percentage of red area (threshold hue: 0–40; threshold saturation: 20–100) was determined in relation to the total area of the fish head and the white background.

The expression of male breeding coloration was quantified by using reflectance measurements of the skin, which were taken on average two days after the photograph (median and quartiles: 2, 2, 4). Shortly before reflectance measurements, males were stimulated with a receptive female for 15 min. Reflectance scans were taken with a spectrophotometer (Avantes AVS-USB2000) connected to a deuterium-halogen light source (Avantes DH-2000) for illumination (see Rick et al.2011 for a detailed description). Measurements were made directly below the eye (A-region, breeding coloration) and at the dorsum below the first dorsal spine (R-region). Data were recorded without changing probe contact using Spectrawin 5.1 (Avantes) and imported into Microsoft Excel. About twenty measurements were taken in succession and averaged for the A-region (median and quartiles: 20, 17, 27) and the R-region (median and quartiles: 18, 16, 19).

The reflectance spectrum of the carotenoid-based breeding coloration of three-spined stickleback males is double-peaked with one peak in the UV-region and an extended plateau at longer wavelengths (Rick and Bakker 2008; Figure 1). Hence, for the A-region the UV chroma ($C_{UV} = R_{300\text{-}400} / R_{300\text{-}700}$; R = reflectance at a given wavelength) and, as a measure of carotenoid pigmentation (e.g. Blount and Pike 2012), carotenoid chroma ($C_{caro} = (R_{700} - R_{450}) / R_{700}$) were calculated. The R_{50} value for the A-region was determined, defined as the wavelength at the halfway reflectance point between the minimum reflectance (400 to 500 nm) and the maximum reflectance (500 to 700 nm). Higher R_{50} values indicate a more red-shifted hue of the measured region (Rick and Bakker 2008 ; Pike et al. 2011). Finally, the total brightness ($R_{300-700}$) was measured for both regions.

Measurement of Testis Traits

Directly after reflectance measurements were taken, males were euthanised quickly by decapitation, both testes were removed, placed separately on a tissue paper and weighed to the nearest milligram (OHAUS, Explorer, E11140) so that the relative testis mass (gonadosomatic index, GSI,) could be calculated after de Vlaming et al. (1982; GSI = (TM_{total} / M) * 100, where TM_{total} is the sum of the absolute mass of both testes).

As the testes of three-spined stickleback males are covered with melanophores and there is striking between-male variation in testicular melanisation and the L*value (brightness) is a good indicator of melanophore density (see Figure 2 a-b; Mehlis et al. 2012), the intensity of melanophore pigmentation was quantified using the same method as described in Mehlis et al. (2012). Melanophores are generally thought to protect the testes from deleterious UV light due to their strong light absorbance (Kaidbey et al. 1979 ; Plonka et al. 2009) and/or to protect males' germ cells from oxidative stress (Galván et al. 2011). Testis brightness was determined for each male's testis (L^*_{left} and L^*_{right}) and finally averaged (L^*_{total}).

Measurements of Sperm Traits

The measurement of sperm number was solely conducted on the left testis because sperm number of left and right testes are highly correlated in sticklebacks (Bakker et al. 2006). Right testes were used for later SEM-preparation (see below) hence they were stored in an Eppendorf tube containing 500 µl 4% formalin. The left testis was pestled in 200 µl of a non-activating medium (for mixture see Fauvel et al. 1999). Ten microlitres of the sperm suspension were diluted in 190 µl of tap water in order to reduce sperm density. Twelve microlitres of this dilution were filled into an improved Neubauer counting chamber (Labor Optik, 0.0025 mm^2, depth 0.1 mm). Sperm were counted in 32 equally distributed cells and averaged, so that the total number of sperm was calculated (see Mehlis et al. 2012).

Sperm morphology was determined by scanning electron microscopy (SEM; Figure 2c). The preparation of sperm followed Mortimer (1994) and was adapted for sticklebacks providing highly repeatable measurements of sperm traits (see Mehlis et al. 2012). Sperm variables were measured using 3000–6000 magnified SEM-images (Leitz AMR 1000), which were digitised using DISS (Digital Image Scanning System, Point Electronic GmbH, Halle, Germany) and DIPS (Digital Image Processing System V 2.5.2.1, Point Electronic GmbH, Halle, Germany). Sperm morphology variables (head length (hl), head width (hw), mid-piece length (ml), mid-piece width (mw) and tail length (tl)) were measured only on images that showed intact sperm (with a well visible head and a complete tail; see Figure 2c) using ImageJ. On average 20 sperm were measured per male (median and quartiles: 20, 19, 22).

Unfortunately, it was not possible to measure sperm motility directly because after dissection testes were stored in 4% formalin. However, in stickleback's fertilisation success is predicted by tail length, mid-piece volume and head to tail length ratio (TCMB et al. unpublished data). Thus, the head to tail length ratio ((hl + ml) / tl) and mid-piece volume ($\varpi * (mw / 2)^2 * ml$) were calculated as a proxy of sperm motility being an indicator of sperm quality.

ACKNOWLEDGEMENTS

We are grateful to the "Bakker" research-group, especially Ingolf P. Rick and Meike Hiermes, for discussion. We thank Jan Hottentot for catching the sticklebacks. Lukas K. Hilke is acknowledged for help with the determination of testis melanisation and Dagmar Wenzel for help in measuring SEM images. Deborah A. McLennan is also kindly acknowledged for language corrections. This research was funded by the Deutsche Forschungsgemeinschaft (DFG) (BA 2885/4-1).

REFERENCES

1. Aitken RJ, Baker M (2006) Oxidative stress, sperm survival and fertility control. Mol Cell Endocrinol 250:66-69

2. Allen JRM, Wootton RJ (1982) Age, growth and rate of food consumption in an upland population of the three-spined stickleback, *Gasterosteus aculeatus* L. J Fish Biol 21:95-105
3. Anderson MJ, Dixson AF (2002) Sperm competition: motility and the midpiece in primates. Nature 416:496-496
4. Anderson MJ, Nyholt J, Dixson AF (2005) Sperm competition and the evolution of sperm midpiece volume in mammals. J Zool 267:135-142
5. Andziak B, O'Connor TP, Qi W, DeWaal EM, Pierce A, Chaudhuri AR, Van Remmen H, Buffenstein R (2006) High oxidative damage levels in the longest-living rodent, the naked mole-rat. Aging Cell 5:463-71
6. Bakker TCM, Milinski M (1993) The advantages of being red: sexual selection in the stickleback. Mar Behav Physiol 23:287-300
7. Bakker TCM, Mundwiler B (1994) Female mate choice and male red coloration in a natural three-spined stickleback (*Gasterosteus aculeatus*) population. Behav Ecol 5:74-80
8. Bakker TCM, Zbinden M, Frommen JG, Weiss A, Largiadèr CR (2006) Slow fertilization of stickleback eggs: the result of sexual conflict? BMC Ecol 6:7
9. Balbontín J, de Lope F, Hermosell IG, Mousseau TA, Møller AP (2011) Determinants of age-dependent change in a secondary sexual character. J Evol Biol 24:440-448
10. Beck CW, Promislow DEL (2007) Evolution of female preference for younger males. PLoS One 2:e939
11. Billard R, Takashima F (1983) Resorption of spermatozoa in the sperm duct of rainbow trout during the post-spawning period. B Jpn Soc Sci Fish 49:387-392
12. Blount J, Pike TW (2012) Deleterious effects of light exposure on immunity and sexual coloration in birds. Funct Ecol 26:37-45
13. Blount JD, Metcalfe NB, Birkhead TR, Surai PF (2003) Carotenoid modulation of immune function and sexual attractiveness in zebra finches. Science 300:125-127
14. Bolger T, Connolly PL (1989) The selection of suitable indices for the measurement and analysis of fish condition. J Fish Biol 34:171-182

15. Borg B (1982) Seasonal effects of photoperiod and temperature on spermatogenesis and male secondary sexual characters in the three-spined stickleback, *Gasterosteus aculeatus*. Can J Zool 60:3377-3386
16. Borg B, Bornestaf C, Hellqvist A, Schmitz M, Mayer I (2004) Mechanisms in the photoperiodic control of reproduction in the stickleback. Behaviour 141:1521-1530
17. Candolin U, Vlieger L (2013) Should attractive males sneak: the trade-off between current and future offspring. PLoS One 8:e57992
18. Cardullo RA, Baltz JM (1991) Metabolic regulation in mammalian sperm: mitochondrial volume determines sperm length and flagellar beat frequency. Cell Motil Cytoskelet 19:180-188
19. Cubillos ER, Guderley HE (2000) Analysis of the factors related with mate choice and reproductive success in male three-spined sticklebacks. J Fish Biol 56:1201-1216
20. Czeczuga B (1970) Some carotenoids in *Chironomus annularius* Meig. larvae (Diptera: Chironomidae). Hydrobiologia 36:353-360
21. de Vlaming V, Grossman GD, Chapman F (1982) On the use of the gonosomatic index. Comp Biochem Physiol 73:31-39
22. Dean R, Cornwallis CK, Lovlie H, Worley K, Richardson DS, Pizzari T (2010) Male reproductive senescence causes potential for sexual conflict over mating. Curr Biol 20:1192-1196
23. DuVal EH (2012) Variation in annual and lifetime reproductive success of lance-tailed manakins: alpha experience mitigates effects of senescence on siring success. Proc R Soc Lond B 279:1551-1559
24. Fauvel C, Savoye O, Dreanno C, Cosson J, Suquet M (1999) Characteristics of sperm of captive seabass in relation to its fertilization potential. J Fish Biol 54:356-369
25. Fitzpatrick JL, Garcia-Gonzalez F, Evans JP (2010) Linking sperm length and velocity: the importance of intramale variation. Biol Lett 6:797-799
26. Frommen JG, Luz C, Mazzi D, Bakker TCM (2008) Inbreeding depression affects fertilization success and survival but not

breeding coloration in threespine sticklebacks. Behaviour 145:425-441

27. Gage MJG, MacFarlane C, Yeates S, Shackleton R, Parker GA (2002) Relationships between sperm morphometry and sperm motility in the Atlantic salmon. J Fish Biol 61:1528-1539
28. Galván I, Møller AP, Erritzøe J (2011) Testicular melanization has evolved in birds with high mtDNA mutation rates. J Evol Biol 24:988-998
29. Gambling SJ, Reimchen TE (2012) Prolonged life span among endemic *Gasterosteus* populations. Can J Zool 90:284-290
30. Garratt M, Stockley P, Armstrong SD, Beynon RJ, Hurst JL (2011) The scent of senescence: sexual signalling and female preference in house mice. J Evol Biol 24:2398-2409
31. Gasparini C, Marino IAM, Boschetto C, Pilastro A (2010) Effect of male age on sperm traits and sperm competition success in the guppy (*Poecilia reticulata*). J Evol Biol 23:124-135
32. Goldschmidt T, Foster SA, Sevenster P (1992) Inter-nest distance and sneaking in the three-spined stickleback. Anim Behav 44:793-795
33. Gomendio M, Roldan ERS (1991) Sperm competition influences sperm size in mammals. Proc R Soc Lond B 243:181-185
34. Gomendio M, Roldan ERS (2008) Implications of diversity in sperm size and function for sperm competition and fertility. Int J Dev Biol 52:439-447
35. Gomez D, Thery M, Gauthier A-L, Lengagne T (2011) Costly help of audiovisual bimodality for female mate choice in a nocturnal anuran (*Hyla arborea*). Behav Ecol 22:889-898
36. Goodwin TW (1984) The Biochemistry of the Carotenoids vol 2. Chapman & Hall, London: Animals
37. Guillette L, Weigel J, Flater G (1983) Unilateral testicular pigmentation in the Mexican lizard*Sceloporus variabilis*. Copeia 1983:155-161
38. Harcourt AH, Harvey PH, Larson SG, Short RV (1981) Testis weight, body weight and breeding system in primates. Nature 293:55-57
39. Harman D (1956) Aging: a theory based on free radical and radiation chemistry. J Gerontol 11:298-300

40. Heckel G, Zbinden M, Mazzi D, Kohler A, Reckeweg G, Bakker TCM, Largiadèr CR (2002) Microsatellite markers for the three-spined stickleback (*Gasterosteus aculeatus* L.) and their applicability in a freshwater and an anadromous population. Conserv Genet 3:79-81
41. Helfenstein F, Losdat S, Møller AP, Blount JD, Richner H (2010) Sperm of colourful males are better protected against oxidative stress. Ecol Lett 13:213-222
42. Hill GE, Inouye CY, Montgomerie R (2002) Dietary carotenoids predict plumage coloration in wild house finches. Proc R Soc Lond B 269:1119-1124
43. Hoffmann E, Walstad A, Karlsson J, Olsson P-E, Borg B (2012) Androgen receptor-beta mRNA levels in different tissues in breeding and post-breeding male and female sticklebacks, *Gasterosteus aculeatus*. Reprod Biol Endocrinol 10:23
44. Holliday R (2006) Aging is no longer an unsolved problem in biology. Ann N Y Acad Sci 1067:1-9
45. Hughes KA, Reynolds RM (2005) Evolutionary and mechanistic theories of aging. Annu Rev Entomol 50:421-445
46. Humphries S, Evans JP, Simmons LW (2008) Sperm competition: linking form to function. BMC Evol Biol 8:319
47. Jamieson IG, Colgan PW (1992) Sneak spawning and egg stealing by male threespine sticklebacks. Can J Zool 70:963-967
48. Johnson SL, Gemmel NJ (2012) Are old males still good males and can females tell the difference? BioEssays 34:609-619
49. Kaidbey K, Agin P, Sayre R, Kligman A (1979) Photoprotection by melanin - a comparison of black and Caucasian skin. J Amer Acad Dermatol 1:249-260
50. Kanuga MK, Benner MJ, Doble JA, Wilson Leedy JG, Robison BD, Ingermann RL (2011) Effect of aging on male reproduction in zebrafish (*Danio rerio*). J Exp Zool 315:156-161
51. Kraak SBM, Bakker TCM, Mundwiler B (1999) Sexual selection in sticklebacks in the field: correlates of reproductive, mating, and paternal success. Behav Ecol 10:696-706
52. Künzler R, Bakker TCM (2001) Female preference for single and combined traits in computer animated stickleback males. Behav Ecol 12:681-685

53. Largiadèr CR, Fries V, Bakker TCM (2001) Genetic analysis of sneaking and egg-thievery in a natural population of the three-spined stickleback (*Gasterosteus aculeatus* L.). Heredity 86:459-468

54. Locatello L, Pilastro A, Deana R, Zarpellon A, Rasotto MB (2007) Variation pattern of sperm quality traits in two gobies with alternative mating tactics. Funct Ecol 21:975-981

55. Louiz I, Ben-Attia M, Ben-Hassine O (2009) Gonadosomatic index and gonad histopathology of*Gobius niger* (Gobiidea, Teleost) from Bizerta lagoon (Tunisia): evidence of reproduction disturbance. Fish Res 100:266-273

56. Lozano GA (1994) Carotenoids, parasites, and sexual selection. Oikos 70:309-311

57. McLennan DA, McPhail JD (1990) Experimental investigations of the evolutionary significance of sexually dimorphic nuptial colouration in *Gasterosteus aculeatus* (L.): the relationship between male colour and female behaviour. Can J Zool 68:482-492 Medawar PB (1952) An Unsolved Problem of Biology. London: H.K. Lewis & Co

58. Medvedev ZA (1990) An attempt at a rational classification of theories of ageing. Biol Rev 65:375-398

59. Mehlis M, Bakker TCM, Frommen JG (2008) Smells like sib spirit: kin recognition in three-spined sticklebacks (*Gasterosteus aculeatus*) is mediated by olfactory cues. Anim Cogn 11:643-650 Mehlis M, Bakker TCM, Engqvist L, Frommen JG (2010) To eat or not to eat: egg-based assessment of paternity triggers fine-tuned decisions about filial cannibalism. Proc R Soc Lond B 277:2627-2635

60. Mehlis M, Frommen JG, Rahn AK, Bakker TCM (2012) Inbreeding in sticklebacks (*Gasterosteus aculeatus* L.): effects on testis and sperm traits. Biol J Linn Soc 107:510-520

61. Milewski LAK (2010) The evolution of ageing. Bioscience Horizons 3:77-84

62. Mortimer D (1994) Preparation of human spermatozoa for electron microscopy. In: Mortimer D (ed) Practical Laboratory Andrology. Oxford: Oxford University Press. pp 168-173

63. Navara KJ, Hill GE (2003) Dietary carotenoid pigments and immune function in a songbird with extensive carotenoid-based plumage coloration. Behav Ecol 14:909-916

64. Parker GA (1982) Why are there so many tiny sperm? Sperm competition and the maintenance of two sexes. J Theor Biol 96:281-294

65. Parker GA (1990) Sperm competition games: raffles and roles. Proc R Soc Lond B 242:120-126

66. Pike TW, Bjerkeng B, Blount JB, Lindstroem J, Metcalfe NB (2011) How integument colour reflects its carotenoid content: a stickleback's perspective. Funct Ecol 25:297-304

67. Pitcher TE, Rodd FH, Rowe L (2007) Sexual colouration and sperm traits in guppies. J Fish Biol 70:165-177

68. Plonka P, Passeron T, Brenner M, Tobin D, Shibahara S, Thomas A (2009) What are melanocytes really doing all day long…? Exp Dermatol 18:799-819

69. Poole A, Lawton C (2009) The translocation and post release settlement of red squirrels *Sciurus vulgaris* to a previously uninhabited woodland. Biodivers Conserv 18:3205-3218

70. Raveh S, Heg D, Dobson FS, Coltman D, Gorrell J (2010) Mating order and reproductive success in male Columbian ground squirrels (*Urocitellus columbianus*). Behav Ecol 21:537-547

71. Rick IP, Bakker TCM (2008) Males do not see only red: UV wavelengths and male territorial aggression in the three-spined stickleback (*Gasterosteus aculeatus*). Naturwissenschaften 95:631-638

72. Rick IP, Mehlis M, Bakker TCM (2011) Male red ornamentation is associated with female red sensitivity in sticklebacks. PLoS One 6:e25554

73. Rico C, Kuhnlein U, FitzGerald GJ (1992) Male reproductive tactics in the threespine stickleback - an evaluation by DNA fingerprinting. Mol Ecol 1:79-87

74. Rose MR, Burke MK, Shahrestani P, Mueller LD (2008) Evolution of ageing since Darwin. J Genet 87:363-371

75. Rowe M, Pruett-Jones S (2011) Sperm competition selects for sperm quantity and quality in the Australien maluridae. PLoS One 6:e15720

76. Rowland WJ (1989) The effects of body size, aggression and nuptial coloration on competition for territories in male threespine sticklebacks, *Gasterosteus aculeatus*. Anim Behav 37:282-289
77. Sasson DA, Johnson SL, Brockmann HJ (2012) The role of age on sperm traits in the American horseshoe crab, *Limulus polyphemus*. Anim Behav 84:975-981
78. Schneider L (1969) Experimentelle Untersuchungen über den Einfluß von Tageslänge und Temperatur auf die Gonadenreifung beim Dreistachligen Stichling (*Gasterosteus aculeatus*). Oecologia 3:249-265
79. Snook RR (2005) Sperm in competition: not playing by the numbers. Trends Ecol Evol 20:46-53
80. Somashekar K, Krishna MS (2011) Evidence of female preference for older males in *Drosophila bipectinata*. Zool Stud 50:1-15
81. Stockley P, Gage MJG, Parker GA, Møller AP (1997) Sperm competition in fishes: the evolution of testis size and ejaculate characteristics. Am Nat 149:933-954
82. Symonds MRE, Moussalli A (2011) A brief guide to model selection, multimodel inference and model averaging in behavioural ecology using Akaike's information criterion. Behav Ecol Sociobiol 65:13-21
83. van Mullem PJ, van der Vlugt JC (1964) On the age, growth and migration of the anadromous stickleback *Gasterosteus aculeatus* L. investigated in mixed populations. Arch Néerl Zool 16:111-139
84. Velando A, Noguera JC, Drummond H, Torres R (2011) Senescent males carry premutagenic lesions in sperm. J Evol Biol 24:693-697
85. Verburgt L, Ferreira M, Ferguson JWH (2011) Male field cricket song reflects age, allowing females to prefer young males. Anim Behav 81:19-29
86. Vlieger L, Candolin U (2009) How not to be seen: does eutrophication influence three-spined stickleback *Gasterosteus aculeatus* sneaking behaviour? J Fish Biol 75:2163-2174
87. Wedekind C, Meyer P, Frischknecht M, Niggli UA, Pfander H (1998) Different carotenoids and potential information content

of red coloration of male three-spined stickleback. J Chem Ecol 24:787-801

88. Williams GC (1957) Pleiotropy, natural selection, and the evolution of senescence. Evolution 11:398-411
89. Wootton RJ (1976) The Biology of the Sticklebacks. London: Academic Press.
90. Yang H, Chryssikos T, Houseni M, Alzeair S, Sansovini M, Iruvuri S, Torigian D, Zhuang H, Dadparvar S, Basu S, Alavi A (2011) The effects of aging on testicular volume and glucose metabolism: an investigation with ultrasonography and FDG-PET. Mol Imag Biol 13:391-398
91. Zbinden M, Largiadèr CR, Bakker TCM (2001) Sperm allocation in the three-spined stickleback. J Fish Biol 59:1287-1297
92. Zbinden M, Mazzi D, Künzler R, Largiadèr CR, Bakker TCM (2003) Courting virtual rivals increase ejaculate size in sticklebacks (*Gasterosteus aculeatus*). Behav Ecol Sociobiol 54:205-209
93. Zbinden M, Largiadèr CR, Bakker TCM (2004) Body size of virtual rivals affects ejaculate size in sticklebacks. Behav Ecol 15:137-140
94. Zieri R, Taboga SR, de Oliveira C (2007) Melanocytes in the testes of *Eupemphix nattereri* (Anura, Leiuperidae): histological, stereological, and ultrastructural aspects. Anat Rec 290:795-800.

chapter 5

Methods for Separation, Recycling and Reuse of Biodegradation Products

Ganapati D. Yadav[1] and Jyoti B. Sontakke[1]

[1]Department of Chemical Engineering, Institute of Chemical Technology, Matunga, Mumbai, India

INTRODUCTION

Thousands of chemicals and materials with varied properties and functionalities are manufactured and used for commercial and day-to-day applications, whose ultimate fate in the environment may not be known. During their manufacture and use, these substances are often discharged into the environment through different routes in air, water and land. Creation of tremendous quantities of solid waste of all kind and its effective disposal has posed innumerable problems that need technological breakthroughs. Many of these substances degrade slowly and exert toxic effects on plants and animals, thus causing large scale environmental degradation [1, 2]. Pollution by abandoned plastic articles is also a matter of great concern [3]. Industrial wastewaters associated with the manufacture of organic chemicals are voluminous and characteristically have concentrations ranging from a few ppm to a thousands of ppm. Biodegradation of such dissolved pollutants is an area of immense interest to various sectors. Emission of volatile organic compounds (VOCs) from various sources has detrimental effects on quality of air we breathe and on environmental phenomena. Biodegradation, either aerobic or anaerobic, can be an approach to cleave big molecules through a series of steps in to smaller molecules from a mosaic of chemicals and materials and some of them can be valorized as pollution abatement strategy and source of energy through biogas generation [2]. Biogas can be produced from nearly all kind of biomass, among which the primary agricultural sectors and various organic waste streams can be properly tapped as renewable source of energy. Untreated or poorly managed animal manure is a major source of air and water pollution. Nutrient leaching, mainly nitrogen and phosphorous, ammonia evaporation and pathogen contamination are some of the foremost threats [3]. A conservative estimate is provided by Steinfeld et al. [4] that the animal production sector is responsible for 18% of the overall greenhouse gas emissions, measured in CO_2 equivalent and for 37% of the anthropogenic methane, which has 23 times the global warming potential of CO_2. Furthermore, 65% of anthropogenic nitrous oxide and 64% of anthropogenic ammonia emission originate from the worldwide animal production sector. Biogas production from anaerobic digestion of animal manure and slurries can be harnessed to alleviate greenhouse gas emissions in particularly ammonia and methane [5].

Plastics are bane and benefactor simultaneously. Over 230 million tons of plastic are produced annually. Plastics are used in all walks of life and provide improved insulation, lighter packaging, are found in cars, aeroplanes, railways, phones, computers, medical devices, etc. but appropriate disposal is often not properly addressed. On one hand, plastic waste and disposal is a hotly debated issue globally whereas on the other, it can contribute to reduce the carbon footprint. Many leading

European countries recover more than 80% of their used plastics, by adopting an integrated waste and resource management strategy to address each waste stream with the best options [6]. Plastic sorting and separation, recycling, depolymerisation, cracking, and production of fuel are some of the strategies used to abate plastic pollution. Development of biopolymers is pursued vigorously. Biodegradation of plastics by microorganisms and enzymes appears to be the most effective process. When plastics are used as substrates for microorganisms, evaluation of their biodegradability should not only be based on their chemical structure, but also on their physical properties such as melting point, glass transition temperature, crystallinity, storage modulus, etc. [7-11].

This chapter has covered the mechanisms of biodegradation, biodegradation of a variety of industrial chemicals, plastics and other biomass, advances in anaerobic digestion technologies and biogas generation, plastic processing, biopolymer synthesis and degradation. Synthesis of biopolymers is covered. The scope for treating municipal organic solid waste, manure and polymers to generate biogas as a renewable energy option, and also as a pollution abatement strategy is discussed including technological aspects. The synthesis of biohydrogen, bioethanol, biobutanol and other biotransformation leading to valuable chemicals, which also involve breaking down of larger molecules, plastics and biomaterials are not addressed [7,10]. Biorefinery is a concept which is akin to petrorefinery, wherein biomass is converted into useful platform chemicals through extraction, controlled pyrolysis, fermentation, enzyme and chemical catalysis [12].

MECHANISMS OF BIODEGRADATION

Cellulose, lignocellulose and lignin are major sources of plant biomass and are polymeric substances; therefore, their recycling is indispensable for the carbon cycle [13]. Each of these polymer is degraded by a variety of microorganisms which produce scores of enzymes that work in tandem. The diversity of cellulosic and lignocellulosic substrates has contributed to the difficulties found in enzymatic treatment. Fungi are the best-known microorganisms capable of degrading these three polymers. Because the substrates are insoluble, both bacterial and fungal degradation occur exo-cellularly, either in association with the outer cell envelope layer or extra-cellularly. Microorganisms have two types of extracellular enzymatic systems, namely, the hydrolytic system, which produces hydrolases and is responsible for cellulose and hemicellulose degradation; and a unique oxidative and extracellular ligninolytic system, which depolymerizes lignin [13]. The man-made chemicals and materials are comprised of different entities and functional groups which need to be degraded effectively by microorganisms and no single microorganism is obviously capable of doing it [1,14].

Growth and co-metabolism are the two mechanisms of biodegradation. In the case of growth, organic substance is used as the sole source of carbon and energy, which leads to complete degradation (mineralization). Archaebacteria, prokaryotes and eukaryotes (like fungi, algae, yeasts, protozoa) play dominant role in mineralization [7]. On the contrary, co-metabolism encompasses the metabolism of an organic compound in the presence of a growth substrate which is used as the primary carbon and energy source. Thus, biodegradation processes and their rates differ greatly depending on the type of substrate and conditions such as temperature, pH, and aqueous phase solubility, but frequently the major final products of the degradation are carbon dioxide and methane [1,7,10].

Growth-Associated Degradation of Aliphatic Compounds

Growth-associated degradation produces CO_2, H_2O, and cell biomass. The cells act as the complex biocatalysts of degradation. Further, cell biomass may be mineralized after exhaustion of the degradable pollutants in a contaminated site. Bulk chemicals like aromatic hydrocarbons such as benzene, toluene, ethylbenzene, xylenes, and naphthalene are widely used as fuels, industrial solvents and feedstock for petrochemical industry. Phenols and chlorophenols are another class of chemicals, employed in a variety of industries. Since all micro-organisms make aromatic compounds such as aromatic amino acids, phenols, or quinines, in large amounts, many microorganisms have evolved catabolic pathways to degrade aromatic compounds. In general, man-made organic chemicals (xenobiotics) can be degraded by microorganisms, when the respective molecules are similar to natural compounds [7,10]. In general, benzene, condensed ring and related compounds are characterized by a higher thermodynamic stability than aliphatic compounds. Benzene oxidation begins with hydroxylation catalyzed by a dioxygenase leading to a diol (Scheme 1) which is then converted to catechol by a dehydrogenase.

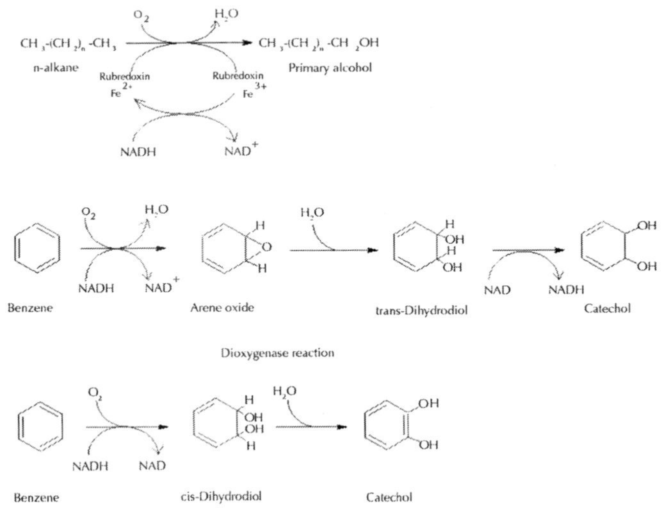

Scheme 1: Monooxygenase and dioxygenase reactions: In this mechanism, monooxygenase initially incorporates one O atom from O_2 into the xenobiotic substrate whereas the other is reduced to H_2O. On the contrary, dioxygenase incorporates both atoms into the substrate [15].

Hydroxylation and dehydrogenation are also common in degradation routes of other aromatic hydrocarbons. The introduction of a substituent group onto the benzene ring renders alternative mechanisms possible to attack side chains or to oxidize the aromatic ring. Many aromatic substrates are degraded by a limited number of reactions such as hydroxylation, oxygenolytic ring cleavage, isomerization, and hydrolysis. The inducible nature of the enzymes and their substrate specificity enable bacteria such as pseudomonads and rhodococci with a high degradation activity, to acclimatize their metabolism to the effective utilization of substrate mixtures in polluted soils and also to grow at a high rate [10,15].

Co-Metabolic Degradation of Organo-Pollutants

Co-metabolism is a common phenomenon of microbial activities and the basis of biotransformation used in biotechnology to convert molecules in to useful modified forms. Microorganisms growing on a particular substrate also oxidize a second substrate. The co-substrate is not incorporated, but the product may be available as substrate for other organisms of a mixed culture. The rudiments of co-metabolic transformation are the enzymes of the growing cells and the synthesis of cofactors necessary for enzymatic reactions; for instance, of hydrogen donors (reducing equivalents, NADH) for oxygenases. Several aromatic substrates can be converted enzymatically to natural intermediates of degradation such as catechol and protecatechuate (Scheme 2) [15].

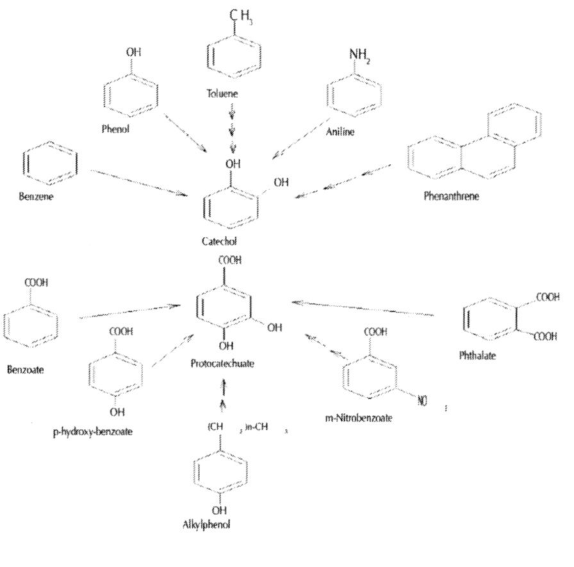

Scheme 2: Degradation of aromatic natural and xenobiotic compounds into two central intermediates, catechol and protocatechuate [15].

Co-metabolism of chloroaromatics is a general activity of bacteria in mixtures of industrial pollutants. The co-metabolic transformation of 2-chlorophenol leads to dead-end metabolites such as 3-chlorocatechol, which may be auto-oxidized or polymerized in soil to humic-like structures. Irreversible binding of dead end metabolites may fulfill the function of detoxification. The accumulation of dead-end products within microbes under selection pressure is the source for the evolution of new catabolic traits. Thus, recalcitrance of organic pollutants increases with increasing halogenation. Substitution of halogen as well as nitro and sulfo groups at the aromatic ring is accomplished by an increasing electrophilicity of the molecule. These compounds resist the electrophilic attack by oxygenases of aerobic bacteria. Compounds that persist under oxic condition are polychlorinated biphenyls (PCBs), chlorinated dioxins and some pesticides like DDT. To overcome the relatively high persistence of halogenated xenobiotics, reductive attack of anaerobic bacteria is of great value. Reductive dehalogenation achieved by anaerobic bacteria is either a gratuitous reaction or a new type of anaerobic respiration. The process reduces the degree of chlorination and, therefore, makes the product more accessible to mineralization by aerobic bacteria [7,15].

Reductive dehalogenation which is the first step of degradation of PCBs requires anaerobic conditions wherein organic substrates act as electron donors. PCBs accept electrons to allow the anaerobic bacteria to transfer electrons to these compounds. Anaerobic bacteria capable of catalyzing reductive dehalogenation seem to be relatively omnipresent in nature. Most dechlorinating cultures are a mixed consortia. Anaerobic dechlorination is always incomplete and the products are di- and monochlorinated biphenyls. These products can be metabolized further by aerobic microorganisms [2,7,15].

The rates of biodegradability of particular substrate is mainly related to accessibility of the substrate for enzymes and can be enhanced by several means as reviewed by van Lier et al. [16] such as (a) mechanical methods: the disintegration and grinding of solid particles present in sludge: releases cell compounds and creates new surface where biodegradation take place, (b) ultrasonic disintegration, (c) chemical methods: the destruction of complex organic compounds by means of strong, mineral acids or alkalis, (d) thermal pretreatment: thermal hydrolysis is able to split and decompose a significant part of the sludge solid fraction into soluble and less complex molecules, (e) enzymatic and microbial pre-treatment: a very promising method for the future for some specific substrates (e.g. cellulose, lignin etc.),(f) stimulation of anaerobic micro-organisms: some organic compounds (e.g. amino acids, cofactors, cell content) act as a stimulating agent in bacteria growth and methane production. Most of the above methods occur at the pre-methanation step and result in a better supply of methanogenic bacteria by suitable substrates.

AEROBIC BIODEGRADATION

Many microorganisms grow under aerobic conditions. The so-called cellular respiration process (CSP) begins with aerobes which employ oxygen to oxidize substrates such as sugars and fats to derive energy. Before the onset of CSP, glucose molecules are degraded into smaller molecules in the cytoplasm of the aerobes. The smaller molecules then enter a mitochondrion, where aerobic respiration takes place. Oxygen is used to break down small entities into water and carbon dioxide, accompanied by release of energy. Aerobic degradation does not produce foul gases, unlike anaerobic process. The aerobic process leads to a more complete digestion of solid waste reducing build-up by more than 50% in most cases [1, 2, 7]. The major enzymatic reactions of aerobic biodegradation are oxidations catalyzed by oxygenases and peroxidases. Oxygenases are oxido-reductases that incorporate oxygen into the substrate as given in Scheme 1. Degradative organisms need oxygen at two metabolic sites, namely, at the initial attack of the substrate and at the end of the respiratory chain. Higher fungi possess a unique oxidative system for the degradation of lignin based on extracellular ligninolytic peroxidases and laccases [13]. This enzymatic system is important for the co-metabolic degradation of persistent organic pollutants. The predominant bacteria of polluted soils belong to a spectrum of genera and species (Table 1) [15].

The most important classes of organic pollutants in the environment are mineral oil constituents and halogenated petrochemicals, for the biodegradation of which the capacities of aerobic microorganisms are of great consequence. The most rapid and complete degradation of the majority of pollutants is brought about under aerobic conditions and these include petroleum hydrocarbons, chlorinated aliphatics, benzene, toluene, phenol, naphthalene, fluorine, pyrene, chloroanilines, pentachlorophenol and dichlorobenzenes. Many cultures of bacteria grow on these chemicals and are capable of producing enzymes which degrade them into non-toxic species. [7,15].

Table 1: Predominant bacteria in soil samples polluted with aliphatic and aromatic hydrocarbons, polycyclic aromatic hydrocarbons, and chlorinated compounds [15]

Gram negative bacteria	**Gram positive bacteria**
Pseudomonas species	Nocardia species
Xanthomonas species	Mycobacteria species
Alcaligenes species	Corynebacterium species
Flavobacterium species	Arthobacter species
Cytophaga group	Bacillus species

There are several essential attributes of aerobic microorganisms degrading organic pollutants amongst which metalobic processes top the list. The chemicals must be accessible to the degrading organisms. For example, hydrocarbons are immiscible in water and their degradation requires the production of biosurfactants in order to have effective biodegradation [14]. The initial intracellular attack of organic pollutants is an oxidative process and therefore, the activation and incorporation of oxygen is the main enzymatic reaction catalyzed by oxygenases and peroxidases. Peripheral degradation pathways convert organic pollutants step by step into intermediates of the central intermediary metabolism, such as the tricarboxylic acid cycle. Biosynthesis of cell biomass from the central precursor metabolites (acetyl-CoA, succinate, pyruvate) is required [14,15]. Sugars needed for various biosyntheses and growth must be synthesized by gluconeogenesis. The predominant degraders of organo-pollutants in the oxic zone of contaminated areas are chemo-organotropic species that are able to use a large number of natural and xenobiotic compounds as carbon sources and electron donors for the generation of energy. Although many bacteria are able to metabolize organic pollutants, a single bacterium does not possess the enzymatic capability to degrade all or even most of the organic pollutants from a heterogeneous mixture originating from particular industries. Thus, mixed microbial communities have the most powerful biodegradative potential. The genetic information of more than one organism is necessary to develop a system which could be used on industrial scale to degrade the complex mixtures of organic compounds present in contaminated areas. The genetic potential and certain environmental factors such as temperature, pH, and available nitrogen and phosphorus sources govern the rate and the extent of degradation [14].

ANAEROBIC BIODEGRADATION

Among biological treatments, anaerobic digestion is frequently the most economical process, due to the high energy recovery linked to the process and its limited environmental impact. Anaerobic biodegradation results when the anaerobic microbes are predominant over the aerobic microbes. Here oxygen does not serve as the final electron acceptor or reactant. Manganese and iron ions, and substances like sulfur, sulfate, nitrate, carbon dioxide, some organic intermediates and pollutants are reduced by electrons originating from oxidation of organic compounds [7]. The common example of anaerobic process is the biodegradable waste in landfill. Paper and other materials degrade more slowly over longer periods of time. Biogas, coming from anaerobic digestion, mainly consists of methane and can be collected efficiently and used for eco-friendly power generation as has been demonstrated on larger scale [3, 16]. Anaerobic digestion is widely used, as part of an integrated waste management system, to treat wastewater sludge and biodegradable waste because it provides volume and mass reduction of the input material. It reduces the emission of landfill gas into the atmosphere [17-20]. Anaerobic digestion is a renewable energy source because the process produces methane and CO_2-rich biogas suitable for energy production helping to replace fossil fuel requirement. Also, the nutrient-rich solids left after digestion can be used as fertilizer [16,21].

There are four major biological and chemical steps of anaerobic digestion: hydrolysis, acidogenesis, acetogenesis, and methanogenesis [17,18] The mechanism commences with bacterial hydrolysis of the organic matter to break down insoluble organic polymers such as carbohydrates and make them available for other bacteria. Acetogenic bacteria convert the sugars and amino acids into carbon dioxide, hydrogen, ammonia, and organic acid. Methanogens then ultimately transform these products in to methane and carbon dioxide [19].

Advances in Anaerobic Digestion Technologies

Thermophilic anaerobic digestion of manure [20] and assessment of biodegradability of macropollutants [21] have demonstrated the prowess of anaerobic digestion which is now a general method used to stabilize municipal wastewater treatment residuals [22,23]. The so-called phased or staged anaerobic digestion is a recent technology for digestion facilities which include four different configurations of reactors: staged mesophilic digestion, temperature-phased digestion, acid/gas phased digestion, and staged thermophilic digestion [24]. Phased or staged configurations are multiple reactor digestion systems. Phased anaerobic digestion is defined as a digestion system having two or more tanks, each with exclusive operating conditions that support unique biomass populations, which may be acid-forming, methane-forming, thermophilic, or mesophilic organism populations. Effective digestion is achieved by manipulating operational parameters such as solids retention time (SRT) and temperature. Temperature phased digestion system is found better than the other systems during each study phase by having higher volatile solids reduction (VSR), higher methane production, and lower residual biological activity [24,25].

On industrial scale, anaerobic digestion of solid waste is considered as a mature technology [16,26]. Around 60% of the plants are reported in Europe to operate at the mesophilic range (40% thermophilic) with continued increase in capacity over the years in most European countries. Yields from the biomethanization process are very much dependent on operating conditions and the kind of substrate used. Digestion of grey wastes or residual refuse after source separation, has caught attention of industry and some of the solutions considered are landfilling or incineration [23]. However, anaerobic digestion is a better option since it gives number of advantages such as greater flexibility, the possibility of additional material recovery (up to 25%), and a more efficient and ecological energy recovery. In this case the low-calorific organic fraction is digested, the high-calorific fraction is treated thermally and the non-energy fractions can be recovered and reused. It is predicted that this residual refuse will be treated by anaerobic digestion [16, 23].

A very high growth potential is expected for the anaerobic digestion of organic fraction of municipal solid waste (OFMSW). Around 50% of MSW is landfilled, with a content of around 30% of organic fraction (without considering paper and cardboard). The growth potential for this technology is very important to reduce greenhouse gases emission as agreed at the Kyoto Summit [23]. Further, the consolidation of anaerobic digestion as a mainstream technology for the OFMSW should occur since the digested residue can be considered quite stable organic matter with a very slow turnover of several decades given adequate soil conditions. Thus, the natural imbalance in CO_2 can be adjusted by restoring or creating organic rich soil. The removal of CO_2 constitutes an extra benefit that would place anaerobic digestion as one of the most relevant technologies in this field. The degradation of chlorinated compounds need to be examined in greater depth, as anaerobic treatment offers high potential in this area [28].

Several novel reactors with high mass transfer rates, such as fluidized bed reactors, expanded granular sludge bed (EGSB) reactors [29-32], and membrane bioreactors [33] with different configurations have been used, in which hydraulic retention times (HRT) are uncoupled from the solids retention time (SRT) to make anaerobic technology economical alternative for conventional wastewater treatment systems. The upflow anaerobic sludge blanket (UASB) reactors [30] and/or related systems are mostly applied, wherein spontaneous formation of granular conglomerates of the anaerobic organisms occurs, leading to anaerobic sludge with an extremely low sludge volume index and optimal settling properties [21]. Besides, several large scale biogas plants have been built which combine waste from agriculture, industry and households and produce both biogas and a liquid fertiliser which is re-circulated back on agri-land. The combination of anaerobic digestion with other biological or physico-chemical processes has led to the development of optimised processes for the combined removal of organic matter, sulphur and nutrients. In conjunction with anaerobic digestion which removes mainly carbon, other processes are used to remove nitrogen and phosphorus (with oxic phase), which mainly use micro-organisms and also physico-chemical processes. For the treatment of municipal wastewater, the ANANOX process [34] takes advantage of sulphate reduction to sulphide to provide an electron donor for the denitrification process [35-37]. The integration of the nitrogen cycle in anaerobic digestion could be maximised with the application of the ANAMMOX process that makes use of particular micro-organisms that are able to oxidise ammonium to N_2 gas with nitrite as electron acceptor [38,39].

BIODEGRADATION OF INDUSTRIAL ORGANIC POLLUTANTS

Knowledge of fate of chemicals discharged in the environment, the life cycle analysis and the mechanisms by which they degrade are of great importance in designing biodegradation systems since many of the industrial chemicals are toxic, recalcitrant and bioaccumulating in organisms [40-42].

Volatile Organic Compounds (VOCS)

There are two classes of VOCs that are responsible for a large number of land and groundwater contamination: (i) petroleum hydrocarbons (PHCs) such as gasoline, diesel, and jet fuel, and (ii) chlorinated hydrocarbon (CHC) solvents such as the dry cleaning agents such as tetrachloroethylene, perchloroethylene (PCE) and the degreasing solvents such as trichloroethylene (TCE), 1,1,1-trichloroethane (TCA), and PCE.

PHCs biodegrade readily under aerobic medium, whereas CHCs characteristically biodegrade much more slowly and under anaerobic conditions [43] Because PHC biodegradation is relatively rapid when oxygen is present, aerobic biodegradation can usually limit the concentration and subsurface migration of petroleum vapours in unsaturated soils. Further, CHC biodegradation can produce toxic moieties, such as dichloroethylene and vinyl chloride, while petroleum degradation usually produces carbon dioxide, water, and sometimes methane or other simple hydrocarbons. A second primary difference is density of pollutant. PHC liquids are lighter than water and immiscible. PHCs can float on the groundwater surface (water table), whereas chlorinated solvents being heavier than water sink through the groundwater column to the bottom of the aquifer. These major differences in biodegradability and density lead to very different subsurface behaviour that often reduces the potential for human exposure.

Petroleum Hydrocarbons (PHCS)

It is known that microorganisms capable of aerobically degrading PHCs are present in nearly all subsurface soil environments [44-49]. Effective aerobic biodegradation of PHCs hinges on the soil having adequate oxygen and water content to provide a habitat for sufficient populations of active microorganisms. If oxygen is present, these organisms will generally consume available PHCs. Furthermore, aerobic biodegradation of petroleum compounds can occur relatively quickly, with degradation half lives as short as hours or days under some conditions [50]. Some petroleum compounds can also biodegrade under anaerobic conditions; however, above the water table, where oxygen is usually available in the soil zone, this process is insignificant and often much slower than aerobic biodegradation. Aerobic biodegradation consumes oxygen and generates carbon dioxide and water. This leads to a characteristic vertical concentration profile in the unsaturated zone in which oxygen concentrations decrease with depth and VOCs including PHCs and methane from anaerobic biodegradation and carbon dioxide concentrations increase with depth [51,52].

Chlorinated Hydrocarbon (CHC) Solvents

Chlorinated solvents such as tetrachloroethylene (TCE), 1,1,2,2-tetrachloroethane, carbon tetrachloride, and chloroform are released as waste products by spills, land-filling, and discharge to sewers during manufacture and their use as solvents in a variety of cleaning processes or as vehicles for solid slurries. TCE is a major pollutant of the industry. It is biodegraded under anaerobic conditions through hydrogenolysis that sequentially produces isomers of 1,2-dichloroethylene (1,2-DCE), vinyl chloride (VC), and ethylene. Some labs have also reported ethane [53,54], methane [55], and carbon dioxide [56] as degradation products.

In addition to anaerobic degradation through reductive dechlorination (hydrogenolysis), TCE and other chlorinated VOCs can be susceptible to co-metabolic oxidation by aerobic microorganisms that have oxygenases with broad substrate specificity. Methanotrophs are microorganisms that primarily oxidize methane for energy and growth using methane monooxygenase (MMO) enzymes and are a group of aerobic bacteria transform TCE through co-metabolic oxidation [57-59]. In contrast to reductive dechlorination, where the degradation rate generally decreases as the degree of chlorination of the aliphatic hydrocarbon decreases, the less-chlorinated VOCs such as 1,2-DCE and VC are more straightforwardly and quickly degraded through aerobic oxidation reactions than the higher chlorinated compounds such as TCE [60]. Methane-oxidizing bacteria are known to convert TCE to its epoxide, which then breaks down immediately in water to form dichloroacetic acid, glyoxylic acid, or one-carbon compounds such as formate or CO. The two carbon acids accumulate in the water phase, while formate and CO are further oxidized by methanotrophic bacteria to CO_2. Hence, coupling of anaerobic and aerobic degradation processes has been recommended as the best possible bioremediation method for chlorinated VOCs such as TCE [60-62].

Quinoline

Quinoline occurs commonly in coal tar, oil shale, and petroleum, and is used as an intermediate and solvent in many industries [63,64]. Due to its toxicity and repulsive odor, quinoline-containing waste is detrimental to human health and environmental quality. The study of quinoline- degrading bacteria not only helps to reveal the metabolic mechanism of quinoline, but also benefits the bio-treatment of quinoline-containing wastewater. Although different genera of bacteria may produce different intermediates, almost all of them transform quinoline into 2-hydroxyquinoline in the first step [63,65]. A quinoline-degrading bacteria strain, Pseudomonas sp. BW003, was isolated from the activated sludge in a coking wastewater treatment plant. Pseudomonas strains degrade quinoline via the 2-hydroxyquinoline and 2,8-hydroquinoline pathway, and then transform 2,8-hydroquinoline into 8-hydrocumarin, which is then transformed into 2,3-dihydroxyphenylpropionic acid, and finally to $CO_2$and H_2O (Scheme 3) [66-69]. Quinoline-N is transformed into ammonia-N, as reported in few genera of bacteria. Thus, quinoline pollution can be eliminated by applying such degrading bacteria in the treatment with bio-augmentation [70-72].

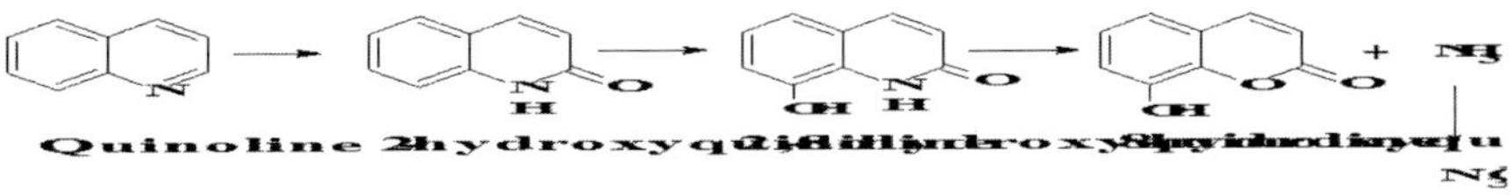

Scheme 3: Degradation products of quinoline [63].

Phenols

Phenols are harmful to organisms at low concentrations and classified as hazardous pollutants because of their potential to harm human health. They exist in different concentrations in wastewaters originated from coking, synthetic rubber, plastics, paper, oil, gasoline, etc. Biological treatment, activated carbon adsorption and solvent extraction are some of the most widely used methods for removing phenol and family compounds from wastewaters [73-76]. Biological treatment is economical, practical, promising and versatile approach for it leads to complete mineralization of phenol. Many aerobic bacteria are capable of using phenol as the sole source of carbon and energy [77]. In recent years, the strain of Pseudomonas putida has been the most widely used to degrade phenol. Under aerobic conditions, phenol may be converted by the bacterial biomass to CO_2; other intermediates such as benzoate, catechol, cis-cis-muconate, -ketoadipate, succinate and acetate are formed during the biodegradation process [77, 78]. p-Nitrophenol (PNP) is one of the most widely used nitrophenolic compounds in industry and finds important applications in agriculture, polymers, pigment and pharmaceutical industries. However, PNP is highly toxic for both the environment and humans and its efficient removal from the environment is required. Hydroquinone (HQ), 4-nitrocatechol (4-NC) and 1,2,4-benzenetriol (1,2,4-BT) are the metabolic intermediates of the PNP biodegradation [80,81].

Chlorinated phenols are common and encountered even in relatively pristine environments [82,83]. These compounds are formed during the bleaching of pulp with chlorine [82-84]. As the pulp accounts only for about 40-45% of the original weight of the wood, these effluents are heavily loaded with organics [85]. Chlorophenols are also used as fungicides and may be formed from hydrolysis of chlorinated phenoxyacetic acid herbicides. Chlorophenols, part of the adsorbable organic halides(AOX), are present in bleaching effluents at concentrations ranging from 0.1 to 2.6 ppm [86]. Aqueous effluents from industrial operations such as polymeric resin production, oil refining and coking plants also contain chlorophenolic compounds. Pentachlorophenol (PCP) is the second most heavily used pesticide in the US. As compared to phenol, chlorophenolic compounds are more persistent in the environment. Toxicity and bioaccumulative potential of chlorophenols increases with the degree of chlorination and with chlorophenol lipophilicity. Haloaromatic compounds are degraded via the formation of halocatechols as intermediates which are subsequently cleaved by dioxygenases, by the mechanism delineated earlier. Dehalogenation then occurs by the elimination of the hydrogen halide, with subsequent double bond formation on the aliphatic intermediate [87]. In anaerobic environments, the biodegradation of chlorinated aromatics takes place through reductive dehalogenation leading to the formation of less toxic and more biodegradable compounds. Reductive dechlorination of 2,4-dichlorophenol is followed by carboxylation, ring fission and acetogenesis, and methanogenesis which finally led to the complete mineralization of 2,4-DCP, which is also biodegraded to 4-chlorophenol in anaerobic sediments. Similarly, biodegradation of PCP under anaerobic conditions occurs through reductive dechlorination [88].

Fluoro Benzenes

Toluene degrading enzymes can transform many 3-fluoro-substituted benzenes to the corresponding 2,3-catechols with the concomitant release of inorganic fluoride. The substrates that induce 2,3-dioxygenase are 3-fluorotoluene, 3-fluorotrifluorotoluene, 3-flurohalobenzene, 3-fluoronisole, and 3-fluorobenzonitrile. While 3-fluorotoluene and 3-fluoronisole produce only deflorinated catechols, other substrates led to catechol products both with and without the toluene substituent [89].

Polycyclic Aromatic Hydrocarbons (PCAHS)

PCAHs are toxic, mutagenic and resist biodegradation [90]. Many strategies have been developed to treat them, including volatilization, photooxidation, chemical oxidation, bioaccumulation, and adsorption on soil particles [91]. Soil clean-up may be achieved using different remediation technologies, among which bioremediation is an effective and low-cost alternative that has garnered widespread use [92]. Two processes have been found to increase the activity of microorganisms during bioremediation: bio-stimulation and bio-augmentation. Bio-stimulation involves the addition of nutrients and/or a terminal electron acceptor to increase the meager activity of indigenous microbial populations. Bio-augmentation involves the addition of external microbial strains (indigenous or exogenous) which have the ability to degrade the desired toxic compounds [93]. The added specific PCAHs degrading strain, which has a competitive capacity to become dominant species with indigenous microbial strains or grow simultaneously with indigenous microbial strains, may greatly enhance the rate of PCAHs biodegradation [94,95]. The ability to degrade PCAHs depends on the complexity of their structure and the extent of enzymatic adaptation by bacteria. In general PCAHs with 2 or 3 aromatic rings are readily degraded, but those with 4 or more are usually recalcitrant and genotoxic. Such examples of PCAHs are acenaphthene, acenaphthylene, anthracene, naphthalene, fluorene, phenanthrene, chrysene, pyrene, etc. The major metabolites are 4-phenanthroic acid and 4-hydroxyperinapthenone. Cinnamic and phthalic acids are ring fission products [96].

Naphthalene is carcinogenic and persistent organic pollutant [97]. Bacteria such as Pseudomonas putida, Rhodococcus opacus, Mycobacterium sp., Nocardia otitidiscaviarum, and Bacillus pumilus are known to biodegrade naphthalene [98-102]. Some metabolites of naphthalene, such as salicylic acid, 1-naphthol and o-phthalic acid could be degraded and support cell growth (Scheme 4). Phenanthrene was used as a model compound for PCAH degradation which shows 1-hydroxy 2-naphthoic acid (1H2NA) as intermediate biodegradation product [103].

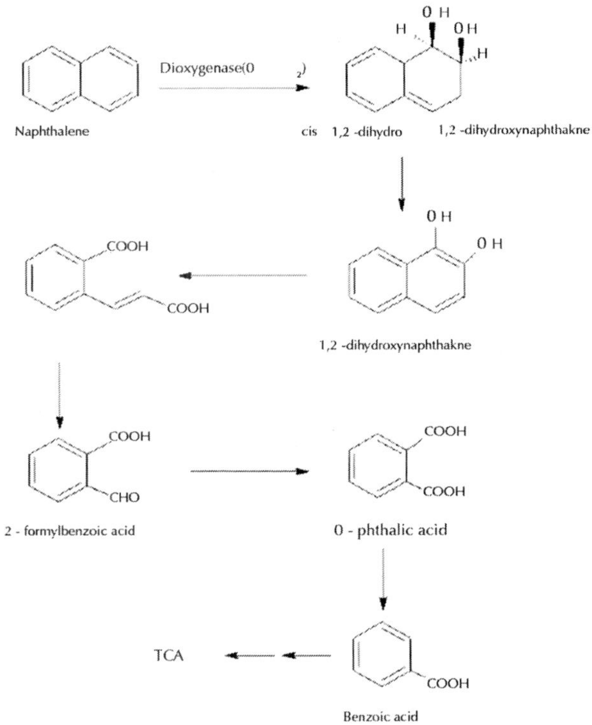

Scheme 4: Proposed pathway for the degradation of naphthalene [103].

Plasticizers

Plasticizers are polymeric additives, used to impart flexibility to polymer materials. The biodegradation of some plasticizers can lead to the formation of metabolites with increased persistence and toxicity relative to the original compounds [104-106]. Use of plasticizers has grown considerably, both with respect to product variety and production volume [107]. Phthalates are the most widely used plasticizers. Presence of phthalates and their metabolites in rats, mice, human plasma and liver are related to adverse health effects such as endocrine disruption and peroxisome proliferation [108,109]. The high production volumes of phthalates and their incomplete biodegradation have led to the presence of these compounds and a number of toxic and stable metabolites in surface waters, groundwater, air, soil and tissue of living organisms [104, 110-113]. Such findings have led to stricter environmental regulations and consequently have broadened the criteria used to evaluate plasticizers. Consequently, dibenzoates have been approved by the European Chemical Agency as alternatives to phthalates [114]. However, the degradation of dipropylene glycol dibenzoate (D(PG)DB) and diethylene glycol dibenzoate (D(EG)DB) by common soil microorganisms such as Rhodotorula rubraand Rhodococcus rhodochrous can lead to the formation and accumulation of monobenzoate metabolites [115,116] that exhibit high acute toxicity [115]. Other compounds including 1,5-pentandiol and 1,6- hexanediol dibenzoates were reported to produce less stable metabolites and have also been tested as potential alternatives to commercial dibenzoate plasticizers [116-118]. Scheme 5 shows the biodegradation products of dibenzoates by R. Rhodochrous, which include 2-[2-(benzoyloxy)propoxy] propanoic acid, 1,3-propanediol monobenzoate and 3-(benzoyloxy) propanoic acid [119].

Plastics

Over the years, plastics have brought economic, environmental and social advantages. Today's material world uses tremendous quantities of plastics of all hue and origins. However, their wide spread use has also increased plastic waste, which brings its own economic, environmental and social problems. The redesign of plastic products, whether individual polymer or product structure, could help alleviate some of the problems associated with plastic waste. Redesign could have an impact at all levels of the hierarchy established by the European Waste Framework Directive: prevention, re-use, recycle, recovery and disposal [120].

Polyethylene, polypropylene and polystyrene, and water-soluble polymers, such as polyacrylamide, polyvinyl alcohol and polyacrylic acid are bulk polymers used in a variety of industries and products. Some of the plastics are not biodegradable and deleterious to the environment due to their accumulation. Plastics can be disposed of by incineration or recycling, but incineration is very difficult, dangerous and expensive whereas recycling is a long process and not very efficient. Some plastics still cannot be recycled or incinerated due to pigments, coatings and other additives during manufacture of materials. Making biodegradable and ecofriendly plastics will avoid accumulation, recycling and incineration [121].

Polyvinyl Alcohol

Polyvinyl alcohol (PVA) is water-soluble but also has thermoplasticity. In addition to its use as a water-soluble polymer, for instance, as a substituent for starch in industrial processes, it can also be molded in various shapes, such as containers and films. PVA can therefore be used to make water-soluble and biodegradable carriers, which may be useful in the manufacture of delivery systems for chemicals such as fertilizers, pesticides, and herbicides. Among the vinyl polymers produced industrially, PVA is the only one known to be mineralized by microorganisms [122]. Extensive use of PVA, in textile and paper industries generates considerable amount of contaminated wastewaters [121]. In aqueous solution, the biodegradation mechanism of PVA involves the random endocleavage of the polymer chains. The initial step is associated with the specific oxidation of methane-carbon bearing the hydroxyl group, as mediated by oxidase and dehydrogenase type enzymes, to give β-hydroxyketone as well as 1,3-diketone moieties. The latter groups are able to facilitate the carbon-carbon bond cleavage as promoted by specific β-diketone hydrolase, leading to the formation of carboxylic and methyl ketone end groups [123,124]. Most of the PVA-degrading microorganisms are aerobic bacteria belonging to Pseudomonas, Alcaligenes, and Bacillus genus. A very moderate PVA biodegradation was reported [125-128].

Polyhydroxyalkanoates

Polyhydroxyalkanoates (PHAs) are degraded to CO_2 and water in aerobic conditions and methane in anaerobic conditions by microbes found in soil, water and other various natural habitats. PHAs are the only proposed replacement polymers that are completely biodegradable [129]. The structures of these polymers have a very similar structure of the petroleum-derived thermoplastics [130].

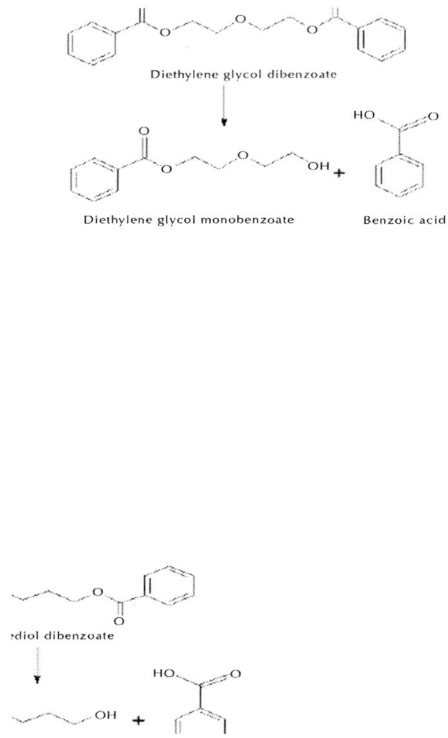

Scheme 5: Proposed biodegradation pathways of diethylene glycol dibenzoate and 1,3-propanediol dibenzoate [116]

PHAs also possess similar physical properties as plastics including the ability to be molded, made into films, and also into fibers. Efforts are underway to identify bacteria, which produce various kinds of PHAs [129] as well as the production of these polyesters or create certain kinds of PHAs by changing the kind of bacteria [130] and/or the substrates given to the bacteria and genetically enhancing bacteria [131].

PROSPECTIVE OF ANAEROBIC DIGESTION AND BIOGAS ENERGY

The foregoing analysis shows that anaerobic digestion technologies have matured so far to treat several organic micro-pollutants, halogenated compounds, substituted aromatics, azo-linkages, nitro-aromatics and the like in industrial effluents and also for municipal effluents containing industrial loads. A very high growth potential is envisaged for the anaerobic digestion of organic fraction of municipal solid waste [27]. Novel reactor and control systems ought to be developed for different purposes depending on the source of pollutants or biomass. Anaerobic digestion of sewage sludge followed by recycling on agricultural land is currently the largest world-wide application of anaerobic processes. Treatment of sludge and slurries targeted at the production of safe end products can be tackled with niche anaerobic technologies [16]. It is predicted that major future process developments will come from the deployment of pre- and post treatment processes, including physical, chemical and biological processes, for the reclamation of the products from the wastewater treatment system. Wastewater treatment for reuse will be effective if anaerobic digestion is adopted for mineralizing organic matter. Hence, anaerobic digestion has the potential to play a major role in closing water, raw materials, and nutrient cycles in industrial processes [37]. Further development is required on the community on-site treatment of domestic sewage under a wide range of conditions, opting for the reuse of the treated water in agriculture and making use of the mineralized nutrients for fertilization purposes. An upstream integration of the anaerobic process with industrial primary production processes under extreme conditions of temperature, pH, salinity, toxic and recalcitrant compounds, and variable load is envisaged in future [39].

There is an emphasis worldwide on renewable energy system among which biogas produced from any biological feedstocks including primary agricultural sectors and from various organic waste streams will come in to prominence in near future [22]. It is estimated [3] that at least 25% of all bioenergy in the future can originate from biogas, produced from wet organic materials like animal manure, slurries from cattle and pig production units as well as from poultry, fish and fur, whole crop silages, wet food and feed wastes, etc. Anaerobic digestion of animal manure offers several environmental, agricultural and socio-economic benefits throughout such as improved fertilizer quality of manure, considerable reduction of odors and inactivation of pathogens and more importantly production of biogas production, as clean, renewable fuel, for multiple utilizations [16]. This biogas can be upgraded to natural gas to mix with the existing natural gas grid which will be cost effective. The potential development of biogas from manure co-digestion includes the use of new feedstock types such as by-products from food processing industries, bio-slurries from biofuels processing industries as well as the biological degradation of toxic organic wastes from pharmaceutical industries, etc. [3,16,22]. This will also call for better reactor systems and careful process control to increase the biogas yield, which will be more attractive if coupled with less capital and operating costs. Integration of biogas production into the national energy grids will eventually be commercially viable since the biogas from anaerobic co-digestion of animal manure and suitable organic wastes would overcome the major environmental and veterinary problems of the animal production and organic waste disposal.

PLASTIC WASTE SEPARATION, REPROCESSING AND RECYCLE

In 2009, around 230 million tonnes of plastic was produced; ~25 % which was used in the European Union [131]. About 50 % plastic is used for single-use disposable applications, such as packaging, agricultural films and disposable consumer items [132]. Although plastics consume approximately 8 % world oil production: 4 % as raw material for plastics and 3-4 % as energy for manufacture [132], supplies are being depleted. Bioplastics make up only 0.1 to 0.2 % total plastics [115]. It is estimated that plastics reduce 600 to 1300 million tonnes of CO_2 through the replacement of less efficient materials, lighter and fuel efficient vehicles, housing sector, contribution to insulation, preservation of food, packaging, use in wind power rotors and solar panels [133]. However, plastic littering and pollution of land and sea have been matters of great concern which should be strategically and technologically solved. Plastics recovery, in addition to increased diversion from disposal, results in significant energy savings (~50-75 MBtu/ton of material recycled) compared with the production of virgin materials, which also leads to reductions in greenhouse gas emissions due to avoided fuel use. Limiting the plastics that enter landfills can lower the costs associated with waste disposal. It is believed that the recycled plastic will fetch as much as 70 % of the typical price for virgin plastics [136].

Waste Reduction Hierarchy

The motto of waste reduction by plastics is by following the principles of (i) prevention, (ii) reuse (iii) recycle, (iv) recovery, and (v) disposal [119].

(i) *Prevention* – Using minimum and as less types of plastic in the product by clever product redesign.

(ii) *Reuse* – Products could be designed for reuse by facilitating the dismantling of products and replacement of parts. This could involve standardizing parts across manufacturers [137].

- *Recycle* – Some types of plastics are easier to recycle than others, for example polyethylene terephthalate (PET). By using fewer types and colors (or colorless) of plastics the recycling process becomes easier. The use of "intelligent" or smart polymers that undergo changes under certain conditions could also reduce disassembly time [138]. For example, a polymer that changes shape when subject to magnetic or electric fields could aid the disassembly of electronic goods.
- *Recovery* – Energy can be recovered from plastics in waste-to-energy plants. By designing products to consider the possibility of energy recovery, plastic may have a greater end-of-life use.
- *Disposal* – Biodegradable plastics are less persistent in the environment than traditional plastics, but need specific and suitable end-of-life treatment.

Bioplastics

Since disposal is one of the important aspect, bioplastics are being favored. There are three main categories of bio-based plastics: (i) Natural polymers from renewable sources, such as cellulose, starch and plant-based proteins, (ii) Polymers synthesised from monomers derived from renewable resources. For example, polylactic acid (PLA) is produced by the fermentation of starch, corn or sugar, (iii) Polymers produced by microorganisms. For example, PHA (polyhydroxyalkanoate) is produced by bacteria through fermentation of sugar or lipids [139].

Biodegradable plastics are not by definition bio-based and bio-based plastics are not always biodegradable, although some fall into both categories, such as PHAs. The term bioplastics is often used to refer to both bio-based and biodegradable plastics. The main applications of bioplastics are disposable plastic bags, packaging and loose fill packaging (beads and chips), dishes and cutlery, electronic casings and car components. However, bioplastics cannot substitute all types of plastic; particularly certain types of food packaging that require gas permeability [135]. Development of novel biodegradable plastic is a solution for the plastic disposal problem since plastics are immiscible in water and are thermo-elastic polymeric materials. Biodegradability of plastics is governed by both their chemical and physical properties. Other factors affecting degradability are the forces associated with covalent bonds of polymer molecules, hydrogen bonds, van der Waals forces, coulombic forces, etc. Enzymatic degradation is an effective way. Lipase and esterase can hydrolyze fatty acid esters, triglycerides and aliphatic polyesters. These lipolytic enzymes have an important role in the degradation of natural aliphatic polyesters such as cutin, suberin and esteroid in the natural environment and animal digestive tract.

As stated earlier, biodegradable plastics decompose in the natural environment from the action of bacteria. Biodegradation of plastics can be achieved through the action of micro-bacteria and fungi in the environment to metabolize the molecular structure of plastic films to produce an inert humus-like material that is less harmful to the environment, along with water, carbon dioxide and/or methane. They may be composed of either bioplastics or petro-plastics. The use of bio-active compounds compounded with swelling agents ensures that, when combined with heat and moisture, they expand the plastic's molecular structure and allow the bio-active compounds to metabolize and neutralize the plastic [140]. Compostable plastics are biodegradable and meet certain criteria, such as rate of biodegradation and impact on the environment. Degradable plastics include biodegradable and compostable plastics, but also plastics that degrade by chemical and physical processes such as the action of sunlight. Purely biodegradable plastics are different from oxy-biodegradable plastics, which contain small amounts of metal salts to speed up degradation. It has been suggested that this process be called "oxo-fragmentation" to avoid confusion [139,140].

It is possible to produce polymers biologically, e.g., PHA grown in genetically modified corn plant leaves, PLA (polylactic acid) produced by the fermentation of sugars extracted from plants, PHA produced by bacteria. Bioplastics could also help alleviate climate change by reducing the use of petroleum for the manufacture of traditional plastics. It is claimed that CO_2 emissions released at the end-of-life of bio-based plastics are offset by absorption of CO_2 during the growth of plants for their production [141].

Sorting Plastic Materials

The technical difficulties and high cost associated with separating plastics have limited recycling in the past. Consumer goods often contain as many as 20 different types of plastic as well as non-plastic materials such as wood, rubber, glass, and fibers. There is upsurge of new products and pigment types, which can pose a challenge to the recycling infrastructure. Consequently, the cost of producing virgin materials is often less than the cost of collecting and processing post-consumer plastics. Used plastic material will contain more than one base polymer, and resins with a variety of additives, including coloring agents and thus technologies for cleaning and separating the materials are an important part of most plastics recycling systems. A particular concern for recycled plastics is their use as food containers requiring stringent regulations to avoid contamination [140].

Separation of different types of polymers from each other is many times a desired part of plastics recycling processes which are classified as macrosorting, microsorting, or molecular sorting.

Macrosorting

Macrosorting involves the sorting of whole or nearly whole objects such as separation of PVC bottles or caps from PET bottles, separation of polyester carpet from nylon carpet, and sorting of automobile components by resin type. Various devices are now commercially available to separate plastics by resin type, which typically rely on differences in the absorption or transmission of certain wavelengths of electromagnetic radiation, or color or resin type. Particularly for recycling of appliances, carpet, and automobile plastics, several IR spectra based equipment are used [135].

Micro sorting

Micro sorting is a size-reduction process to reduce the plastic material in to small pieces which is then separated by resin type or color; for instance, separation of high-density polyethylene (HDPE) base cups from PET soft drink bottles using a sink-float tank. More modern separation processes, such as the use of hydrocyclones, also rely primarily on differences in the density of the materials for the separation. A number of other characteristics have also been used as the basis for microsorting systems, including differences in melting point and in triboelectric behavior. In many of these systems, proper control over the size of the plastic flakes is important in being able to reliably separate the resins. Some systems rely on differences in the grinding behavior of the plastics combined with sieving or other size-based separation mechanisms for sorting. Sometimes cryogenic grinding is used to facilitate grinding and to generate size differences [135]. Three new separation technologies, developed by MBA Polymers, Argonne National Laboratory, and Recovery Plastics International (RPI), could break down these barriers and increase plastics recycling [138].

Automated Separation

According to the process developed by MBA Polymers, plastic scraps from computers and other electronics are first ground into small pieces. Magnets and eddy-current separators then extract ferrous and non-ferrous metals. Paper and other lighter materials are removed with jets of air. Finally, a proprietary sorting, cleaning, and testing process involving various technologies, allows the separation of different types of plastics and compound them into pelletized products comparable to virgin plastics [138].

Froth Flotation

Argonne National Laboratory (ANL) has developed a process to separate acrylonitrile-butadiene styrene (ABS) and high-impact polystyrene (HIPS) from recovered automobiles and appliances. The froth flotation process separates two or more equivalent-density plastics by modifying the effective density of the plastics. There is a careful control of the chemistry of the aqueous "froth" so that small gas bubbles adhere to the solid surface and facilitate the plastic to float to the top [135].

Skin Flotation

Recovery Plastics International (RPI) has developed an automated process capable of recovering up to 80 % plastics found in automobile shredder residue (ASR). The process starts with the separation of light lint materials, followed by the removal of rocks and metals, granulation, washing, and, finally, automated skin flotation separation. This final step adds a skin of plasticizer to make the surface of the targeted plastic hydrophobic. Air bubbles then can attach to the plastic, allowing it to float above denser, uncoated pieces. It is estimated this new skin flotation technology could be used to treat about one-third of the estimated 7 million tons of ASR disposed off each year [141].

Molecular Sorting

Molecular sorting deals with sorting of materials whose physical form has been completely disrupted, such as by dissolving the plastics in solvents using either a single solvent at several temperatures or mixed solvents, followed by reprecipitation. There is a need to control emissions and to recover the solvents, without any residual solvent in the recovered polymer to avoid leaching in stored material. There are at present no commercial systems using this approach. Some research effort has focused on facilitating plastics separation by incorporating chemical tracers into plastics, particularly packaging materials, so that they can be more easily identified and separated.

It has become obvious that many of the difficulties of recycling plastics are related to difficulties in separating plastics from other wastes and in sorting plastics by resin type. Design of products can do a lot to either aggravate or minimize these difficulties [134,135]. The concept of green product embeds recycling at the design stage itself.

Plastic Reprocessing and Recycling

For plastics recycling to be effective, it is necessary to have (i) a system for collecting the targeted materials, (ii) a facility capable of processing the collected recyclables into a form which can be utilized to make a new product and, (iii) new products made in whole or part from the recycled material must be manufactured and sold.

Processing of recyclable plastics is necessary to transform the collected materials into raw materials for the manufacture of new products. Three general categories of processing can be identified: (1) physical recycling, (2) chemical recycling, and (3) thermal recycling, wherein the particulars of the processing are often specific to a given plastic or product.

Physical Processes

Physical recycling, the most popular option, covers size and shape alteration, removing contaminants, blending in additives if desired, and similar approaches that change the appearance of the recycled material, but do not alter its basic chemical structure. Plastic containers, for example, are processed including grinding, air classification to remove light contaminants, washing, gravity-separation, screening, rinsing, drying, and often melting and pelletization, accompanied by addition of colorants, heat stabilizers, or other ingredients, depending on type of plastic [132].

Chemical Reactions

Chemical recycling of plastics deals with chemical reactions using catalysis or solvents such as methanol, glycols or water leading to depolymerization or breaking polymers into monomers or useful chemicals, or fuels [134]. The products of the reaction then can be separated and reused to produce either the same or a related polymer. An example is the glycolysis process sometimes used to recycle polyethylene terephthalate (PET), in which the PET is broken down into monomers, crystallized, and repolymerized. Condensation polymers, such as PET, nylon, and polyurethane, typically much more amenable to chemical recycling than are addition polymers such as polyolefins, polystyrene, and polyvinyl chloride (PVC). Most commercial processes for depolymerization and repolymerization are restricted to a single polymer, which is usually PET, nylon 6, or polyurethane. Methanolysis is another common reaction using methanol [134].

Thermal Cracking

Thermal cracking or recycling also involves cracking of the chemical structure of the polymer using heat in the absence of sufficient oxygen for combustion. At these elevated temperatures, the polymeric structure breaks down. Thermal recycling can be applied to all types of polymers. However, the typical yield is a complex mixture of products, even when the feedstock is a single polymer resin. If reasonably pure compounds can be recovered, products of thermal recycling can be used as feedstock for new materials. When the products are a complex mixture which is difficult to separate, they are most often used as fuel. There are relatively few commercial operations today which involve thermal recycling of plastics. Some European nations have such feedstock recycling facilities. Many plastic resin companies use fluidized bed cracking to produce a waxlike material from mixed plastic waste [134-136, 139]. The product, when mixed with naptha, can be used as a raw material in a cracker or refinery to produce feedstocks such as ethylene and propylene. In certain case, syn gas can be produced and used in Fisher-Tropsch synthesis to produce valuable chemicals.

In landfill, both synthetic and naturally occurring polymers do not get the necessary exposure to UV and microbes to degrade. The discarded plastics occupy space and none of the energy put into making them is being reclaimed. Reclaiming the energy stored in the polymers can be done through incineration, but this can cause environmental damage by release of toxic gases into the atmosphere. Therefore, recycling is a viable alternative in getting back some of this energy in the case of some polymers. With ever increasing petroleum prices, it would be financially viable to recycle polymers rather than produce them from raw materials [141].

CONCLUSIONS

The modern society needs thousands of chemicals and materials of all sorts which are produced annually and used in all sectors of economy. However, their fate in the environment is of great concern since some are toxic, recalcitrant and bioacumulating and hence their discharge into the environment must be regulated. Better understanding of the mechanism of biodegradation has a high ecological significance that depends on indigenous microorganisms to transform or mineralize the organic contaminants. Thus, biodegradation processes differ greatly depending on conditions, but frequently the main final products of the degradation are carbon dioxide and/or methane. Microorganisms have enzyme systems to degrade and utilize different hydrocarbons as a source of carbon and energy. Slow and partial biodegradation of chlorophenolic compounds under aerobic as well as anaerobic natural environment has been observed. Aerobic degradation takes place via formation of catechols while anaerobic degradation occurs via reductive dechlorination. Acclimatization of biomass to chlorophenols markedly enhances their ability to degrade such compounds, both by reducing the initial lag phase as well as by countering biomass inhibition. Aerobic processes as well as anaerobic processes partially remove chlorophenols. However, enhanced removal efficiency can be obtained by operating anaerobic and aerobic treatment processes in combination. Thus microbial degradation can be a key component for clean-up strategy of organopollutants and plastics.

Renewable energy system among which biogas produced from biological feedstocks will play a major role in energy sector. Anaerobic digestion of animal manure, slurries from cattle and pig production units as well as from poultry, fish and fur, whole crop silages, wet food and feed wastes, etc offers several environmental, agricultural and socio-economic benefits by improved fertilizer quality of manure, considerable reduction of odors, inactivation of pathogens and production of biogas production, as clean and renewable fuel. This biogas can be upgraded to natural gas to inject in to the existing natural gas grid which will be cost effective. Biogas from anaerobic co-digestion of animal manure and suitable organic wastes would overcome the major environmental and veterinary problems of the animal production and organic waste disposal.

The recycling of plastics is environmentally beneficial because plastics reduce millions of tonnes of CO_2 emissions through the replacement of less efficient materials, development of lighter and fuel efficient transport systems, housing material, energy saving insulation, food preservation and storage, energy efficient packaging, use in wind power rotors and solar panels. Processing of recyclable plastics is necessary to transform the collected materials into raw materials for the manufacture of new products. Bioplastics offer a very good solution to environmentally deleterious materials. Biodegradation of plastics can be achieved through the action of micro-bacteria and fungi.

REFERENCES

1. Alexander M. Biodegradation and Bioremediation. Academic Press: New York; 1999.
2. Lily Y, Young LY, Cerniglia CE. Microbial Transformation and Degradation of Toxic Organic Chemicals. Wiley-Liss Inc. New York, NY; 1995.
3. Holm-Nielsen JB, Al Seadi T, Oleskowicz-Popiel P. The future of anaerobic digestion and biogas utilization. Bioresource Technology 2009; 100: 5478–5484.
4. Steinfeld H, Gerber P, Wasenaar T, Castel V, Rosales M, de Haan C. Livestock's long shadow. Environmental Issues and Options. Food and Agriculture Organization (FAO) of United Nations; 2006.
5. Nielsen LH, Hjort-Gregersen K, Thygesen P, Christensen J. Samfundsøkonomiske analyser af biogasfllesanlg. Rapport 136; 2002. Fødevareøkonomisk Institut, København (Summary in English).
6. http://www.unesco.org/new/en/natural-sciences/ (accessed December 2012)
7. Van Agteren MH, Keuning S, Janssen D, Handbook on Biodegradation and Biological Treatment of Hazardous Organic Compounds. Kluwer, Dordrecht, The Netherlands; 1998.
8. Tokiwa Y, Calabia BP, Ugwu CU, Aiba S. Biodegradability of Plastics. International Journal of Molecular Science 2009; 10: 3722–3742.
9. Griffin GJL. Chemistry and Technology of Biodegradable Polymers, Springer, London; 1994.
10. Schmidt M., editor. Synthetic Biology: Industrial and Environmental Applications, Wiley-Blackwell; 2012.
11. NIIR Board of Consultants and Engineers (Ed.), Medical, Municipal and Plastic Waste Management Handbook. National Institute of Industrial Research, New Delhi; 2009.

12. Stuart PR, El-Halwagi MM., editor. Integrated Biorefineries: Design, Analysis and Optimization, CRC Press; 2012.
13. Perez JJ, Munoz-Dorado J, de la Rubia TJ, Martınez J. Biodegradation and biological treatments of cellulose, hemicelluloses and lignin: an overview. International Microbiology 2002; 5: 53-63.
14. Berna JL, Cassani G, Hager CD, Rehman N, Lopez I, Schowanek D, Steber J, Taeger K, Wind T. Anaerobic Biodegradation of Surfactants-Scientific Review. Tenside Surfactants Detergents 2007; 44: 312-347.
15. Fritsche W, Hofrichter M. Aerobic Degradation by Microorganisms: Principles of Bacterial Degradation. In: Rehm HJ, Reed G, Puhler A, Stadler A. (eds.) ,Biotechnology, environmental processes II, vol IIb. Wiley-VCH, Weinhein. p145-167.
16. Lier JB van, Tilche A, Ahring BK, Macarie H, Moletta R, Dohanyos M, Hulshoff Pol LW, Lens P, Verstraete W. New perspectives in anaerobic digestion. Water Science and Technology 2001; 43(1): 1-18.
17. Rozzi A, Remigi E. Anaerobic biodegradability: Conference Proceeding. In: 9th World Congress, Anaerobic digestion 2001, Workshop 3 Harmonisation of anaerobic activity and biodegradation assays, 9-2-2001, Belgium.
18. Dolfing J, Bloemen GBM. Activity measurement as a tool to characterize the microbial composition of methanogenic environments. Journal of Microbiological Methods 1985; 4: 1-12.
19. Soto M, Mendez R, Lema JM. Methanogenic activity tests. Theoretical basis and experimental setup. Water Research 1993; 27: 850–857.
20. Angelidaki I, Ahring BK. Thermophilic anaerobic digestion of livestock waste: the effect of ammonia. Applied Microbiology Biotechnology 1993; 38: 560–564.
21. Angelidaki I. Sanders W. Assessment of the anaerobic biodegradability of macropollutants. Reviews in Environmental Science and Biotechnology 2004; 3: 117–129.
22. Holm-Nielsen JB, Oleskowicz-Popiel P, 2007. The future of biogas in Europe: Visions and targets until 2020. In: Proceedings: European Biogas Workshop-Intelligent Energy Europe, 14–16

June 2007, Esbjerg, Denmark. Mata-Alvarez J, Macé S, Llabrés P, Anaerobic digestion of organic solid wastes. An overview of research achievements and perspectives. Bioresource Technology 2000; 74: 3-16.

23. Reusser S, Zelinka G. Laboratory-scale comparison of anaerobic-digestion alternatives. Water Environment Research 2004; 76(4): 360-379.
24. David C, Inman DC. Comparative studies of alternative anaerobic digestion technologies. M.S. (Environ. Eng.) Thesis, Virginia Polytechnic Institute and State University; 2004.
25. Riggle D. Acceptance improves for large-scale anaerobic digestion. Biocycle 1998; 39 (6): 51-55.
26. Mata-Alvarez, J., Tilche, A., Cecchi, F., editor. The treatment of grey and mixed solid waste by means of anaerobic digestion: future developments. Proceedings of the Second International Symposium on Anaerobic Digestion of Solid Wastes, Barcelona, vol. 2. Graphiques 92, 15-18 June, 1999. p302-305.
27. Christiansen N. Hendriksen HV, Jarviene KT, Ahring B. Degradation of chlorinated aromatic compounds in UASB reactors. Water Science and Technology 1999; 31: 249-259.
28. Man AWA de, Last ARM van der, Lettinga G. The use of EGSB and UASB anaerobic systems or low strength soluble and complex wastewaters at temperatures ranging from 8 to 30°C. Proceedings of the 5th International Symposium on Anaerobic Digestion. Bologna, Italy, 1988. p197-211.
29. Driessen WJBM, Habets LHA, Groeneveld N. New developments in the design of Upflow Anaerobic Sludge Bed reactors. 2nd Specialised IAWQ conference on Pretreatment of Industrial Wastewaters, October 16-18,1996.
30. Zoutberg GR, Been P de. The biobed EGSB (Expanded Granular Sludge Bed) systems covers short comings of the upflow anaerobic sludge blanket reactors in the chemical industry. Water Science and Technology 1997; 35(10): 183-188.
31. Collins AG, Theis TL, Kilambi S, He L, Pavlostathis SG. Anaerobic treatment of low strength domestic wastewater using an anaerobic expanded bed reactor. Journal of Environmental Engineering 1998: 652-659.

32. Nagano A, Arikawa E, Kobayashi H. Treatment of liquor wastewater containing high strength suspended solids by membrane bioreactor system. Water Science and Technology 1992; 26(3-4): 887-895.

33. Garuti G, Dohanyos M, Tilche A. Anaerobic-aerobic wastewater treatment system suitable for variable population in coastal are: the ANANOX process. Water Science and Technology 1992; 25(12):185-195.

34. Oude Elferink SJWH, Visser A, Hulshoff Pol LW, Stams AJM. Sulfate reduction in methanogenic bioreactors. FEMSMicrobiology Reviews 1994; 15: 119-136.

35. Boopathy R, Kulpa CF, Manning J. Anaerobic biodegradation of explosives and related compounds by sulfate-reducing and methanogenic bacteria: a review. Bioresource Technoology 1998; 63(1): 81-89.

36. Houten RT van, Lettinga G. Biological sulphate reduction with synthesis gas: microbiology and technology. In: Wijffels RH., Buitelaar RM., Bucke C., Tramper J. (eds.) Progress in Biotechnology. Elsevier, Amsterdam, The Netherlands; 1996. pp. 793-799..

37. Jetten MSM, Strous M, Pas-Schoonen KT Van de, Schalk J, Van Dongen UGJM, Van De Graaf AA, Logemann S, Muyzer G, Van Loosdrecht MCM, Kuenen JG. The anaerobic oxidation of ammonium. FEMS Microbiology Reviews 1999; 22: 421-437.

38. Lier JB van, Lettinga, G. Appropriate technologies for effective management of industrial and domestic wastewaters: the decentralised approach. Water Science and Technology 1999; 40 (7): 171-183.

39. Abrahamsson K, Klick S. Degradation of Halogenated Phenols in Anoxic Marine Sediments. Marine Pollution Bulletin 1991; 22: 227-233.

40. Suflita JM, Horowitz A, Shelton DR, Tiedje JM. Dehalogenation: A Novel Pathway for the Anaerobic Biodegradation of Haloaromatic Compounds. Science 1982; 218: 1115-1117.

41. Annachhatre AP, Gheewala SH. Biodegradation of Chlorinated Phenolic Compounds. Biotechnology Advances 1996; 14(1): 35-56.

42. Howard PH. Handbook of Environmental Degradation Rates. Lewis Publishers: Chelsea MI; 1991.
43. Zobell CE. Action of microorganisms on hydrocarbons. Bacteriological Reviews 1946; 10(1-2): 1-49.
44. Atlas RM. Microbial degradation of petroleum hydrocarbons: an environmental perspective. Microbiological Reviews 1981; 45(1): 180–209.
45. Wilson JT, Leach LE, Henson M, Jones JN. In situ biorestoration as a ground water remediation technique. Ground Water Monitoring Review 1986; 6: 56–64.
46. Leahy JG, Colwell RR. Microbial degradation of hydrocarbons in the environment. Microbiological Reviews 1990; 54(3): 305–315.
47. Bedient PB, Rifai HS, Newell CJ. Ground Water Contamination: Transport and Remediation. PTR Prentice-Hall Inc. Englewood Cliffs, NJ; 1994.
48. EPA (Environmental Protection Agency). Monitored Natural Attenuation of Petroleum Hydrocarbons. Remedial Technology Fact Sheet. EPA/600/F-98/021. Office of Research and Development, Washington, DC; May 1999.
49. DeVaull G. Indoor vapor intrusion with oxygen-limited biodegradation for a subsurface gasoline source. Environmental Science and Technology 2007; 41(9): 3241–3248.
50. Roggemans S, Bruce CL, Johnson PC. Vadose Zone Natural Attenuation of Hydrocarbon Vapors: An Empirical Assessment of Soil Gas Vertical Profile Data. API Technical Bulletin No. 15. American Petroleum Institute, Washington, DC, 2002.
51. http://apiep.api.org/environment (accessed December 2012)
52. EPA (Environmental Protection Agency). Petroleum Hydrocarbons And Chlorinated Hydrocarbons Differ In Their Potential For Vapor Intrusion. Office of Underground Storage Tanks, Washington, D.C. 20460. 2011. p1-11.
53. www.epa.gov/oust (accessed December 2012)
54. Belay N, Daniels L. Production of Ethane, Ethylene, and Acetylene from Halogenated Hydrocarbons by Methanogenic Bacteria. Applied Environmental Microbiology 1987; 53(7): 1604-1610.

55. de Bruin WP, Kotterman MJJ, Posthumus MA, Schraa G, Zehnder AJB. Complete Biological Reductive Transformation of Tetrachloroethene to Ethane. Applied Environmental Microbiology 1992; 58(6): 1996-2000.
56. Bradley PM, Chapelle FH. Methane as a Product of Chloroethene Biodegradation under Methanogenic Conditions. Environmental Science Technology 1999; 33(4): 653-656.
57. Vogel TM, McCarty PL. Biotransformation of Tetrachloroethylene to Trichloroethylene, Dichloroethylene, Vinyl Chloride, and Carbon Dioxide under Methanogenic Conditions. Applied Environmental Microbiology 1985; 49: 1080-1083.
58. Little, CD, Palumbo AV, Herbes SE, Lidstrom ME, Tyndall RL, Gilmer PJ. Trichloroethylene Biodegradation by a Methane-Oxidizing Bacterium. Applied Environmental Microbiology 1988; 54(4): 951-956.
59. Tsien H, Brusseau GA, Hanson RS, Wackett LP. Biodegradation of Trichloroethylene by Methylosinus trichosporium OB3b. Applied Environmental Microbiology 1989; 55(12): 3155-3161.
60. Wilson JT, Wilson BH. Biotransformation of Trichloroethylene in Soil. Applied Environmental Microbiology 1985; 49(1): 242-243.
61. Pfaender FK. Biological Transformations of Volatile Organic Compounds in Groundwater. In: Ram NM, Christman RF, Cantor KP (eds.) Significance and Treatment of Volatile Organic Compounds in Water Supplies. Lewis Publishers: Chelsea, MI 1990. p205–226.
62. Bouwer EJ. Bioremediation of Organic Contaminants in the Subsurface. In: Mitchell R. (Eds.) Environmental Microbiology. John Wiley & Sons: New York 1992. p287–318.
63. Lorah MM, Olsen LD, Capone DG, Baker JE. Biodegradation of Trichloroethylene and Its Anaerobic Daughter Products in Freshwater Wetland Sediments. Bioremediation Journal 2001; 5(2): 101–118.
64. Fetzner S. Bacterial degradation of pyridine, indole, quinoline, and their derivatives under different redox conditions. Applied Environmental Microbiology 1998; 49: 237–250.
65. Shukla OP. Microbial transformation of quinoline by a Pseudomonas species. Applied Environmental Microbiology 1986; 51: 1332–1442.

66. Kaiser JP, Feng YC, Bollag JM. Microbial metabolism of pyridine, quinoline, acridine, and their derivatives under aerobic and anaerobic conditions. Microbiological Reviews 1996; 60: 483–498.

67. Carl B, Arnold A, Hauer B, Fetzner S. Sequence and transcriptional analysis of a gene cluster of Pseudomonas putida 86 involved in quinoline degradation. Gene 2004; 331: 177–188.

68. Kilbane JJ, Ranganathan R, Cleveland L, Kayser KJ, Ribiero C, Linhares MM, Selective removal of nitrogen from quinoline and petroleum by Pseudomonas ayucida IGTN9m. Applied Environmental Microbiology 2000; 66: 688–693.

69. Shukla OP. Microbiological degradation of quinoline by Pseudomonas stutzeri: the coumarin pathway of quinoline catabolism. Microbios 1989; 59: 47–63.

70. Shukla OP. Microbiological transformation of quinoline by Pseudomonas sp. Applied Environmental Microbiology 1986; 51: 1332-1442.

71. O'Loughlin EJ, Kehrmeyer SR, Sims GK, Isolation, characterization, and substrate utilization of a quinoline-degrading bacterium. International Biodeterioration and Biodegradation 1996; 38: 107–118.

72. Sugaya K, Nakayama O, Hinata N, Kamekura K, Ito A, Yamagiwa K, Ohkawa A. Biodegradation of quinoline in crude oil. Journal of Chemical Technology Biotechnology 2001; 76: 603–611.

73. Sun Q, Bai Y, Zhao C, Xiao Y, Wen D, Tang X. Aerobic biodegradation characteristics and metabolic products of quinoline by a Pseudomonas strain. Bioresource Technology 2009; 100: 5030-5036.

74. Annadurai G, Juang R, Lee DJ. Microbial degradation of phenol using mixed liquors of Pseudomonas putida and activated sludge. Waste Manage 2002; 22: 703–710.

75. Mohan D, Chander S. Single component and multi-component adsorption of phenols by activated carbons. Colloids and Surfaces A: Physicochemical &. Engineering Aspects 2001; 177: 183–196.

76. Dursun G, Cicek HC, Dursun AY. Adsorption of phenol from aqueous solution by using carbonised beet pulp. Journal of Hazardous Materials B 2005; 125: 175–182.

77. Patterson JF. Industrial Wastewater Treatment Technology, Second ed., Butterworths, London, 1985.
78. Tepe O, Dursun AY. Combined effects of external mass transfer and biodegradation rates on removal of phenol by immobilized Ralstonia eutropha in a packed bed reactor. Journal of Hazardous Materials 2008; 151: 9-16.
79. Knoll G, Winter J. Anaerobic degradation of phenol in sewage sludge: benzoate formation from phenol and carbon dioxide in the presence of hydrogen. Applied Environmental Microbiology 1987; 25(4): 384–391.
80. El-Naas MH, Al-Muhtaseb SA, Makhlouf S. Biodegradation of phenol by Pseudomonas putida immobilized in polyvinyl alcohol (PVA) gel. Journal of Hazardous Materials 2009; 164: 720–725.
81. Carrera J, Martín-Hernández M, Suárez-Ojeda ME, Pérez J. Modelling the pH dependence of the kinetics of aerobic p-nitrophenol biodegradation. Journal of Hazardous Materials 2011; 186: 1947–1953.
82. Ye J, Singh A, Ward O. Biodegradation of nitroaromatics and other nitrogen containing xenobiotics. World Journal Microbiology Biotechnology 2004; 20: 117–135.
83. Abrahamsson K, Klick S. Degradation of Halogenated Phenols in Anoxic Marine Sediments. Marine Pollution Bulletin 1991; 22: 227-233.
84. Hakulinen R, Woods S, Ferguson J, Benjamin M. The Role of Facultative Anaerobic Microorganisms in Anaerobic Biodegradation of Chlorophenols. Water Science & Technology 1985; 17: 289-301.
85. Jain V, Bhattacharya SK, Uberoi V. Degradation of 2,4-Dichlorophenol in Methanogenic Systems. Environmental Technology 1994; 15: 577-584.
86. Leuenberger C, Giger W, Coney R, Graydon JW, Molnar-Kubica E. Persistent Chemicals in Pulp Mill Effluents. Water Research 1985; 19: 885-894.
87. Sierra-Alvarez R, Field JA, Kortekaas S, Lettinga G. Overview of the Anaerobic Toxicity caused by Organic Forest Industry Wastewater Pollutants. Water Science Technology 1994; 29: 353-363.

88. Wood JM. Chlorinated Hydrocarbons: Oxidation in the Biosphere. Environmental Science & Technology 1982: 16: 291A-297A.

89. Annachhatre AP, Gheewala SH. Biodegradation of Chlorinated Phenolic Compounds. Biotechnology Advances 1996; 14 (1): 35-56.

90. Cheremisinoff NP. Biological Degradation of hazardous Waste. In: Biotechnology for Waste and Wastewater Treatment. Noyes Publications: Westwood, New Jersey, USA. 1996. p37-110.

91. Smith MJ, Lethbrideg G, Burns RG. Bioavailability and biodegradation of polycyclic aromatic hydrocarbons in soils. FEMS Microbiology Letters 1997; 152: 141–147.

92. Yuan SY, Wei SH, Chang BV. Biodegradation of polycyclic aromatic hydrocarbons by a mixed culture. Chemosphere 2002; 41: 1463–1468.

93. Ulrici W. Contaminated soil areas, different countries and contaminants, monitoring of contaminants, In: Rehm HJ., Reed G., Puhler A., Stadler P. (Eds.) Environmental Processes II Soil Decontamination Biotechnology: A Multi Volume Comprehensive Treatise, In: J. Klein (Ed.), Second Ed., vol. 11b, Wiley–VCH,Weihheim, FRG, 2000. p5-42.

94. Odokuma LO, Dickson AA, Bioremediation of a crude oil polluted tropical rain forest soil. Global Journal of Environmental Science 2003; 2: 29–40.

95. Cheung KC, Zhang JY, Deng HH, Ou YK, Leung HM, Wu SC, Wong MH. Interaction of higher plant (jute), electrofused bacteria and mycorrhiza on anthracene biodegradation. Bioresource Technology 2008; 99: 2148–2155.

96. Somtrakoon K, Suanjit S, Pokethitiyook P, Kruatrachue M, Lee H, Upatham S. Enhanced biodegradation of anthracene in acidic soil by inoculated Burkholderia sp. VUN10013. Current Microbiology 2008; 57: 102–107.

97. Li X, Lin X, Li P, Liu W, Wang L, Ma F, Chukwuka KS. Biodegradation of the low concentration of polycyclic aromatic hydrocarbons in soil by microbial consortium during incubation. Journal of Hazardous Materials 2009; 172: 601–605.

98. Santos EC, Rodrigo JS, Jacques Bento FM, Peralba MDCR, Selbach PA, Enilso LSS, Camargo FAO. Anthracene biodegradation

and surface activity by an iron-stimulated Pseudomonas sp. Bioresource Technology 2008; 99: 2644–2649.

99. Zeinali M, Vossoughi M, Ardestani SK. Naphthalene metabolism in Nocardia otitidiscaviarum strain TSH1, a moderately thermophilic microorganism. Chemosphere 2008; 72: 905–909.

100. Hwang G, Park SR, Lee CH, Ahn IS, Yoon YJ, Mhin BJ. Influence of naphthalene biodegradation on the adhesion of Pseudomonas putida NCIB 9816-4 to a naphthalene-contaminated soil. Journal of Hazardous Materials 2009; 171: 491–493.

101. Gennaro PD, Rescalli E, Galli E, Sello G, Bestetti G, Characterization of Rhodococcus opacus R7, a strain able to degrade naphthalene and o-xylene isolated from a polycyclic aromatic hydrocarbon-contaminated soil. Research in Microbiology 2001; 152: 641–651.

102. Calvo C, Toledo FL, González-López J. Surfactant activity of a naphthalene degrading Bacillus pumilus strain isolated from oil sludge. Journal of Biotechnology 2004; 109: 255–262.

103. Kelley I, Freeman JP, Evans FE, Cerniglia CE. Identification of metabolites from degradation of naphthalene by a Mycobacterium sp. Biodegradation 1990; 1: 283–290.

104. Lin C, Gan L, Chen ZL. Biodegradation of naphthalene by strain Bacillus fusiformis (BFN). Journal of Hazardous Materials 2010; 182: 771–777.

105. Staples CA, Peterson DR, Parkerton TF, Adams WJ. The environmental fate of phthalate esters: a literature review. Chemosphere 1997; 35: 667–749.

106. Nalli S, Cooper DG, Nicell JA. Biodegradation of plasticizers by Rhodococcus rhodochrous. Biodegradation 2002; 13: 343–352.

107. Nalli S, Cooper DG, Nicell JA. Metabolites from the biodegradation of di-ester plasticizers by Rhodococcus rhodochrous. Science of the Total Environment Journal 2006; 366: 286–294.

108. Rahman M, Brazel CS. The plasticizer market: an assessment of traditional plasticizers and research trends to meet new challenges. Progress in Polymer Science 2004; 29: 1223–1248.

109. Tickner JA, Schettler T, Guidotti T, McCally M, Rossi M. Health risks posed by use of di-2-ethylhexyl phthalate (DEHP) in PVC

medical devices: a critical review. American Journal of Industrial Medicine 2001; 39: 100–111.

110. Onorato TM, Brown PW, Morris P. Mono-(2-ethylhexyl)phthalate increase spermatocyte mitochondrial peroxiredoxin 3 and cyclooxygenase 2. Journal of Andrology 2008; 29: 293–303.

111. Horn O, Nalli S, Cooper DG, Nicell JA. Plasticizer metabolites in the environment. Water Research 2004; 38: 3693–3698.

112. Nalli SS, Horn OJ, Grochowalski AR, Cooper DG, Nicell JA. Origin of 2- ethylhexanol as a VOC. Environmental Pollution Journal 2006; 140: 181–185.

113. Barnabé S, Beauchesne I, Cooper DG, Nicell JA. Plasticizers and their degradation products in the process streams of a large urban physicochemical sewage treatment plant. Water Research 2008; 42: 153–162.

114. Beauchesne I, Barnabé S, Cooper DG, Nicell JA. Plasticizers and related toxic degradation products in wastewater sludges. Water Science & Technology 2008; 57: 367–374.

115. Deligio T. Phthalate Alternative Recognized by ECHA. 2009.

116. http://www. plasticstoday.com/articles/phthalate-alternative-recognized-echa/ (accessed December 2012)

117. Gartshore J, Cooper DG, Nicell JA. Biodegradation of plasticizers by Rhodotorula Rubra. Environmental Toxicology & Chemistry 2003; 22: 1244–1251.

118. Pour AK, Cooper DG, Mamer OA, Maric M, Nicell JA. Mechanism of biodegradation of dibenzoate plasticizers. Chemosphere 2009; 77: 258–263.

119. Firlotte N, Cooper DG, Maric M, Nicell JA. Characterization of 1,5-pentanediol dibenzoate as a potential green plasticizer for poly(vinyl chloride). Journal of Vinyl Additive Technology 2009; 15: 99–107.

120. Pour AK, Mamer OA, Cooper DG, Maric M, Nicell JA. Metabolites from the biodegradation of 1,6-hexanediol dibenzoate, a potential green plasticizer, by Rhodococcus rhodochrous. Journal of Mass Spectrometry 2009; 44: 662–671.

121. Pour AK, Roy R, Coopera DG, Maric M, Nicell JA. Biodegradation kinetics of dibenzoate plasticizers and their metabolites.

Biochemical Engineering Journal 2013; 70: 35-45.

122. http://ec.europa.eu/environment/waste/framework/index.htm (accessed December 2012)

123. Shimao M. Biodegradation of plastics. Current Opinion in Biotechnology 2001; 12: 242–247.

124. Chiellini E, Corti A, D'Antone S, Solaro R. Biodegradation of poly(vinylalcohol) based materials. Progress in Polymer Science 2003; 28: 963-1014.

125. Sakai K, Hamada N, Watanabe Y. Studies on the poly(vinyl alcohol)-degrading enzyme. Part VI. Degradation mechanism of poly(vinyl alcohol) by successive reactions of secondary alcohol oxidase and -diketone hydrolase from Pseudomonas sp. Agricultural & Biological Chemistry 1986; 50: 989-996.

126. Suzuki T. Degradation of poly(vinyl alcohol) by microorganisms. Journal of Applied Polymer Science Applied Polymer Symposium 1979; 35: 431-437.

127. Hatanaka T, Kawahara T, Asahi N, Tsuji M. Effects of the structure of poly(vinyl alcohol) on the dehydrogenation reaction by poly(vinyl alcohol) dehydrogenase from Pseudomonas sp. 113P3. Bioscience Biotechnology Biochemistry 1995; 59: 1229-1231.

128. Bloembergen S, David J, Geyer D, Gustafson A, Snook J, Narayan R. Biodegradation and composting studies of polymeric materials. In: Doi Y, Fukuda K. (Eds.) Biodegradable plastics and polymers. Amsterdam: Elsevier; 1994. p601-609.

129. David C, De Kesel C, Lefebvre F, Weiland M. The biodegradation of polymers: recent results. Angewandte Makromolekulare Chemie 1994; 216: 21-35.

130. Chiellini E, Corti A, Sarto GD, D'Antone S. Oxo-biodegradable polymers e Effect of hydrolysis degree on biodegradation behaviour of poly(vinyl alcohol). Polymer Degradation and Stability 2006; 91: 3397-3406.

131. Khanna S, Srivastava AK, Recent Advances in microbial polyhydroxyalkanoates. Process Biochemistry 2005; 40: 607-619.

132. Ghatnekar MS, Pai JS, Ganesh M. Production and recovery of poly-3-hydroxybutyrate from Methylobacterium sp.V49. Journal of Chemical Technology and Biotechnology 2002; 77: 444-448.

133. DeMarco S. Advances in polyhydroxyalkanoate production in bacteria for biodegradable plastics. MMG 445. Basic Biotechnology eJournal 2005; 1: 1-4.
134. Mudgal S, Lyons L, Bain, J. Plastic Waste in the Environment – Final Report for European Commission DG Environment. BioIntelligence Service; 2010. http://www.ec.europa.eu/environment/ (accessed December 2012)
135. Hopewell J, Dvorak R, Kosior E. Plastics recycling: challenges and opportunities. Philosophical Transactions of the Royal Society B 2009; 364: 2115-2126.
136. Plastics Europe. An analysis of European Plastics production, demand and recovery for 2009. Plastics - the Facts 2010.
137. http://www.plasticseurope.org/ (accessed December 2012)
138. The Encyclopedia of Polymer Science and Technology, 4th Edition, John Wiley and Sons, New York; 2012.
139. Selke SE. Plastics recycling In: Harper CA. (Ed.), Handbook of plastics, elastomers and composites, 4th edition, McGraw-Hill, New York; 2002. p693–757.
140. Fact sheet, Recycling the hard stuff. U.S. Environmental Protection Agency, Solid Waste and Emergency Response, 2002 EPA 530-F-02-023 Washington, D.C. http://www.docstoc.com/docs (accessed December 2012)
141. Hendrickson CT, Matthews DH, Ashe M, Jaramillo P, McMichael FC. Reducing environmental burdens of solid-state lighting through end-of-life design. Environmental Research Letters 5. 2010. Doi: 10.1088/1748-9326/5/1/014016.
142. Cerdan C, Gazulla C, Raugei M, Martinez E, Fullana-i-Palmer P. Proposal for new quantitative eco-design indicators: a first case study. Journal of Cleaner Production 2009; 17: 1638-1643.
143. Plastic Waste: Redesign and Biodegradability. Science for Environmental Policy, Future Brief, 2001; 1: 1-8.
144. Tokiwa Y, Calabia BP, Ugwu CU, Aiba S. Biodegradability of Plastics. International Journal of Molecular Science 2009; 10: 3722–3742.
145. Jackson S, Bertényi T. Recycling of Plastics. ImpEE Project. 2006. p1-27
146. http://www-g.eng.cam.ac.uk/ (accessed December 2012)

Chapter 6

Peyronie's Disease Cell Culture Models: Phenotypic, Genotypic and Functional Analyses

J P Mulhall[1, 2], M S Anderson[1, 2], T Lubrano[1], and T V Shankey[1, 2]

[1]Andrology Research Laboratory, Hines VA, Hines, Illinois, USA

[2]Department of Urology, Weill Medical College of Cornell University, The New York Hospital, 525 East 68th St, New York, NY 10021

ABSTRACT

Peyronie's disease is a fibromatosis of the tunica albuginea. While trauma is believed to be the inciting event, the exact pathophysiology of this condition is unknown. In vitro analysis of cell biology can shed light on the pathogenesis of medical conditions and has been used for many decades as a research tool. We have established a cell culture model, which we have used to study the pathobiology of cells derived from Peyronie's disease plaque tissue. In 10 separate cell cultures derived from different individuals, these cells have demonstrated consistent phenotypic, genotypic and functional alterations. In neither of the control cell cultures, neonatal foreskin fibroblasts and normal tunica-derived fibroblasts have any of the above aberrations been demonstrated. The cells studied have been shown to be fibroblasts in nature with a sub-population of myofibroblasts present in culture. The Peyronie's disease plaque tissue-derived fibroblasts have demonstrated (i) consistent morphologic transformation (ii) increased S-phase on flow cytometry (iii) decreased dependence on culture medium (iv) cytogenic instability (v) excess production of fibrogenic cytokines and (vi) stabilization and dysfunctionalization of p53. Further refinement of this model and future analyses may permit an increased understanding of the pathogenesis of this condition and allow the development of therapeutic strategies.

INTRODUCTION

Peyronie's diseases is a fibromatosis affecting approximately 3% of men.[1,2,3,4,5] It is characterized by scar (plaque) formation in the tunica albuginea of the corpora cavernosa. This plaque, the result of a fibrotic process, leads to penile curvature with functional shortening of the penis and erectile dysfunction.[2,3,6,7] Presenting symptoms include penile pain, curvature and inability to accomplish penetrative sexual relations. Peyronie's disease primarily affects men aged 45-60 y but may affect men of all ages. The psychosocial implications of Peyronie's disease can be remarkable, with as many as three-quarters of patients reporting psychological disturbances.[3] The condition is associated with other fibromatoses, including Dupuytren's contracture (aponeurotic palmar fibrosis) of the hand and Ledderhose's disease (aponeurotic plantar fibrosis) of the foot, and at a cellular level it shares some features with benign neoplasms such as ovarian fibromata.[4, 8, 9, 10, 11]

The pathogenesis of Peyronie's disease appears to be multifactorial and has not been fully elucidated. As torqueing of the penis occurs in all men during penetrative sexual relations, one of the conundrums concerning Peyronie's disease is, why is it that such a small population of men manifest plaque formation? While trauma is believed to be the inciting event,[12] many theories have been proposed for the pathogenesis of Peyronie's disease, including, auto-immune factors,[11,12,13,14] excess production of fibrogenic cytokines,[15,16] impaired fibrin clearance within the tunica 4,5 and cytogenetic aberrations.[4,5,17,18,19,20] The microscopic appearance of a Peyronie's plaque reveals an increased number of fibroblasts, inflammatory cells and increased amounts of collagen deposited in a disorganized fashion.[21,22,23] The concept that some patients may be predisposed to the development of excessive fibromatosis while others are not has led to more recent interest in alterations of the cellular and molecular mechanisms which may play a role in Peyronie's disease. Cell culture models have permitted a more in-depth exploration of such mechanisms. Expanding the knowledge case on a disease process is based in part, upon basic research using either animal or cell culture models. El-Sakka et al have developed a rat model for the study of Peyronie's disease. Injecting cytomodulin, a synthetic heptapeptide with TGF-beta-like properties into the rat penis has been shown to induce an intense fibrotic reaction in both the tunica albuginea and corpus cavernosum.[15, 24] This model is heavily predicated upon the role the TGF-beta plays in the pathogenesis of Peyronie's disease and does not take into account any upstream factors that may play a role in the development of Peyronie's disease plaque. However, the development of such a model permits the research investigator to explore the fundamental mechanisms involved in the fibrogenesis in Peyronie's disease and also enables the evaluation of therapeutic strategies for this condition. A cell culture model, while not perfectly replicating the in vivo environment does ensure that the cells studied are derived from and representative of actual Peyronie's disease tissue. Furthermore, such models allow the ready and reproducible study of Peyronie's disease plaque-derived cells in both a cost-efficient and time-efficient manner. Finally, cell culture models allow the study of different cell lines derived from multiple individuals, thus, permitting investigators to identify any inter-individual variance in the pathobiology of the derived cells.

Cell Culture Methodology

It is hoped that this treatise will serve as a guide to those workers who are interested in developing cell culture models of Peyronie's disease. The methodology outlined here has served us well and has allowed excellent cell production with reliability and reproducibility of the results presented later.

Patient Population

The patients enrolled in these studies and from whom tissue is excised have documented clinically significant Peyronie's disease of greater than 12 months duration. They were enrolled according to an approved Institutional Review Board protocol, prior to the date of their operation for correction of penile curvature or prosthesis placement. They were informed that the amount of tissue excised is approximately the size of a match-stick head and will not interfere with the operation or their post-operative care.

Tissue Acquisition

Two tunical samples are taken from each patient, one from the plaque itself and the other from an area of 'normal' tunica remote from the plaque. Using loupe magnification, all fascial tissue and corporal smooth muscle is stripped from both specimens to ensure that the source tissue represents the tunica albuginea alone. The plaque specimen is generally a partial-thickness shave biopsy, while the normal tunical specimen is a full-thickness tunical specimen excised from either the corporotomy site (if prosthetic surgery is being performed) or from the site of the plication surgery (if Nesbit surgery is being performed). The specimens are placed immediately into transport media (RPMI, 10% fetal bovine serum, 10 mM HEPES, ciprofloxacin) and transported directly to the laboratory. Ciprofloxacin has been chosen as the antibiotic because of mycoplasma contamination of some of our early cell cultures. Two types of control tissue has been utilized, neonatal foreskins and tunical tissue excised at the time of reconstructive surgery from young men with congenital penile curvature. All control tissues are handled in an identical manner to the Peyronie's disease tunical tissue.

Cell Isolation and Culture

Using sterile technique, the tissue is sharply divided into 1 mm^2 fragments. Fragments from normal and plaque tissue are placed into separate 50 ml sterile centrifuge tubes containing -MEM (JRH Scientific). The cells are then incubated overnight at 37°C in 5% humidified CO_2. The cells and tissue fragments are collected by centrifugation and washed in fresh tissue culture media. Pieces of digested tissue are placed into 25 cm^2 sterile tissue culture flasks along with cells from the pellet and incubated in tissue culture medium (-MEM+10% fetal bovine serum, 1% glutamine, ciprofloxacin) at 37°C in 5% CO_2. Tissue culture media is changed at 48 h and every 5-6 days thereafter. Once they have formed confluent monolayers, the cells are harvested using trypsin/EDTA. After washing, cells for continuous cultures are split 1:3 and grown to confluence. At various passages, cells are stored in RPMI/15% fetal bovine serum/7.5% DMSO at -90°C.

Phenotypic Analyses

The cells derived from Peyronie's disease plaque tissue have been categorically defined as fibroblasts by a number of authors. The original description was published by Somers et al in 1982[20] and this has been confirmed by our laboratory as well as by the UCLA workers. Defining the phenotype of cultured cells is based, in part, upon microscopic morphologic criteria as well as the expression of intracellular antigens.

In our laboratory, cells established in tissue culture have been characterized by analysis of the expression of intermediate filament proteins, and actin-containing microfilaments using indirect immunofluorescence. Cells at early passage (as soon as sufficient cells were available for freezing and for continuation of the culture) and at selected later passages were cultured in sterile multi-chamber slides (Corning Inc., Corning, NY, USA) and grown until nearly confluent (observed using an inverted tissue-culture microscope). Slides were washed three times with cold PBS, and were then ixed using either 100% cold methanol (4°C) or 2% paraformaldehyde (15 min at 4°C, freshly prepared in PBS). The cells were then washed in cold (4°C) PBS, and underwent cell permeabilization (100% cold methanol). Slides were again washed three times with cold PBS. Individual chambers were incubated with antibodies to either vimentin (Dako, Carpenteria, CA, USA), cytokeratin (BD Bioscience, San Jose, CA, USA), or smooth muscle specific actin (Dako). All experiments included chambers incubated with appropriate mouse isotope controls at the same final protein concentration as used for primary monoclonal antibodies. Primary antibodies were incubated at 4°C for 60 min, followed by washing three times with cold PBS containing 5% BSA, and incubation with secondary antibody (FITC-goat anti-mouse Ig, final dilution 1:20) (BD Bioscience) for 30 min. Following washing (three times with cold PBS/5% BSA), nuclei were counterstained using propidium iodide (1 µg/ml), and slides were cover-slipped following the addition of anti-fade solution. Chamber slides were viewed using a Zeiss Axioscope fluorescence microscope using epifluorescence illumination. Control cells used for all immunofluorescence experiments included human foreskin fibroblasts at early passage number, derived from several different individuals.

To date, 10 separate and distinct cell cultures have been successfully established from Peyronie›s plaques and eight cell cultures from normal tunical tissue from the same patients with Peyronie›s disease. Multiple neonatal foreskin and congenital penile curvature tunica-derived cultures have also been established. Cells with fibroblast-like morphology typically grow out from varying numbers of tissue fragments from neonatal foreskins

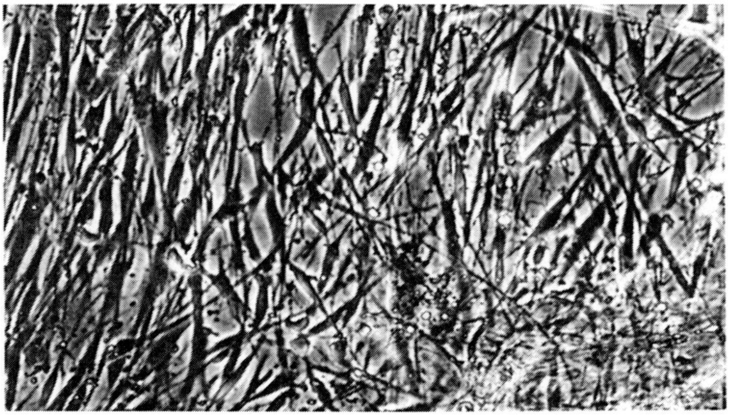

Figure 1: Representative phase-contrast photomicrograph of cultured cells derived from foreskin (´200). See text for description.

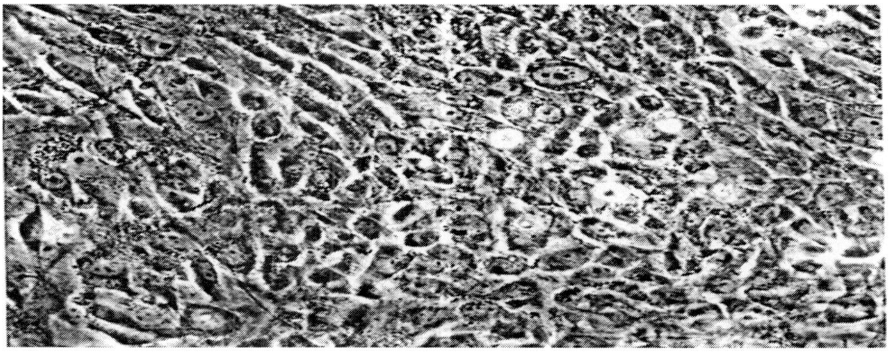

Figure 2: Representative phase-contrast photomicrograph of cultured cells derived from Peronei's disease plaque tissue (´200). See text for description.

(Figure 1), plaque (Figure 2) and normal tunical tissues from Peyronie's patients.

In low passage, plaque-derived cultures, the cells typically demonstrate plump cell bodies with cytoplasmic extensions, and generally grow in a more random fashion, in contrast to the pattern seen for foreskin fibroblasts cultured under identical conditions, which grow in parallel, closely packed cell clusters with a 'swirling' appearance. Cells from later passages of Peyronie's disease plaque-derived tissue exhibited considerable pleomorphism, but underwent consistent morphologic transformation between passages eight and 12, resulting in loss of cytoplasmic extensions, and failure to exhibit contact inhibition with the development of cell foci within culture.

Immunofluorescence analysis has been performed to characterize cells isolated from Peyronie's patients with an emphasis on antigenic markers characteristic of fibroblasts. The results have demonstrated strong staining with anti-vimentin antibodies

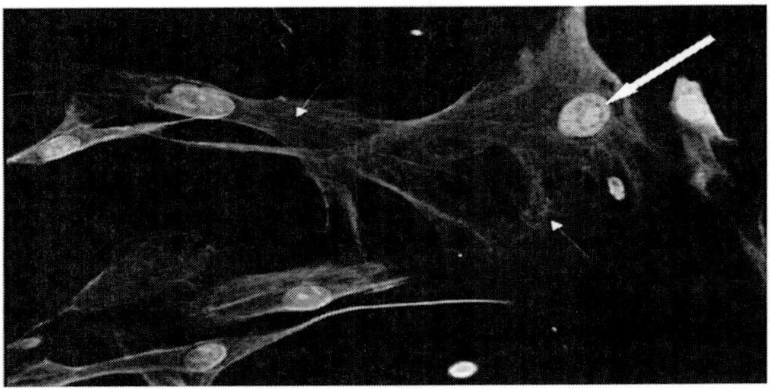

Figure 3: Indirect immunofluorescent staining of intracellular vimentin (fine arrows) in cultured fibroblasts derived from Peyronie's plaque tissue. The nuclei are counter-stained with propidium iodide (large arrow).

(Figure 3) for normal tunical and plaque-derived fibroblast-like cells. Staining was characterized by a thin web-like pattern extending from the cell membrane to the nucleus, a pattern characteristic of intermediate filaments. Similar staining patterns were seen for normal tunical and plaque-derived fibroblast-like cells, which was similar to the staining pattern seen for foreskin-derived fibroblasts stained with anti-vimentin antibodies using identical fixation conditions. Low levels of cytoplasmic staining with antibodies to smooth muscle actin was seen in plaque and normal Peyronie's derived cells

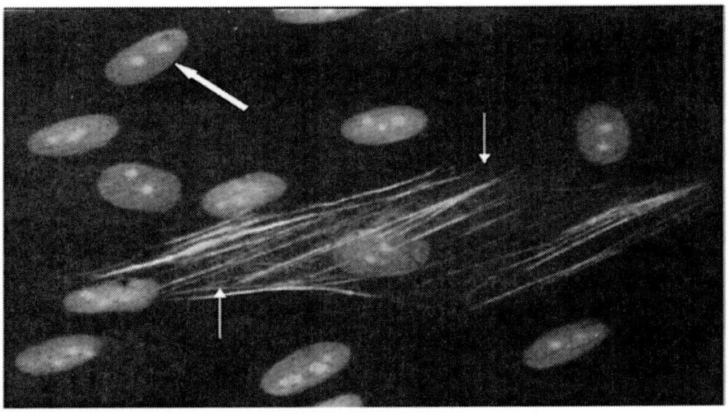

Figure 4: Indirect immunofluorescent staining of intracellular smooth muscle alpha-actin (fine arrows) in cultured fibroblasts derived from Peyronie's plaque tissue. The nuclei are counter-stained with propidium iodide (large arrow).

(Figure 4), but not in cells derived from foreskin. Actin immunofluorescence was characterized by a diffuse cytoplasmic staining pattern in most cells, with occasional cells demonstrating organized actin microfilaments in both plaque and normal Peyronie's derived cells. Neonatal foreskin-derived fibroblasts were negative for smooth muscle actin expression. Similar patterns of smooth muscle actin expression were seen in Peyronie's derived cells fixed in either para-formaldehyde followed by cold methanol, or in cold ethanol alone, suggesting that the antigen expression patterns seen here were unlikely to be the result of fixation technique. All cells (tunica and foreskin-derived fibroblasts) were negative for cytokeratin and desmin expression by immunofluorescence. Together, these results suggest that the cells cultured from both plaque and normal Peyronie's tissues are myofibroblasts, and agree with previously reported results by Somers et al, [20] who used similar techniques to obtain cells from Peyronie's tissues.

This work has been confirmed and extended by the UCLA group, [25] which has recently used Western blotting techniques to confirm the presence of vimentin and alpha-smooth muscle actin in fibroblast cultures derived from normal human tunica. Furthermore, they showed the presence of a novel growth and differentiation factor from the TGF-beta family, myostatin. The number of cells expressing myostatin increased with passage number. These processes appeared to be inducible by incubating cells with TGF-beta.

Genotypic Analyses

Since previous experiments by others in Peyronie's disease and the associated Dupuytren's contracture have indicated macroscopic changes in specific chromosomes,[20,26,27,28] we undertook studies of numerical changes in specific chromosomes using flourescent in situ hybridization (FISH).[18,19] For these studies, we have used probes to chromosomes 7, 8, 17, 18, X and Y (Vysis, Downers Grove, IL, USA). FISH was accomplished using simultaneous hybridization with two different fluorochrome-labeled probes FITC (green) plus Cy5 (red). In summary, the number of centromere-specific probes was determined using fluorescence microscopy. On FISH microscopy, control fibroblasts isolated from neonatal foreskins contained two copies of chromosomes 7, 8 17 and 18 (Figure 5).

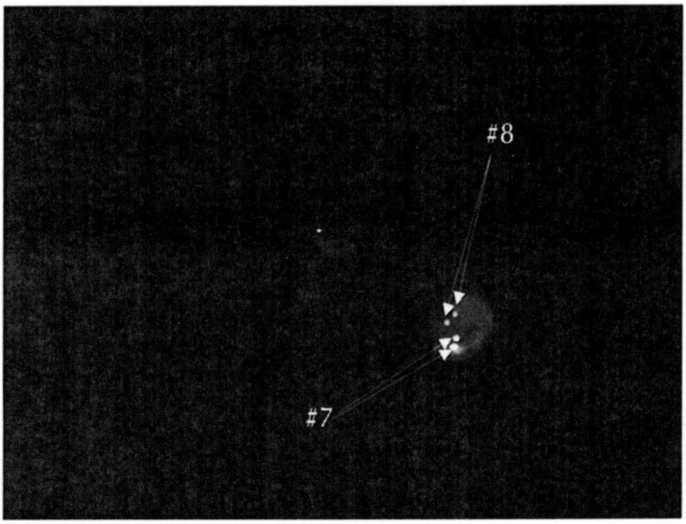

Figure 5: FISH photomicrograph of neonatal foreskin derived fibroblasts demonstrating disomy of chromosomes 7 and 8.

In contrast, all Peyronie's disease plaque-derived fibroblasts studied were aneusomic for chromosomes 7, 8, 17, 18 (Figure 6). Foreskin fibroblasts typically had one copy of chromosomes X and Y.

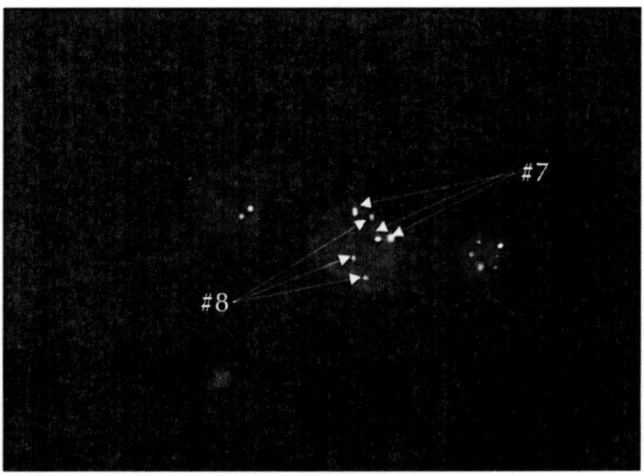

Figure 6: FISH photomicrograph of Peyronie's disease plaque-derived fibroblasts (passage three) demonstrating trisomy of chromosomes 7 and 8.

In general, plaque-derived fibroblasts had no copies of the Y chromosome and were often tetrasomic for the other autosomes that were probed. These chromosomal aberrations were present in plaque-derived fibroblasts in very early passages, as low as passage three. Thus, using Poisson statistics, it is probable that these alterations were present at the commencement of cell culture. The presence of aneusomies in early passage plaque-derived cells, combined with the absence of any cytogenetic instability in either foreskin or normal tunica-derived fibroblasts, suggests that chromosomal instability in Peyronie's disease plaque-derived fibroblasts is not the result of culture artifact and, is therefore, likely to be of significance.

Recently, Yamanaka et al assessed DNA isolated fom Peyronie's disease plaque tissue for loss of heterozygosity (LOH) and microsatellite alterations (MSI).[17] Using PCR technology, chromosomes 3, 8 and 9 were selected and 20 different polymorphic markers were used to assess for MSI and LOH. Forty per cent of the patients demonstrated MSI on at least one locus. Likewise, 40% of patients demonstrated LOH on at least one locus. These data confirm that cytogenetic instability is prevalent in Peyronie's disease tissue and that it is probably more widespread throughout the genome than previously demonstrated. Of course, whether, these finding are a cause of an effect in the disease process is currently unknown.

Functional Analyses

We have utilized this model to assess Peyronie's disease plaque-derived fibroblasts for: (i) proliferation profiles; (ii) basic FGF (bFGF) expression; (iii) the inhibitory effect of biologic agents; and (iv) cell cycle regulator expression.

Fibroblast Proliferation Profiles

Determination of cell growth rates has been performed using the MTT assay (Vybrant ™ cell proliferation assay, Molecular Probes, Eugene, OR, USA), with slight modifications. This assay, originally developed by Mossman, [29] is based on the reduction of soluble MTT dye to an insoluble compound (formazan) by mitochondrial dehydrogenases, with subsequent dye solubilization by the addition of SDS (sodium dodecyl sulfate). While the assay generally measures the total number of viable cells present, other enzymes that can retain activity after loss of cell viability (for example, glutathione-S-transferase) can reduce the specificity of this assay.

For the cell growth assays, confluent cells were harvested, counted, and the viability determined by trypan blue dye exclusion. Cells were plated into flat-bottomed microtiter (96-well) plates at a final density of 5×10^3 viable cells in 200 µl culture media (MEM+10% FCS, ciprofloxacin). This cell concentration was chosen based on preliminary experiments using cell densities between 10^3 and 5×10^5 per well, which demonstrated that optimal growth was obtained using this initial cell concentration. All experiments were performed in triplicate, with cells incubated at 37°C in 5% CO_2 in a humidified atmosphere for periods of up to 96 h. Four hours before the termination of cultures, 150 µl of tissue culture media was carefully removed, and replaced with 100 µl phenol-free (RPMI/10%FCS) tissue culture medium and 10 µl of MTT stock solution (12 mM MTT), and incubated for an additional 4 h at 37°C in 5% CO_2. The times indicated for growth, thus represent the total time of viable culture conditions, as MTT at the concentration used, and has minimal effect on cell viability. MTT stock solution (12 mM) was prepared by first dissolving 5 mg MTT in 400 µl methanol. This solution, which was stored at 4°C, was diluted in sterile PBS to a final concentration of 5 mg MTT/ml immediately before addition to cell cultures. Cells in each well were carefully mixed, and the MTT reaction product was solubilized by the addition of 100 µl HCl-SDS solution (1 g SDS in 10 ml 0.01 M HCl). Following overnight incubation at 37°C, absorbance was measured at 595 nm using a microplate reader (Fisher Biotech BT 2000, Pittsburgh, PA, USA).

Low passage Peyronie›s disease plaque-derived fibroblasts and neonatal foreskin fibroblasts were plated at increasing cell concentrations from 10^3 to 5×10^5 cells per well for periods from 24 to 96 h (Figure 7).

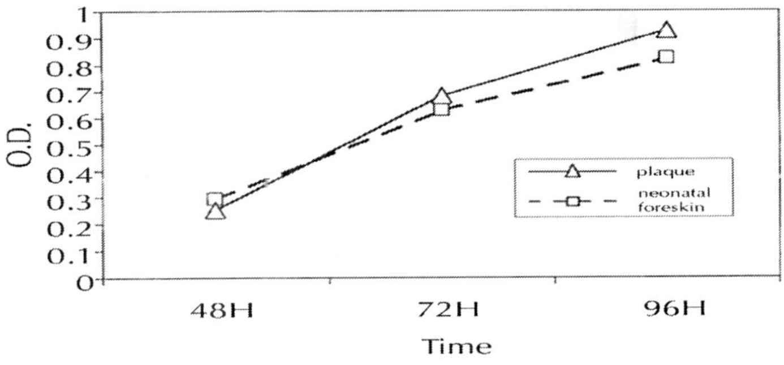

Figure 7: MTT assay: proliferation of fibroblasts as measured by optical density (OD) plotted against time (48-96 h). The graphs represent the mean OD values from multiple experiments.

At initial concentrations of 10^3 cells, insignificant levels of MTT dye metabolism were detected, which did not change during the 96 h the cells were in culture. These results suggest that Peyronie's derived cells, like normal fibroblasts, will not grow below a minimal cell density. With increasing initial cell concentration, both plaque-derived and control fibroblasts showed higher levels of MTT dye metabolism, with the former demonstrating significantly higher cell concentrations. With increasing initial cell concentration, cultures of plaque-derived cells reached a growth plateau, consistent with contact inhibition, which was also seen in foreskin fibroblasts. Overall, these results demonstrate two growth characteristics Peyronie's disease plaque-derived fibroblasts, namely lack of growth below a critical cell concentration, and growth arrest at high cell densities, both classic properties of cells in culture.

In order to evaluate growth requirements by Peyronie's fibroblast-like cells, control foreskin fibroblasts, as well as cells derived from plaque were seeded at an initial concentration of 10^4 cells per microtiter well in different concentrations of fetal calf serum (FCS) from 1% to 10% (final concentration). Cultures were evaluated for overall growth using the MTT assay after a total of 72 h in culture. Both plaque and control fibroblasts demonstrated a pattern of decreased cell growth which was directly proportional to the concentration of FCS in the growth media, with growth in 1% FCS only 50% of that in media supplemented with 10% FCS. Finally, Peyronie's disease plaque-derived fibroblasts have been grown in 0.1% FCS medium further supporting the concept that these cells are biologically transformed. We have never been able to grow neonatal foreskin-derived fibroblasts in 0.1% FCS cell culture medium.

Basic FGF Expression

With the demonstration by El-Sakka et al that Peyronie's disease plaques expressed TGF-beta, we were interested in defining the role that other fibrogenic cytokines might play in the pathogenesis of Peyronie's disease. For a detailed methodological outline, we refer the reader to our previously published work.[16] the amount of bFGF was compared between supernatant fluids obtained from plaque, normal tunical tissue, foreskin fibroblasts and culture medium (containing 10% FCS) cultured under similar conditions without cells. Multiple analyses (minimum of three independent replicates) were conducted on all specimens including plaque-derived cell lines from five different individuals (Figure 8).

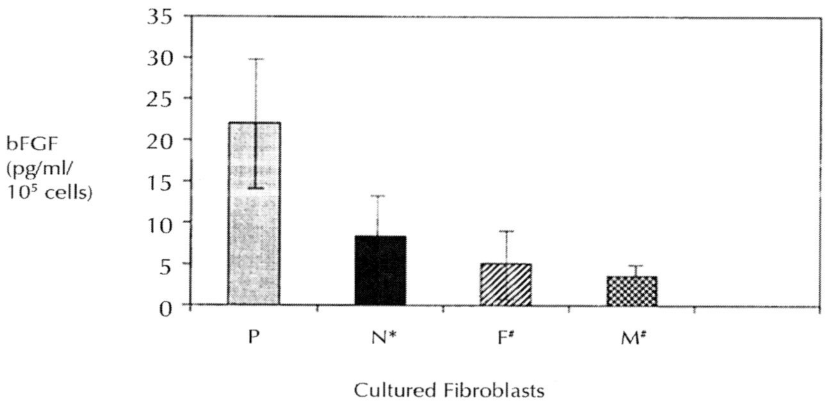

Figure 8: bFGF production by cultured fibroblasts. P, plaque; N, normal tunica; F, foreskin; M, culture medium. *Denotes statistical significance at the 0.02 level (P vs N). # denotes statistical significance at the 0.01 level (P vs F, P vs M).

ELISA analysis demonstrated that plaque-derived cells produced more bFGF (22±7.5 pg/ml per 10^5 cells) than either normal tunica-derived cells (8.4±5.5 pg/ml per 10^5 cells) or foreskin fibroblast-derived cells (5.1±4.2 pg/ml per 10^5 cells). Tissue culture medium cultured for

48 h at 37°C contained 3.53±0.6 pg/ml of bFGF. The mean amount of bFGF produced by the five plaque derived cell lines was significantly greater than that produced by foreskin fibroblast cell lines (P=0.013), conditioned tissue culture media (P=0.01), and non-plaque tunica-derived cells (P=0.02). While the levels of bFGF produced by foreskin fibroblasts are greater than those found in conditioned tissue culture medium, this difference did not reach statistical significance. Thus, these data suggested a role for bFGF in the development of Peyronie's disease plaque.

The Inhibitory Effect of Biologic Agents

Because the pathophysiology of Peyronie's disease is so poorly understood, there is no clear consensus on how it should be treated. Numerous conservative (oral and intralesional) therapies have been used in the treatment of Peyronie's disease, including verapamil, colchicine, steroids, and alpha-interferon.[30, 31, 32] the effectiveness of these agents has not been clearly proven. We utilized, the previously outlined model for the culture and quantification of proliferation of fibroblasts to investigate the in vitro effects of prostaglandin E_1 (PGE_1), verapamil, colchicine, and alpha-interferon on the proliferation rates of fibroblasts derived from Peyronie's disease tissue.[33] Cell viability was assayed separately by co-incubating cells for 96 h at a concentration of 5000 cells/ml with each biologic agent and staining with trypan blue. For this purpose, PGE_1, verapamil, colchicine, and interferon were added in concentrations of 7.5 μg/ml, 100 μg/ml, 2.5 μg/ml, and 10^5 IU/ml, respectively. Cells and biological agents were placed into a 10 ml flask and brought to a final volume of 10 ml with 10% FCS. Following trypan blue staining, cells were counted using a hemocytometer. As controls, identical cells were incubated without the addition of biologic agents.

The effects of the various agents on plaque-derived fibroblasts are reported in Figure 9.

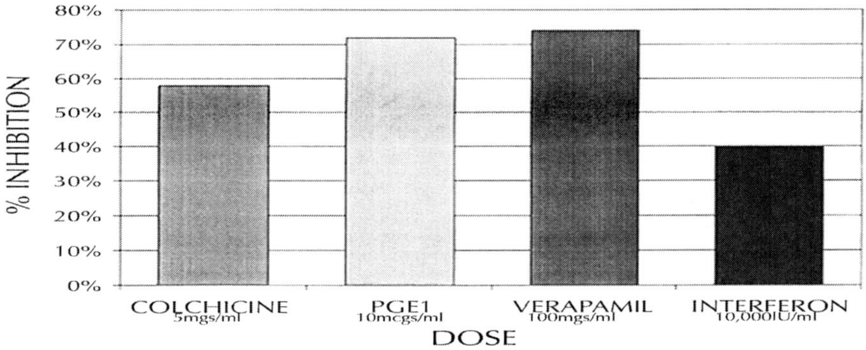

Figure 9: Percentage inhibition of fibroblasts in response to colchicines, verapamil, and PGE_1 and interferon α-2b at the doses listed. Per cent inhibition is defined as the percentage reduction in optical density (OD) on spectrophotometry at 96 h when compared to control cells (plaque-derived fibroblasts in culture medium alone).

Inhibition is expressed as the percentage reduction in optical density (OD) on spectrophotometry at 96 h when compared to control cells, that is, cells cultured in culture medium alone without biologic agents. Maximum inhibition occurred at 96 h in all cases. Culture of plaque fibroblasts with PGE_1 resulted in inhibition of growth of 72±15% at 10 μg/ml, 60±11% at 7.5 μg/ml and 32±19% at 5 μg/ml. No significant effect was seen at 1 and 0.1 μg/ml. Culture with verapamil resulted in a 75% inhibition of cells at 1000 μg/ml and 74±15% at 100 μg/ml. No significant effect was seen at 50, 25, and 10 μg/ml, respectively. Culture with alpha-IFN resulted in 40% inhibition at a concentration of 10^5 IU/ml, 36% at 10^4 IU/ml, and 17±5% at 10^3 IU/ml. Culture with colchicine resulted in a 58±19% growth inhibition at 2.5 μg/ml and 58±24% at 0.5 μg/ml. The viability of those cells not co-incubated with biologic agents (controls) was 88%. Viability was 87% when co-incubated with colchicine, 70% with PGE_1, and 65% with interferon-alpha 2b. Cell viability after co-incubation with verapamil was significantly less at 40%. These post co-incubation viabilities represent 99% of controls for colchicines, 80% of controls for PGE_1, and 75% of controls for IFN and 45% of controls for verapamil.

Cell Cycle Regulator Expression

Cell over-proliferation, such as that occurring in malignant neoplasms and Peyronie's disease, may result from promotion by activators, failure of suppressors, or the failure to promote cell death (apoptosis). p [53] is intrinsically involved in cell cycle regulation, apoptosis and DNA damage repair pathways. Aberrant p53 function leading to cell proliferation and immortalization has been implicated in several human malignancies.[34,35,36,37,38] Absence, alteration or loss of function of this protein may allow damaged cells, normally halted from passage through the cell cycle, to pass and proliferate, resulting in unregulated cell replication. In certain circumstances, this may lead to the development of non-malignant conditions such as fibromatoses. Recent work has explored the function of p53 in fibromatoses and although controversy exists in this literature a number of workers have implicated aberrations in the p[53] pathway in the etiogenesis of certain benign conditions.[35,37,39,40,41,42,43] In the normal state, the detection of the p[53] protein is difficult due to its very short half-life.[37] Furthermore, p53 does not act in isolation but is under negative feedback control through the action of a variety of downstream elements, two of which are mdm2 and p[21].[36] The methods used for these experiments are outlined in our previously published work.[44]

Cells from all plaque cultures isolated in these experiments expressed variable but clearly measurable levels of p[53] protein (Figure 10).

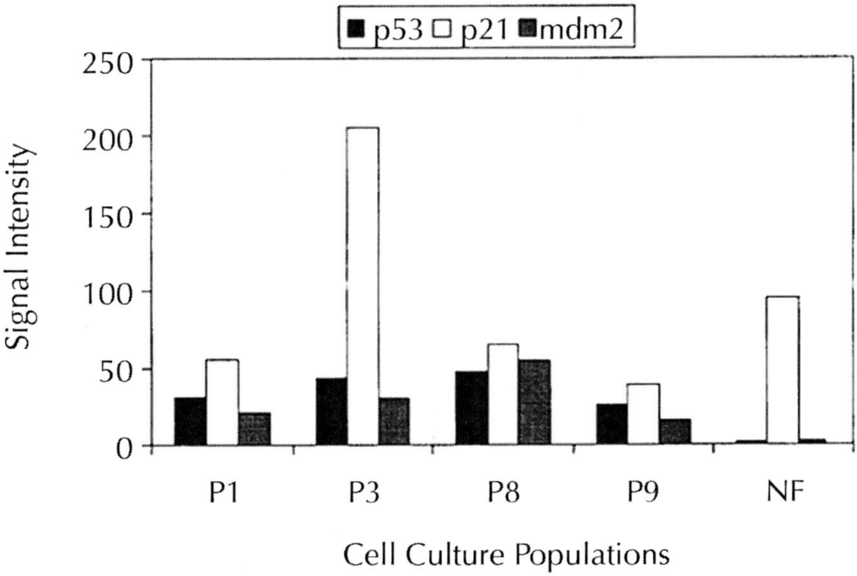

Figure 10: Baseline cell cycle regulator levels. Signal intensity was measured by flow cytometry and figures represent mean signal intensity above background (isotype control). P1, P3, P8, P9 represent four discrete populations of plaque-derived fibroblasts. NF represents neonatal foreskin fibroblasts. Note the presence of all three cell cycle regulators in the four plaque cell cultures at baseline compared to an absence of p53 and mdm2 in foreskin cell cultures.

The immunofluorescence pattern seen for fibroblasts stained with anti-p^{53} antibodies demonstrated predominantly cytoplasmic p^{53} protein expression, although nuclear staining was also demonstrated at lower frequency. Neonatal foreskin fibroblasts showed no discernible levels of immunofluorescence above background level when stained with anti-p^{53} antibodies. While there was some heterogeneity in the expression of cell cycle regulators, all four plaque-derived cultures demonstrated clear p^{53}, p^{21} and mdm2 expression. Foreskin fibroblasts demonstrated measurable levels of p^{21} but no detectable levels of mdm2. The difference in p^{53} expression between each individual plaque-derived cell culture and foreskin cells was highly statistically significant ($P<0.001$).

SUMMARY

Peyronie's disease involves a multifactorial process, which probably involves penile trauma as the inciting event, leading to alterations in cellular and/or molecular pathways which cause excessive scarring and fibrosis. The elucidation of these cellular and molecular pathways is paramount in completing our understanding of the pathophysiology of Peyronie's disease and has significant implications for the development of effective conservative treatments. To date, numerous local and oral therapies have been investigated with varying results. The basic science behind these therapies remains poorly understood. Consequently, surgical procedures for correction of curvature and insertion of penile prosthesis remain the mainstay of effective treatment for significant long-standing Peyronie's disease. We have established fibroblast cultures derived from Peyronie's and normal tunical tissue, which can be reliably studied using a variety of microscopic, immunohistochemical, flow cytometric and molecular biologic techniques. It is hoped that these and future analyses will lead to a more comprehensive understanding of the pathophysiology of Peyronie's disease, specifically, a more enlightened understanding of those factors that render a sub-population of men more susceptible to this disease process.

ACKNOWLEDGEMENTS

Experiments outlined in this paper that were conducted at the Andrology Research Laboratory were funded by a Veterans Administration Career Development Award to Dr Mulhall.

REFERENCES

1. Schwarzer U et al. Prevalence of Peyronie's disease: results of an 8000 man survey. J Urol 2000; 163: 167.
2. Jordan G. Peyronie's disease. In: Walsh PC, ed Campbell's urology WB Saunders: Philadelphia, 1992, pp 2204-2222.
3. Gelbard MK, Dorey F, James K. The natural history of Peyronie's disease. J Urol 1990; 144: 1376-1382. MEDLINE

4. Devine CJJ, Somers RD, Lagoda LE. Peyronie's disease: pathophysiology. Prog Clin Biol Res 1991; 370: 355-358.
5. Devine CJJ, Jordan GH, and Somers RD. Peyronie's disease: cause and surgical treatment. AUA Today 1989; 2: 1-7.
6. Chilton CP, Castle WM, Westwood CA, Pryor JP. Factors associated in the etiology of Peyronie's disease. Br J Urol 1982; 54: 748-751. MEDLINE
7. Weidner W, Schroeder-Printzen I, Weiske W, Vosshenrich R. Sexual dysfunction in Peyronie's disease: an analysis of 222 patients without previous local plaque therapy. J Urol 1997; 157: 325-328.
8. Alman RA et al. Aggressive fibromatosis. J Pediatr Orthop 1992; 12: 1-10. MEDLINE
9. Vande Berg JS, Devine CJ Jr, Horton CE. Mechanisms of calcification in Peyronie's disease. J Urol 1982; 127: 52-54.
10. Liang SB et al. Tetrasomy 12 in ovarian tumors of the coma-fibroma group: a fluorescence in situ hybridization analysis using paraffin sections. Pathol Int 2001; 51: 37-42.
11. Ralph DJ, Mirakian R, Pryor JP, Bottazzo GF. The immunological features of Peyronie's disease. J Urol 1996; 155: 159-162.
12. Devine CJJ, Somers KD, Jordan GH, Scholssberg SM. Proposal: trauma as the cause of Peyronie's lesion. J Urol 1997; 157: 285-290.
13. Leffell MS et al. Non-association of Peyronie's disease with HLA B7 cross-reactive antigens. J Urol 1982; 127: 1223-1224.
14. Nachsteim DA, Rearden A. Peyronie's disease is associated with an HLA class II antigen HLA-DQ5, implying an autoimmune etiology. J Urol 1996; 156: 1330.
15. El-Sakka AI et al. An animal model of Peyronie's-like condition associated with an increase of TGF beta mRNA and protein expression. J Urol 1997; 158: 2284-2290.
16. Mulhall JP, Thom J, Lubrano T, Shankey TV. Basic fibroblast growth factor expression in Peyronie's disease. J Urol 2001; 165: 419-423.
17. 17 Yamanaka M et al. Genetic instability in Peyronie's disease. J Urol 2001; 165: 201.

18. Pierpaoli S et al. Chromosomal instability in Peyronie's disease plaques: preliminary data. J Urol 1998; 159: 362A.
19. Mulhall JP, Thom J, Lubrano T, Shankey TV. Cytogenetic evidence in support of Peyronie's disease being a tunical field defect process. J Urol 2000; 163: 747A.
20. Somers KD et al. Cell culture of Peyronie's disease plaque and normal penile tissue. J Urol 1982; 127: 585-588.
21. Smith BH. Peyronie's disease. Am J Clin Path 1966; 45: 670-674.
22. Brock G et al. The anatomy of the tunica albuginea in the normal penis and Peyronie's disease. J Urol 1997; 151: 276-281.
23. Devine CJJ, Angemeir RW. Anatomy of the penis and male perineum. AUA Update 1993; 12: 1-6.
24. El-Sakka AI et al. Histological and ultrastructural alterations in an animal model of Peyronie's disease. Br J Urol 1998; 81: 445-452.
25. Vernet D et al. Differentiation phenotype of myofibroblasts from penile tuncia albuginea. J Urol 2001; 165: 200.
26. Bridge JA et al. Clonal chromosomal abnormalities in desmoid tumors. Implications for histopathogenesis. Cancer 1992; 69: 430-436.
27. Rudolph R, Vande Berg J. The myofibroblast in Dupuytren's contracture. Hand Clin N Am 1991; 7: 683-692.
28. Bowser-Riley S, Bain AD, Noble J, Lamb DW. Chromosome abnormalities in Dupuytren's disease. Lancet 1975; 2: 1282-1283.
29. Mosmann T. Rapid colorimetric assay for cellular growth and survival: application to proliferation and cytotoxicity assays. J Immun Methods 1983; 65: 55-58.
30. El-Sakka A et al. The effects of colchicine on a Peyronie's-like condition in an animal model. J Urol 1999; 161: 1980-1983.
31. Levine LA. Treatment of Peyronie's disease with intralesional verapamil injection. J Urol 1997; 158: 1395-1399.
32. Wegner HE, Andersen R, Knipsel HH, Miller K. Treatment of Peyronie's disease with local interferon-alpha 2b. Eur Urol 1995; 28: 236-240.
33. 33 Anderson MS, Shankey TV, Lubrano T, Mulhall JP. Inhibition of Peyronie's plaque fibroblast proliferation by biologic agents. Int J Impot Res 2000; 12: ((Suppl 3)) S25-31.

34. Cross SM et al. A p53-dependent mouse spindle checkpoint. Science 1995; 267: 1353-1356. MEDLINE

35. Ioakim-Liossi A et al. p53 Protein expression and oestrogen and progesterone receptor status in invasive ductal breast carcinomas. Cytopathology 2001; 12: 197-202.

36. Leite KR et al. Abnormal expression of mdm2 in prostate carcinoma. Mod Pathol 2001; 14: 428-436.

37. Levine AJ. p53, the cellular gatekeeper for growth and division. Cell 1997; 88: 323-331.

38. Cordon-Cardo C et al. p53 Mutations in human bladder cancer genotypic versus phenotypic patterns. Int J Biochem Cell Biol 1994; 56: 347-350.

39. Campomenosi P et al. p53 Mutants can often transactivate promoters containing a p21 but not Bax or PIG3 responsive elements. Oncogene 2001; 20: 3573-3579.

40. Hoos A et al. Characterization of molecular abnormalities in human fibroblastic neoplasms: a model for genotype-phenotype association in soft tissue tumors. Cancer Res 2001; 61: 3171-3175.

41. Halberg RB et al. Tumorigenesis in the multiple intestinal neoplasia mouse: redundancy of negative regulators and specificity of modifiers. Proc Natl Acad Sci USA 2000; 97: 3461-3466. Article MEDLINE

42. Moffatt EJ, Kerns BJ, Madden JM, Layfield LJ. Prognostic factors for fibromatoses: a correlation of proliferation index, estrogen receptor, p53, retinoblastoma, and src gene products and clinical features with outcome. J Surg Oncol 1997; 65: 117-122.

43. Muller E et al. Molecular genetics and immunohistochemical analysis of the tumor suppressor genes Rb and p53 in palmar and aggressive fibromatosis. Diagn Mol Pathol 1996; 5: 194-200.

44. Mulhall JP, Branch J, Lubrano T, Shankey TV. Perturbations of cell cycle regulators in Peyronie's disease. Int J Impot Res 2001; 13: ((Suppl 5)) S21-S28.

Chapter 7

Comprehensive Proteomic Analysis of Bovine Spermatozoa of Varying Fertility Rates And Identification of Biomarkers Associated With Fertility

Divyaswetha Peddinti[1,4†], Bindu Nanduri[1,4†], Abdullah Kaya[2], Jean M Feugang, Shane C Burgess[1,4,5] and Erdogan Memili[3*†]

[1]Department of Basic Sciences, Mississippi State University, Mississippi State, MS 39762, USA

[2]Alta Genetics, Inc., Watertown, WI, USA

[3]Department of Animal and Dairy Sciences, Mississippi State University, Mississippi State, MS 39762, USA

[4]Institute for Digital Biology, Mississippi State University, Mississippi State, MS 39762, USA

[5]Mississippi Agricultural and Forestry Experimental station, Mississippi State, MS 39762, USA

ABSTRACT

Background

Male infertility is a major problem for mammalian reproduction. However, molecular details including the underlying mechanisms of male fertility are still not known. A thorough understanding of these mechanisms is essential for obtaining consistently high reproductive efficiency and to ensure lower cost and time-loss by breeder.

Results

Using high and low fertility bull spermatozoa, here we employed differential detergent fractionation multidimensional protein identification technology (DDF-Mud PIT) and identified 125 putative biomarkers of fertility. We next used quantitative Systems Biology modeling and canonical protein interaction pathways and networks to show that high fertility spermatozoa differ from low fertility spermatozoa in four main ways. Compared to sperm from low fertility bulls, sperm from high fertility bulls have higher expression of proteins involved in: energy metabolism, cell communication, spermatogenesis, and cell motility. Our data also suggests a hypothesis that low fertility sperm DNA integrity may be compromised because cell cycle: G_2/M DNA damage checkpoint regulation was most significant signaling pathway identified in low fertility spermatozoa.

Conclusions

This is the first comprehensive description of the bovine spermatozoa proteome. Comparative proteomic analysis of high fertility and low fertility bulls, in the context of protein interaction networks identified putative molecular markers associated with high fertility phenotype.

BACKGROUND

Male infertility is a major problem for mammalian reproduction. The nature of sub-fertility due to the male is as complex as that of the female [1]. Infertility due to male factor contributes approximately 40% of the infertility cases in humans. For this reason it is very important to investigate the factors that affect male fertility. Here we used bovine spermatozoa to model human male fertility because cattle provide several advantages as a model for male factor infertility. These include good breeding records fertility data records and progeny records. In cattle breeding, Artificial insemination (AI), a common breeding technique, utilizes semen from genetically superior sires to inseminate cows. In the United States more than ~70% of cows are bred by AI but only ~50% of these matings result in successful full term pregnancy [2]. The underlying molecular events/mechanisms that determine the fertilizing potential of a semen sample are not well defined. A thorough understanding of these mechanisms is essential for obtaining consistently high reproductive efficiency and to ensure lower cost and time-loss by breeder.

Fertility traits of semen can be categorized as compensable or uncompensable [1, 3-7]. Defects in compensable traits (motility and morphology) can be overcome by increasing the number of spermatozoa per insemination [1]. Defects in uncompensable traits affect the function of spermatozoa during the later stages of fertilization and in embryonic development [1, 8] and as such cannot be compensated. Uncompensable traits include nuclear vacuoles [9], morphological deficiencies that do not suppress movement [4], defective chromatin structure [10]. Low fertility in bulls has an uncompensable component that includes reduced cleavage rate and delayed pronuclear formation following in vitro fertilization [1, 11]. Currently available fertility assays assess the defects that affect functional competence of spermatozoa (i.e. capacitation, acrosome reaction, sperm-oocyte interaction) [8, 12], however these cannot definitively predict fertility. At present, the molecular nature of sperm fertility defects or biomarkers for accurate fertility prediction is not known [13].

Spermatozoa are transcriptionally inactive so the only comprehensive method to understand the molecular functions in spermatozoa is via proteomics [13]. Published proteomic studies with bull spermatozoa described the sub-proteome of the sperm and functions of proteins from its surrounding cells. Accessory gland (AG) proteins were shown to modulate important sperm functions after ejaculation and in the female reproductive tract such as capacitation, acrosome reaction, sperm-oocyte interaction, and sperm protection [14]. It is known that fertile associated antigen (FAA), a heparin binding protein from seminal vesicles and prostate glands, binds to spermatozoa membrane and modulates heparin-sperm interactions that are indicative of fertility [15]. Two seminal plasma proteins such as, prostaglandin-D-synthetase and osteoponin were more abundant in the semen of high fertility bulls when compared to low fertility bulls [16, 17].

Here we describe a comprehensive proteomic analysis of bull sperm using differential detergent fractionation (DDF) two-dimensional liquid chromatography followed by electrospray ionization tandem mass spectrometry (DDF 2-LC ESI MS^2; [18]). We compared protein expression profiles of sperm from high and low fertility bulls to characterize the differences in fertility at the protein level. Our results show that expression of 2051 and 2281 proteins was specific to high and low fertility bull spermatozoa, respectively and 1518 proteins were common to both. Differential expression of 125 proteins was significant between high and low fertility bull spermatozoa and these proteins are potential biomarkers for bovine male fertility. Biological systems utilize highly complex, interrelated metabolic and signaling pathways to function. Therefore, to identify signaling pathways involved in fertility, we carried out systems modeling of our proteomic datasets using Gene Ontology (GO) and Ingenuity Pathway Analysis (IPA). We identified differences in the signaling pathways between high and low fertility bull spermatozoa and found that EGF and PDGF signaling pathways were specific to high fertility.

RESULTS

Proteome Profiles of Spermatozoa from High and Low Fertility Bulls

We identified 3569 and 3799 proteins in high and low fertility group spermatozoa respectively. Among these 1518 (20.4%) were common to both groups and 2051 and 2281 proteins were unique to high and low fertility groups respectively (Figure 1). Only those proteins identified by at least three peptides were included in the analysis for differential expression and we identified 125 proteins as differentially-expressed between the high and low fertility spermatozoa. Compared to low fertility bull spermatozoa, expression of 74 proteins increased and there was a decrease in the expression of 51 proteins in high fertility spermatozoa (Table 1). Only a small proportion of proteins identified in this study have been previously described (15.1% of the high fertility group specific and 14.3% of the low fertility group specific proteins (Figure 1)). The majority of the identified proteins are 'predicted' (i.e. predicted based on sequence similarity to known proteins in other species and are frequently found in NRPD database for species that have had their genomes sequenced [19]). We contributed to the annotation of the newly sequenced bovine genome by experimentally confirming the in vivo expression of 4,313 electronically predicted proteins We also identified 10.6% and 9.8% 'hypothetical' (i.e. proteins predicted from nucleic acid sequences and that have not been shown to exist by experimental protein chemical evidence [20]) proteins specific to high fertility and low fertility spermatozoa respectively.

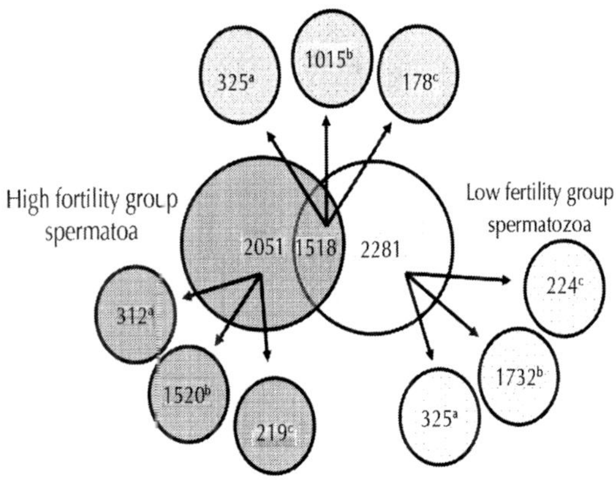

Figure 1: Comparison of proteins identified in high fertility and low fertility spermatozoa. Distribution of predicted, known and hypothetical proteins is shown. [a] known proteins, [b] predicted proteins, [c] hypothetical proteins.

Table 1: Differentially expressed proteins

Accesion	Name	Peptides		ΣXcorr		P-value	Regulation
		HF	LF	HF	LF		
115496714	Actin-like 7B	16	7	60.06	42.11	0.02243	up
77736067	Acyl-CoA thioesterase 9	14	4	39.23	16.48	2.11E-04	up
41386786	A-kinase anchor protein 4	679	581	2581.8	2424.3	0.001694	up
30794280	Albumin	7	1	27.09	5.24	1.49E-04	up
60302887	Aldose reductase	1	3	3.03	12.82	0.03293	down
27807289	Annexin A2	4	10	29.17	26.46	0.04155	down
84490369	ATP synthase, H+ transporting, mitochondrial	16	8	48.01	31.88	0.0333	up
28603752	ATP synthase, H+ transporting, mitochondrial F0	7	1	18.99	7.14	0.005907	up
28461221	ATP synthase, H+ transporting, mitochondrial F1 complex	201	174	765.55	700.71	0.006727	up
28461251	ATPase inhibitory factor 1 precursor	18	10	45.95	30.03	0.01581	up
27807145	Casein kinase 2, alpha prime polypeptide	3	0	11.25	0	5.01E-04	up
60101831	Cytochrome c oxidase subunit III	5	4	17.45	11.47	0.01008	up
84000107	Glycoprotein (transmembrane) nmb	0	3	6.9	8.98	0.0133	down
84000035	Hypothetical protein LOC504736	3	1	8.66	2.04	0.03204	up
115497288	Hypothetical protein LOC506544	4	7	13.54	18.39	0.04931	down
78369248	Hypothetical protein LOC509274	18	10	77.94	51.72	0.01217	up
115496338	Hypothetical protein LOC516024	27	22	109.76	67.93	1.54E-05	up

115495377	Hypothetical protein LOC520260	44	58	201.9	232.07	0.04396	down
114052468	Hypothetical protein LOC532785	8	19	32.19	55.25	0.003313	down
115496742	Hypothetical protein LOC534599	27	11	88.93	61.57	0.02739	up
84000301	Hypothetical protein LOC534927	9	3	32.16	14.67	0.01593	up
115495951	Hypothetical protein LOC540767	20	12	62.88	41.8	0.004421	up
94966950	Hypothetical protein LOC614199	4	0	10.84	1.66	0.007311	up
84000391	Hypothetical protein LOC615316	11	5	35.17	24.34	0.02524	up
115497750	Hypothetical protein LOC617117	19	12	58.06	44.14	0.03432	up
116004271	Hypothetical protein LOC767959	4	0	12.9	3.03	0.04429	up
27805989	Lysyl oxidase-like 4	1	3	1.59	7.16	0.03124	down
27806307	Mitochondrial ATP synthase, O subunit	13	8	51.79	34.78	0.03731	up
28461275	NADH dehydrogenase (ubiquinone) 1 alpha subcomplex	13	3	48.9	27.96	0.05046	up
28461255	NADH dehydrogenase (ubiquinone) 1 beta subcomplex	2	4	3.67	13.56	0.01051	down
62751972	Potassium voltage-gated channel shaker-related	3	0	5.86	0	1.21E-04	up
119891540	PREDICTED: glutathione S-transferase kappa 1	3	3	10.97	8.47	0.01147	up
119887606	PREDICTED: hypothetical protein	1	3	2.03	8.02	0.04382	down
119903031	PREDICTED: hypothetical protein	5	15	25.57	46.02	2.23E-04	down
119908822	PREDICTED: hypothetical protein	3	1	7.23	1.65	0.03051	up
119888977	PREDICTED: hypothetical protein	11	3	37.09	22.02	0.03232	up
119905186	PREDICTED: hypothetical protein	0	3	0	6.3	1.90E-05	down
76661674	PREDICTED: hypothetical protein	1	4	2.22	9.87	0.01595	down
119901076	PREDICTED: hypothetical protein	1	5	9.84	11.22	0.04157	down
119918378	PREDICTED: hypothetical protein	3	15	16.31	36.68	5.24E-04	down

61843441	PREDICTED: hypothetical protein	0	4	0	9.99	4.37E-05	down
119901737	PREDICTED: hypothetical protein	4	6	20.4	18.24	0.02245	down
119904572	PREDICTED: hypothetical protein	3	0	6.15	4.95	0.01124	up
119884876	PREDICTED: hypothetical protein	3	2	9.65	2.72	0.03549	up
76631114	PREDICTED: hypothetical protein	35	15	106.7	81.25	0.02224	up
119923822	PREDICTED: hypothetical protein	63	51	205.06	170.94	0.001919	up
76644873	PREDICTED: hypothetical protein isoform 2	3	0	7.78	1.83	0.03381	up
76645752	PREDICTED: hypothetical protein isoform 4	1	4	1.62	9.68	0.003268	down
119912558	PREDICTED: hypothetical protein isoform 6	4	0	10.87	0	7.37E-12	up
119893872	PREDICTED: hypothetical protein LOC535130	5	1	14.93	12.61	0.03256	up
76687954	PREDICTED: hypothetical protein, partial	3	0	7.7	1.95	0.04264	up
119925886	PREDICTED: hypothetical protein, partial	3	0	6.76	5.69	0.01623	up
119895251	PREDICTED: profilin 3	2	4	12.89	19.46	0.01716	down
119922439	PREDICTED: similar to 1700016M24Rik protein	3	0	8.17	0	1.04E-04	up
119879571	PREDICTED: similar to AAT1-alpha	22	12	69.77	50.74	0.01412	up
119912554	PREDICTED: similar to Ace protein	15	4	55.74	20.29	8.69E-06	up
61878077	PREDICTED: similar to Actin-related protein T1	7	2	16.82	7.44	0.02775	up
119928361	PREDICTED: similar to ADAM metallopeptidase	7	2	23.85	10.3	0.01155	up
119913547	PREDICTED: similar to ADAM metallopeptidase with thrombospondin type 1 motif, 17 preproprotein	5	0	12.58	0	1.24E-07	up

119903267	PREDICTED: similar to ALMS1 protein	4	0	10.2	2.89	0.02294	up
119892487	PREDICTED: similar to Ankyrin repeat domain-containing	1	3	1.88	7.82	0.03473	down
76657564	PREDICTED: similar to calmodulin	10	5	23.53	16.83	0.04331	up
119901005	PREDICTED: similar to centrosomal protein 110kD	3	0	8.38	2.06	0.03921	up
119893858	PREDICTED: similar to chromosome 13 open reading	0	3	0	6.84	4.35E-04	down
61814552	PREDICTED: similar to Cytochrome c oxidase subunit	13	10	41.99	47.17	0.01639	up
119904416	PREDICTED: similar to diaphanous homolog 3	0	3	0	7.64	3.85E-04	down
119915202	PREDICTED: similar to DNAH8, partial	12	3	33.72	16.39	0.001961	up
119927503	PREDICTED: similar to DNAH8, partial	6	1	22.2	8.36	0.04519	up
119911633	PREDICTED: similar to EF-hand calcium binding domain 5	0	3	0	7.52	3.23E-05	down
119888835	PREDICTED: similar to EPH receptor A8	4	0	9.46	1.9	0.009866	up
119895747	PREDICTED: similar to FAT tumor suppressor 2	12	3	28.56	32.84	1.15E-04	up
119919673	PREDICTED: similar to ferritin L subunit isoform	1	4	0.57	10.42	3.74E-05	down
119909426	PREDICTED: similar to fertilin alpha	12	27	63.45	89.9	0.003791	down
119919953	PREDICTED: similar to filamin	0	3	0	6.94	4.54E-04	down
76662361	PREDICTED: similar to GFHL3075 isoform 3	3	0	8.3	7.63	0.01657	up
61820991	PREDICTED: similar to GK2 protein	16	9	54.86	31.79	0.01383	up
119901324	PREDICTED: similar to HECT domain and ankyrin repeat containing, E3 ubiquitin protein ligase 1 isoform 1	2	3	6.09	6.74	0.01418	down

119895512	PREDICTED: similar to HIST1H4I protein	3	0	6.36	1.06	0.007699	up
119915532	PREDICTED: similar to histone H2b-616	4	10	17.41	34.08	0.005828	down
76613952	PREDICTED: similar to histone H4	2	2	7.48	5.88	0.02561	down
76642199	PREDICTED: similar to Izumo sperm-egg fusion 1	39	24	133.67	99.29	0.005314	up
119890207	PREDICTED: similar to KIAA0191	18	26	70.99	64.29	0.01024	down
119891377	PREDICTED: similar to KIAA0225 isoform 1	1	4	1.01	9.43	5.50E-04	down
119890395	PREDICTED: similar to KIAA0467 protein	0	3	0	7.91	3.74E-06	down
119902048	PREDICTED: similar to KIAA1305 protein	0	3	0	7.91	0.001712	down
119906772	PREDICTED: similar to KIAA1429 protein isoform	0	3	0	6.98	4.55E-04	down
119912552	PREDICTED: similar to KIAA1636 protein	3	0	7.44	0	1.53E-04	up
119891313	PREDICTED: similar to KIAA1793 protein	12	8	52.91	37.11	0.0228	up
119909205	PREDICTED: similar to KIAA2017 protein isoform	6	0	17.51	6.69	0.01123	up
76664109	PREDICTED: similar to LOC505732 protein	4	6	14.08	12.97	0.01832	down
76641602	PREDICTED: similar to LOC507431 protein isoform	10	7	31.93	36.41	0.03413	up
119902010	PREDICTED: similar to LOC512571 protein	47	34	189.9	155.47	0.03649	up
119905900	PREDICTED: similar to NDRG3	0	3	0	7.3	1.80E-04	down
76612380	PREDICTED: similar to nestin	0	3	0	6.85	1.25E-04	down
119911939	PREDICTED: similar to netrin-1	2	4	2.84	8.74	0.01328	down
119894490	PREDICTED: similar to obscurin, cytoskeletal calmodulin and titin-interacting RhoGEF, partial	1	3	1.45	7.16	0.03376	down

119905455	PREDICTED: similar to Pitrilysin metallopeptidase	1	6	2.49	22.6	3.23E-05	down
76618065	PREDICTED: similar to Pou6f1 protein	4	1	15.92	11.31	0.006931	up
119894859	PREDICTED: similar to Protein KIAA1543 isoform	1	3	1.36	8.01	0.008488	down
119893105	PREDICTED: similar to protein kinase A binding protein	135	113	480.21	392.89	2.35E-05	up
76627105	PREDICTED: similar to RAB2B, member RAS oncogene	7	16	29.46	52.58	0.004367	down
119912290	PREDICTED: similar to RIKEN cDNA 4121402D02	3	0	7.29	0	2.00E-07	up
119914167	PREDICTED: similar to RIKEN cDNA A530050D06 gene	6	8	12.57	21.82	0.007372	down
119903563	PREDICTED: similar to RNA polymerase I polypept	3	6	7.15	15.59	0.03155	down
119910233	PREDICTED: similar to sca1	3	0	7.43	1.65	0.0301	up
119916698	PREDICTED: similar to Septin 12	0	3	0	8.2	2.26E-07	down
119903556	PREDICTED: similar to sulfotransferase K1	0	3	0	6.79	1.49E-04	down
119902145	PREDICTED: similar to telomerase-associated protein	3	0	8.27	0	8.45E-06	up
119914302	PREDICTED: similar to trans-Golgi p230	4	0	8.82	2.85	0.01983	up
119917225	PREDICTED: similar to TRRAP protein	2	5	2.92	11.86	0.002132	down
119917582	PREDICTED: similar to TUBA	3	1	9.42	3.39	0.03158	up
119912117	PREDICTED: similar to Tumor necrosis factor receptor	7	0	17.77	0	6.66E-12	up
119903686	PREDICTED: similar to ubiquitin specific protease 34 isoform1	1	4	2.31	9.99	0.01666	down
77736091	Prohibitin	7	3	22.59	9.08	0.03313	up
114052901	Rhabdoid tumor deletion region gene 1	10	2	31.71	15.41	0.009593	up

84000339	Sperm associated antigen 6	4	1	13.76	2.2	0.02495	up
87196516	Sperm mitochondria-associated cysteine-rich protein	3	0	9.82	3.51	0.03455	up
115495195	Tektin 1	27	19	107.5	76.3	0.0155	up
84000201	Transmembrane protein 5	3	1	6.27	6.97	0.004588	up
61888856	Triosephosphate isomerase	40	26	158.4	122.55	0.005981	up
27807143	Ubiquinol-cytochrome c reductase core protein II	7	2	33.24	16.14	0.02472	up

List of differentially expressed proteins in high fertility (HF) group spermatozoa when compared to low fertility group. (LF) spermatozoa In this table we provided the information about number of peptides, Sequest cross correlation (∑Xcorr) score and P value for each protein in high and low fertility group spermatozoa respectively.

Predicted and hypothetical proteins do not have any functional annotation associated with them and they represent ~80% of differentially expressed proteins between high and low fertility spermatozoa (Table 1). This poses a problem for meaningful biological modeling of our data without carrying out some functional annotation first. Therefore, we annotated all differentially expressed proteins in our data sets using AgBase GO resources.

Membrane and Nuclear Proteins

Membrane and nuclear proteins are fundamental for inter and intra cellular signaling and are thus fundamental for modeling cell-cell interactions. Sperm oocyte fusion is a key element for fertilization. This process is facilitated by sperm surface proteins and leads to specific binding of the sperm surface-active component with the egg zona pellucida and, ultimately sperm-egg fusion [21]. To identify proteins from the sperm membrane and the nucleus which function in cell fusion, we focused on membrane and nuclear proteins identified in our datasets. Based on the GO associations of known proteins, 40.6% (395) are membrane proteins. We also identified 112 nuclear proteins based on GO associations. Biological process annotation of membrane proteins revealed that majority of membrane proteins involved in transport (33%), cell communication (18%) and metabolism (17%).

We GO annotated all differentially expressed proteins and applied the generic GO Slim [22] to identify 7 functional super-categories represented in differentially expressed proteins in high fertility spermatozoa. Most GO Slim categories, including processes such as metabolism, cell communication and cell motility showed overall up regulation of protein expression in the high fertility group while transport proteins showed an overall down regulation in the high fertility group (Figure 2).

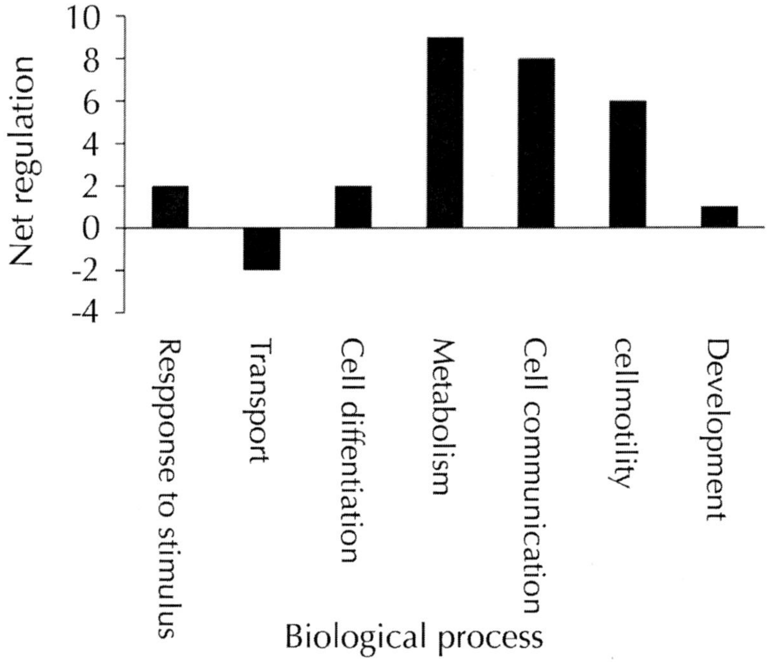

Figure 2: Overall effects in GO Slims of differentially expressed proteins of high and low fertility spermatozoa. Biological process GO annotations of all significantly altered proteins between high and low fertility spermatozoa were used to generate GO Slims. For each GO Slim, the difference in the numbers of proteins with increased expression and the number of proteins with decreased expression (relative to low fertility spermatozoa) was calculated to estimate the net regulatory effect.

High Fertility and Low Fertility Sperm Proteomes: Molecular Network and Pathway Analysis

Protein identification from biological samples on a global scale is important. However, there is a need to move beyond this level of analysis; Instead of simply enumerating a list of proteins, the analysis needs to include their interactions as parts of complexes, pathways and biological networks. To achieve this level of analysis with our high fertility and low fertility spermatozoa proteomic datasets we used Ingenuity Pathway Analysis (IPA). At IPA thresholds for significance, 71, and 73 networks and 68, and 73 functions/diseases were significantly represented in the proteomes of high fertility and low fertility spermatozoa respectively. The top 10 functions/diseases (ranked based on significance), and the associated signaling pathways are shown in Table 2 and Table 3 for proteomes of high and low fertility groups respectively. Analysis of the top 10 functions revealed that functions like cellular movement, cell to cell signaling and interaction were identified only in the high fertility sperm proteome (Table 2). Whereas, functions like cell death and reproductive system disease were identified only in the low fertility sperm proteome (Table 3).

Table 2: Top ten functions/diseases and their respective top ten signaling pathways in high fertility group spermatozoa

	Signaling Pathways									
Functions & diseases	EGF signaling	PDGF signaling	Integrin signaling	Amyloid processing	Complement and Coagulation cascade	PPAR signaling	Neurotrophin signaling	Huntingtons disease signaling	IGF1 Signaling	Apoptosis signaling
Cell cycle	12	14	13	10	4	11	11	13	14	10
Cellular movement	9	12	25	10	11	13	9	12	11	14
Connective tissue development and function	3	4	7	5	2	2	3	2	5	2
Cellular assembly and Organization	3	5	15	9	3	4	4	5	4	7
Cell morphology	15	17	31	10	6	10	15	16	14	12
Cardio-vascular disease	4	5	3	5	3	2	3	7	3	7
Lipid metabolism	2	2	2	2	1	2	2	3	2	2
Small molecule Biochemistry	9	10	12	12	1	6	8	9	12	12
Cell to cell signaling and interaction	6	8	22	3	13	3	5	6	7	7
Post translational modification	8	10	14	13	1	7	7	9	9	10

EGF: Epidermal Growth Factor; PDGF: Platelet Derived Growth Factor; IGF1: Insulin Growth Factor-1.

Table 3: Top ten functions/diseases and their respective top ten signaling pathways in low fertility group spermatozoa

Signaling Pathways										
Functions & Diseases	Cell cycle:G2/M DNA damage check point regulation	Integrin signaling	Apoptosis signaling	MAPK signaling	Amyloid Processing	VEGF signaling	G-protein coupled receptor signaling	PTEN signaling	Actin Cyto-skeleton signaling	Axonal guidance signaling
1.Cell cycle	10	11	11	10	5	8	8	10	10	7
2. Cell morphology	3	26	13	18	7	11	18	14	31	26
3. Post translational modification	9	12	9	11	9	5	11	9	14	11
4.Cellular assembly and Organization	3	18	4	10	5	5	7	4	23	20
5. Lipid metabolism	0	2	3	5	5	3	5	2	2	4
6. Small molecule biochemistry	5	9	10	11	8	4	13	7	11	11
7.Connective tissue disorder	1	12	1	11	2	4	10	6	11	1
8. Gene Expression	8	6	8	16	6	5	16	11	6	8
9.Cell death	7	17	14	17	8	8	14	13	15	18
10.Reproductive system disease	9	5	6	9	2	7	4	8	14	12

MAPK: Mitogen Activated Protein Kinase; VEGF: Vascular Endothelial Growth Factor; PTEN: Phosphatase and tensin homolog deleted on chromosome ten.

Compared to low fertility sperm proteome (9), the high fertility sperm proteome (20) had a 2-fold enrichment in signaling pathways. However, the number of significant metabolic pathways represented was comparable between the low (8) and high (9) fertility spermatozoa. Epidermal growth factor (EGF) signaling was the most prominent signaling pathway specific to high fertility sperm (Figure 3). EGF signaling is known to promote proliferation, survival, and differentiation of a wide variety of mammalian cells [23]. In addition to the EGF signaling pathway, platelet derived growth factor (PDGF) signaling, peroxisome proliferated activator receptor (PPAR) signaling, interleukin(IL) -4 signaling, NF-k signaling, chemokine signaling, and insulin growth factor (IGF)-1 signaling were identified only in high fertility spermatozoa. In low the fertility group, Cell cycle: G2/M DNA damage check point regulation was the most significant pathway followed by integrin signaling.

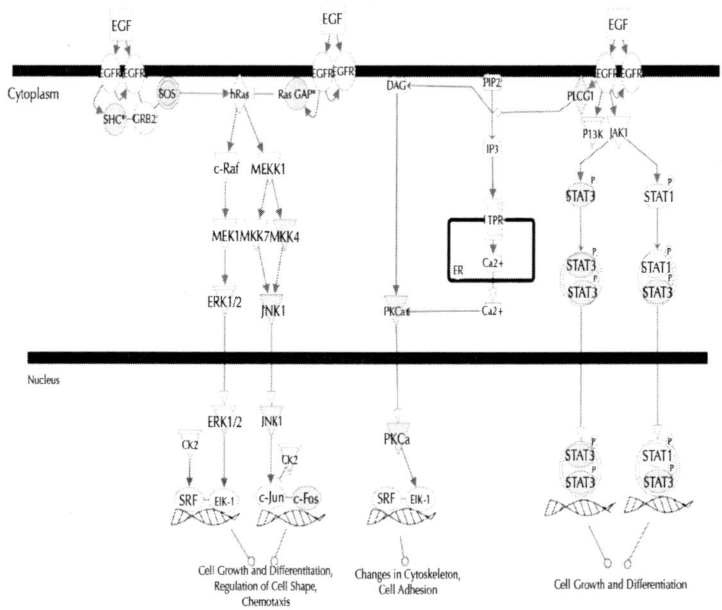

Figure 3: EGF signaling pathway generated by the Ingenuity Pathway Analysis (IPA) software. EGF and PDGF signaling pathways were the top two pathways in the top 10 functions/diseases associated with the high fertility spermatozoa

(Table 2). Each node represents a protein; proteins in shaded nodes were found in the high fertility spermatozoa dataset while proteins in clear nodes were not found in the high fertility spermatozoa dataset.

Proteins with Significantly Altered Expression: Molecular Network and Pathway Analysis

Systems analysis of global proteomes revealed that some signaling pathways are differentially represented between the high and low fertility group spermatozoa. To further analyze these differentially expressed pathways, we carried out IPA analysis with just the 125 differentially expressed proteins. In high fertility spermatozoa, expression of 74 proteins was increased when compared to low fertility spermatozoa. IPA analysis identified three significant networks with scores of 22, 19, and 13 respectively. Proteins identified in the top three networks are participants in EGF signaling, PDGF signaling, oxidative phosophorylation, and pyruvate metabolism pathways. Expression of two proteins, ATP synthase, H+ transporting, mitochondrial F1 complex (ATP5B), and cytochrome c oxidase subunit III (COX3) involved in oxidative phosphorylation and casein kinase II involved in EGF signaling and PDGF signaling were higher in the high fertility spermatozoa compared to low fertility spermatozoa (Table 1). IPA also identified pyruvate metabolism as the most significant pathway in up regulated proteins of high fertility spermatozoa. In the low fertility sperm proteome, expression of 51 proteins increased when compared to high fertility spermatozoa. IPA analysis identified two significant networks in highly expressed proteins of low fertility sperm. Proteins identified in the top two significant networks are participants in integrin signaling and estrogen receptor signaling.

DISCUSSIONS

Male fertility can be described as the success by spermatozoa to fertilize oocytes and of the resulting zygotes continue on through embryonic and fetal development until birth [11]. In this study we used bovine spermatozoa to study fertility as it can serve as a model for understanding human male infertility and reproductive diseases. Studying Bovine male fertility on its own merit has implications in agro-economics involving cattle industry worldwide.

A spermatozoon must reach the site of fertilization and be capacitated for successful fertilization to occur. A subsequent step is the acrosome reaction characterized by fusion of a spermatozoon outer acrosomal membrane with overlying plasma membrane [8]. The molecular mechanisms and signal transduction pathways mediating the processes of capacitation and acrosome reaction have been partially defined [8]. Bull sperm cytosolic fraction proteomic analysis showed enrichment for tyrosine kinases which are essential for phosphorylation of specific sperm proteins during capacitation [24]. The abundance of a variety of proteins from cells surrounding the sperm has been proposed to indicate male fertility [2, 14, 15]. Most of the studies used 2-dimensional electrophoresis (2-DE) for isolation and identification of sperm proteins [13, 25-28]. To our knowledge this is the first comprehensive non-electrophoretic proteomic study of bull sperm proteome. The aim of our study was to identify proteins that were differentially expressed between high and low fertility bull spermatozoa and interrelated metabolic and signaling pathways that have a role in fertility.

We identified 125 proteins as differentially expressed in between the high and low fertility sperm even though 1518 proteins were common to both groups and about 2000 were unique to each. The reasons for this apparent discrepancy are that we took a conservative approach to the statistical analysis: only proteins identified by at least three peptides were included in the analysis for differential expression and the statistical method used in *ProtQuant* is very conservative. *ProtQuant* specifically address the issue of "missing" mass spectra that occurs in all 2-D LC MS^2 -based expression proteomics methods. No other published method (either non-isotopic or isotopic) addresses this issue. Missing mass spectra are due to the inherent limitations of the mass spectrometers, the probabilistic nature of sampling and the cutoffs used to determine "true" assignments of peptides to mass spectra [29]. *ProtQuant* is highly conservative method which is based on sum of Xcorr method itself increases the specificity of spectral counting and reduce the type I errors of differential expression. Regardless, proteins were analyzed from each of three of the areas represented in Figure 1 and differentially-expressed proteins occurred in all three (i.e. proteins unique to the high and low fertility sperm as well as those common to both).

From proteome profiles of specific cells or tissues, one acquires large datasets that are inherently complex. As a result we consider it beneficial to model our bovine sperm proteome data sets using GO and IPA. From GO associations of differentially expressed proteins we found that there was a comparative up regulation of three biological processes in high fertility spermatozoa: metabolism, cell communication and cell motility (Fig 2).

Up regulation of metabolism is consistent with the fact that capacitation is coupled to a specific type of metabolism, that is glycolysis or oxidative respiration [30]. Pyruvate metabolism and glycolysis were the top most significant metabolic pathways represented in high fertility sperm proteome by IPA. In glycolysis, expression of pyruvate kinase (PKM2) was higher in high fertility spermatozoa. PKM2 catalyzes the production of pyruvate and ATP from phosphoenol pyruvate. Pyruvate formed in this process serves as an energy source for cells [31]. Impaired or lower pyruvate metabolism could limit the cell's ability to produce energy and this could be one of the reasons for reduced fertility in the low fertility group.

Expression of COX 3 and ATP5B involved in oxidative respiration was higher in high fertility spermatozoa compared to low fertility spermatozoa. COX3 is a member of the large transmembrane protein complex found in the mitochondrion and is the last protein in the electron transport chain. Coupling of electron transport to oxidative respiration maintains the high mitochondrial transmembrane potential required for mitochondrial ATP production [32]. ATP5B catalyzes the production of ATP from ADP in the presence of a proton gradient across the mitochondrial membrane and this ATP is utilized for the motility of sperm and capacitation [33].

Communication between sperm and oocyte is critical for successful fertilization. We found that there was up regulation of cell communication in the high fertility sperm proteome when compared to low fertility sperm proteome (Figure 2). To bring about cell to cell communication several signaling pathways are necessary. EGF signaling and PDGF signaling were the top two significant signaling pathways identified in high fertiliy spermatozoa. EGF and PDGF signaling pathways stimulate tyrosine phosphorylation of various MAP kinases and their upstream activators MEK1, MEK2 and MEKK [34, 35]. EGF signaling has an important role in sperm capacitation as it stimulates tyrosine phosphorylation of many proteins [36]. In addition, EGF signaling also activates phospholipase C (PLC) [36] (Figure 3). PLC is important for the acrosome reaction (AR), fertilization and embryo development. PLC catalyzes the production of inositol 1, 4, 5-triphosphate (IP3) from phosphatidylinositol 4, 5-biphosphate. IP3 generated by PLC activates the extra cellular calcium influx required for the AR via binding to the IP3 receptor (IP3R) gated calcium channel located on the acrosome membrane [37]. Mutations in mouse PLCB1 reduced the AR rate, fertilization rate and embryo development [38]. EGF signaling was specific to high fertility bull sperm. Defects in EGF signaling in low fertility spermatozoa may prevent capacitation.

Expression of casein kinase 2 (CKII) prime poly peptide in EGF signaling was higher in high fertility spermatozoa compared to low fertility spermatozoa (Table 1). CKII is preferentially expressed in late stages of spermatogeneis and is involved in sperm chromatin decondensation after sperm oocyte fusion [39, 40]. CKII deficient mice are infertile with oligospermia and globozoospermia[40]. EGF signaling also induces actin polymerization in bovine sperm capcitation [41]. Actin polymerization is essential for incorporation of sperm into egg cytoplasm [42] and for sperm nuclei decondensation [43].

Comparing the proteome profiles of bull sperm of high and low fertility showed some molecular features associated with low fertility. Cell cycle: G2/M DNA damage check point regulation was the topmost significant signaling pathway followed by integrin signaling in low fertility bull sperm (Table3). The G2/M DNA damage checkpoint could help in maintaining the integrity of the genome during different stages of development. Progression through different phases of the cell cycle requires the sequential activation of various cyclin dependent kinases and these kinases in turn are regulated by integrin signaling. Integrin signals are necessary for cells to traverse the cell division cycle [44]. These two pathways may be a compensatory response for reproductive system disease function which was identified only in low fertility sperm (Table 3).

In addition to differences in signaling and metabolic pathways between high and low fertility spermatozoa, we identified differences in protein expression that had implications in sperm motility. Expression of A-kinase anchor protein-4 (AKAP4) was significantly higher in high fertility spermatozoa (Table 1). AKAP4 is a major fibrous sheath protein of the principal piece of the sperm flagellum. AKAP4 recruits Protein kinase A to the fibrous sheath and facilitates local phosphorylation to regulate flagellar function in humans [45]. It also serves as a scaffolding protein for signaling proteins and proteins involved in metabolism. Higher expression of AKAP4 in the high fertility group sperm could result in higher motility.

CONCLUSIONS

In summary, this is the first comprehensive description of the spermatozoa proteome of bovine. Comparative proteomic analysis of high fertility and low fertility bulls, in the context of protein interaction networks identified putative molecular markers associated with high fertility phenotype. We observed marked differences in signaling and metabolic pathways between high fertility and low fertility spermatozoa that have implications in sperm capacitation, acrosomal reaction and sperm-oocyte communication.

METHODS

Selection of High and Low Fertility Bulls

Frozen semen samples and bull fertility data from six mature and progeny tested Holstein bulls with satisfactory semen quality were provided by Alta Genetics (Watertown, WI).

Sample and Data Sources

The fertility data were established by a progeny testing program named Alta Advantage®, which is the industry›s most reliable source of fertility information. It consisted of insemination records collected from 180 well managed partner dairy farms located in different geographical regions across the United States. This breeding program provided the advantages of DNA verification of the paternity of the offspring, and diagnosed pregnancies by veterinary palpation, instead of just relying on non-return rates 60–90 days after breeding.

Bull Fertility Prediction

To predict fertility of the bulls from the given source, a sub-set of data were generated consisting of 962,135 insemination records from 934 bulls with an average of 1,030 breedings ranging from 300 to 15,194. The environmental and herd management factors that influence fertility performance of sires were adjusted using threshold models which were similar to previously published models by Zwald et al [46, 47]. Parameters estimation and fertility prediction were obtained using Probit.F90 software developed by Y. M. Chang [48].

Therefore, for the definition of fertility, instead of relying only on the number of pregnant cows (verified using palpation by a veterinarian or ultrasound examination) divided by the total number of cows examined for pregnancy, we considered the outcome of each breeding event and adjusted the environmental factors such as the effects of herd-year-month, parity, cow, days in milk, sire proven status (young, proven, colored) in order to rank the bulls based on their breeding values for fertility. Further, the fertility of each bull was calculated and expressed as the percent deviation of its conception from the average conception of all bulls having at least 300 breeding in the data set.

Selection of High and Low Fertility Bulls

For this study, we used an arbitrary threshold for classifying high and low fertility bulls. However, the bulls scoring highest and lowest fertility deviation from average with highest reliability (>1,000 breeding/bull) were selected for this study. The differences in the average fertility indexes between high and low fertility groups were 5.46% which was obtained from bulls having adequate records for higher reliability. While three bulls which were scored 5.3% above the average were considered high fertile, three bulls which were scored 10.76% below the average were defined as low fertility Two separated pools of sperm cells (3×10^8) were constituted by mixing equal amounts of sperm cells from either three low or three high fertility bulls. The experiment was replicated three times.

Isolation of Pure Sperm Cells

Spermatozoa were collected from high and low fertility bulls and frozen in 0.25 ml straws. For each bull, the total spermatozoa collected were purified by Percoll gradient centrifugation: 90% Percoll solution in water was prepared with DL-Lactate (19 μM), $CaCl_2$ (2 μM), $NaHCO_3$ (25 mM), $MgCl_2$ (400 μM), KCl (3 μM), NaH_2PO_4 (310 μM), NaCl (2 mM) and Hepes (10 mM). 90% Percoll solution was diluted to 45% with sperm diluent medium (1 mM pyruvate, 10 mM Hepes, 0.021 mM DL-Lactate in Tyrode›s salt solution, pH 7.4). A density gradient of Percoll was prepared in an Eppendorf tube (0.1 ml of 90% fraction under 1 ml of the 45% fraction). Spermatozoa were thawed at 35°C for 1 min and layered on top of the percoll gradient. The spermatozoa were pelleted by centrifugation (956 *g*; 15 min) followed by two washes in phosphate-buffered solution (PBS) (956 *g*; 5 min,). The total sperm count was obtained using an Improved Neubauer Hemacytometer and 10^8 sperm cells were aliquoted and stored at -80°C.

Protein Extraction by DDF

DDF sequentially extracts proteins from different cellular compartments using a series of detergents and this off-line pre-fractionation step in sample preparation increases the proteome coverage. Another advantage of using DDF is that based on the DDF fractions from which proteins are identified, proteins can be found in different cellular locations. Proteins were isolated using DDF as previously described [18]. Cytosolic proteins were extracted by six sequential incubations in a buffer containing digitonin (10 min each); next a fraction containing predominantly membrane proteins was isolated by incubating the cells in 10% Triton X-100 buffer for 30 min and then removing the soluble protein. Nuclear DDF buffer containing deoxycholate (DOC) was then added to the remaining insoluble material and subjected to freeze-thawing to disrupt the nucleus. Nuclear proteins were collected from the resulting soluble fraction and the sample was then aspirated through an 18 g needle and treated with a mixture of DNase I (50U, Invitrogen, Carlsbad CA;) and RNase A (50 mg; Sigma-Aldrich, St Louis, MO) at 37°C for 1 h) to digest nucleic acids. Any remaining pellet, containing the least soluble proteins, was treated with a buffer containing 5% SDS.

Proteomics

Proteomic analysis was carried out with triplicate samples of spermatozoa from the high fertility group and low fertility group spermatozoa as described [19]. Proteins were precipitated with 25% tricholoroacetic acid to remove salts and detergents. Protein pellets were resuspended in 0.1 M ammonium bicarbonate with 5% HPLC grade acetonitrile (ACN), reduced (5 mM, 65°C, 5 min), and alkylated (iodoacetamide, 10 mM, 30°C, 30 min) and then trypsin digested until there was no visible pellet (sequencing grade modified trypsin, Promega; 1:50 w/w 37°C, 16 h). Peptides were desalted using a peptide macrotrap (Michrom BioResources, Inc., Auburn, CA) and eluted using a 0.1% trifluoroacetic acid, 95% ACN solution. Desalted peptides were dried in a vacuum centrifuge and resuspended in 20 μL of 0.1% formic acid and 5% ACN. LC analysis was accomplished by strong cation exchange(SCX) followed by reverse phase liquid chromatography (RP-LC) coupled directly in line with an ESI ion trap mass spectrometer (LCQ Deca XP Plus; ThermoElectron Corporation; San Jose, CA). Samples were loaded into a LC gradient ion exchange system (Thermo Separations P4000 quaternary gradient pump coupled with a 0.32 × 100 mm BioBasic strong cation exchange column). A flow rate of 3 μL/min was used for both SCX and RP columns.

A salt gradient was applied in steps of 0, 10, 15, 20, 25, 30, 35, 40, 45, 50, 57, 64, 90, and 700 mM ammonium acetate in 5% ACN, 0.1% formic acid, and the resultant peptides were loaded directly into the sample loop of a 0.18 × 100 mm BioBasic C18 reverse phase liquid chromatography column of a Proteome X workstation (ThermoElectron). The reverse phase gradient used 0.1% formic acid in ACN and increased the ACN concentration in a linear gradient from 5% to 30% in 20 min and then 30% to 95% in 7 min, followed by 5% for 10 min for 0, 10, 15, 25, 30, 45, 64, 90, and 700 mM salt gradient steps. For 20, 35, 40, 50 and 57 mM salt gradient steps ACN concentration was increased in a linear gradient from 5% to 40% in 65 min 95% for 15 min and 5% for 20 min.

The mass spectrometer was configured to optimize the duty cycle length with the quality of data acquired by alternating between a single full MS scan followed by three tandem MS scans on the three most intense precursor masses (as determined by Xcalibur software in real time) from the full scan. The collision energy was normalized to 35%. Dynamic mass exclusion windows were set at 2 min, and all of the spectra were measured with an overall mass/charge (m/z) ratio range of 300–1700.

All searches were done using TurboSEQUEST™ (Bioworks Browser 3.2; ThermoElectron). Mass spectra and tandem mass spectra were searched against an *in silico* trypsin-digested database of bovine RefSeq proteins downloaded from the National Center for Biotechnology Institute [NCBI; 12/26/2006; 24,853 entries]. Trypsin digestion including mass changes due to cysteine carbamidomethylation (C, 57.02 Da) and methionine mono- and di-oxidation (15.99 Da and 32 Da), was included in the search criteria. The peptide (MS precursor ion) mass tolerance was set to 1.5 Da and the fragment ion (MS^2) mass tolerance was set to 1.0 Da. Rsp Value less than 5.

As a primary filter we first limited our Sequest search output to include only peptides ≥ 6 amino acids long, with Cn ≥ 0.08 and Sequest cross correlation (Xcorr) scores of 1.5, 2.0 and 2.5 for +1, +2, and +3 charge states, respectively. We next used a decoy database search strategy [49] (using the same primary filter for the real database search) to calculate P values for peptide identifications as this allows us to assign the probability of a false identification based on the real data from the experiment itself[49-52]. Since the accuracy of peptide identification depends on the charge state we calculated P values for +1, +2, and +3 charge states separately. The probability that peptide identification from the original database is really a random match (P value) is estimated based on the probability that a match against the decoy database will achieve the same Xcorr [51, 53]. Protein probabilities were calculated exactly as described [54, 55] using only peptides with a $P < 0.05$ and only those proteins were used for further modeling. All protein identifications and their associated MS data have been submitted to the PRoteomics IDEntifications database (PRIDE; [56]) and PRIDE accession numbers are 1883–1888.

Differential Protein Expression

Label free quantification approaches design to quantify relative protein abundances directly from high throughput proteomic analyses without labeling techniques. Here, we used *ProtQuant* [29], a java based tool for label free quantification that uses a spectral counting method with increased specificity (and thus decreased false positive i.e. type I errors). This increased specificity is achieved by incorporating the quantitative aspects of the Sequest cross correlation (XCorr) into the spectral counting method. *ProtQuant* also computes the statistical significance of differential expression of control and treatment for each protein using one-way ANOVA (≤ 0.05). This method requires at least 3 peptides for each protein from the combination of the control and treatment before to calculate a p-value.

Gene Ontology Annotation

We used Gene Ontology (GO) resources and tools available at AgBase [57] to identify the molecular functions and biological processes represented in differentially expressed proteins in our datasets. We used *GORetriver* tool to obtain all existing GO annotations available for known proteins in our datasets. We first GO-annotated differentially expressed proteins in our datasets using existing annotations from probable orthologs with ≥90% sequence identity using the UniRef 90 database. Proteins without annotation at UniRef 90, but between 70–90% sequence identities to presumptive orthologs with GO annotation were GO-annotated using *GOanna tool* [22]. Biological process annotations for these proteins were grouped into more generalized categories using *GOSlim viewer* [22].

Modeling Using Ingenuity Pathway Analysis

To gain insights into the biological pathways and networks that are significantly represented in our proteomic datasets we used Ingenuity Pathways Analysis (IPA; Ingenuity Systems, California). Currently IPA accepts gene/protein accession numbers from human, mouse, and rats only. Therefore, to use IPA, we mapped bovine proteins from our datasets to their corresponding human orthologs by identifying reciprocal-best-BLAST hits and uploaded these accession numbers into IPA. IPA selects "focus genes" to be used for generating biological networks. Focus genes are based on proteins from our datasets that are mapped to corresponding gene objects in the Ingenuity Pathways Knowledgebase (IPKB) and are known to interact with other genes based on published, peer reviewed content in the IPKB. Based on these interactions IPA builds networks with a size of no more than 35 genes or proteins. A P-value for each network and canonical pathway is calculated according to the fit of the user's set of significant genes/proteins. IPA computes a score for each network from P-value and indicates the likelihood of the focus genes in a network being found together due to chance. We selected networks scoring ≥ 2, which have > 99% confidence of not being generated by chance [58, 59].

Biological functions are assigned to each network by using annotations from scientific literature and stored in the IPKB. Fisher exact test is used to calculate the P-value determining the probability of each biological function/disease or pathway being assigned by chance. We used P ≤ 0.05 to select highly significant biological functions and pathways represented in our proteomic datasets [58].

AUTHORS' CONTRIBUTIONS

DP performed the proteomics sample preparation, data generation, analyzed and interpreted proteomic data, systems biology modeling and analysis and wrote the draft of the manuscript. BN developed the biomarker discovery computational tools, participated in design of this study and helped to interpret the systems biology modeling. AK and JF did sample collection and pre-proteomic sample preparation. EM facilitated sample collection, contributed to design of the study, provided expert knowledge and interpretation in reproductive biology and helped to draft the manuscript. SCB conceived of the study, participated in its design and coordination, helped analyze and interpret the statistical analysis of the proteomics data and helped to draft the manuscript. All authors read and approved the final manuscript.

ACKNOWLEDGEMENTS

This study was the result of collaboration between the Laboratories of Drs. Burgess and Memili.

This study was funded by the Life Sciences and Biology Institute & Mississippi Agricultural and Forestry Experiment Station, Mississippi State University (Manuscript number: J-11138), and by Alta Genetics, Inc. We would like to acknowledge Dr. Susan M Bridges and Bryce

Magee for helping us with Biomarker discovery tool and Dr. Tibor Pechan for MS/MS analysis.

REFERENCES

1. Saacke RG, Dalton JC, Nadir S, Nebel RL, Bame JH: Relationship of seminal traits and insemination time to fertilization rate and embryo quality. Animal reproduction science 2000, 60–61:663-677.
2. Killian GJ: High – Fertility Proteins Enhance Reproduction Rates in Dairy Cattle. 1999.
3. Watson PF: The causes of reduced fertility with cryopreserved semen. Animal reproduction science 2000, 60–61:481-492.
4. DeJarnette JM, Saacke RG, Bame J, Vogler CJ: Accessory sperm: their importance to fertility and embryo quality, and attempts to alter their numbers in artificially inseminated cattle. Journal of animal science 1992, 70(2):484-491.
5. Dejarnette JM: The effect of semen quality on reproductive efficiency. The Veterinary clinics of North America 2005, 21(2):409-418.
6. Love CC: The sperm chromatin structure assay: a review of clinical applications. Animal reproduction science 2005, 89(1–4):39-45.
7. Evenson DP: Loss of livestock breeding efficiency due to uncompensable sperm nuclear defects. Reproduction, fertility, and development 1999, 11(1):1-15.
8. Braundmeier AG, Miller DJ: The search is on: finding accurate molecular markers of male fertility. Journal of dairy science 2001, 84(9):1915-1925.
9. Saacke RG, DeJarnette JM, Bame JH, Karabinus DS, Whitman SS: Can spermatozoa with abnormal heads gain access to the ovum in artificially inseminated super- and single-ovulating cattle? Theriogenology 1998, 50(1):117-128.
10. Ballachey BE, Evenson DP, Saacke RG: The sperm chromatin structure assay. Relationship with alternate tests of semen quality and heterospermic performance of bulls. Journal of andrology 1988, 9(2):109-115.

11. Eid LN, Lorton SP, Parrish JJ: Paternal influence on S-phase in the first cell cycle of the bovine embryo. Biology of reproduction 1994, 51(6):1232-1237.

12. Aitken RJ: Sperm function tests and fertility. International journal of andrology 2006, 29(1):69-75. discussion 105–108.

13. Pixton KL, Deeks ED, Flesch FM, Moseley FL, Bjorndahl L, Ashton PR, Barratt CL, Brewis IA: Sperm proteome mapping of a patient who experienced failed fertilization at IVF reveals altered expression of at least 20 proteins compared with fertile donors: case report. Human reproduction (Oxford, England) 2004, 19(6):1438-1447.

14. Moura AA, Koc H, Chapman DA, Killian GJ: Identification of proteins in the accessory sex gland fluid associated with fertility indexes of dairy bulls: a proteomic approach. Journal of andrology 2006, 27(2):201-211.

15. McCauley TC, Zhang H, Bellin ME, Ax RL: Purification and characterization of fertility-associated antigen (FAA) in bovine seminal fluid. Molecular reproduction and development 1999, 54(2):145-153.

16. Gerena RL, Irikura D, Urade Y, Eguchi N, Chapman DA, Killian GJ: Identification of a fertility-associated protein in bull seminal plasma as lipocalin-type prostaglandin D synthase. Biology of reproduction 1998, 58(3):826-833.

17. Henault MA, Killian GJ: Effect of homologous and heterologous seminal plasma on the fertilizing ability of ejaculated bull spermatozoa assessed by penetration of zona-free bovine oocytes. Journal of reproduction and fertility 1996, 108(2):199-204.

18. McCarthy FM, Burgess SC, van den Berg BH, Koter MD, Pharr GT: Differential detergent fractionation for non-electrophoretic eukaryote cell proteomics. Journal of proteome research 2005, 4(2):316-324.

19. McCarthy FM, Cooksey AM, Wang N, Bridges SM, Pharr GT, Burgess SC: Modeling a whole organ using proteomics: the avian bursa of Fabricius. Proteomics 2006, 6(9):2759-2771.

20. Lubec G, Afjehi-Sadat L, Yang JW, John JP: Searching for hypothetical proteins: theory and practice based upon original data and literature. Progress in neurobiology 2005, 77(1–2):90-127.

21. Bhattacharyya AK, Kanjilal S: Assessment of sperm functional competence and sperm-egg interaction. Molecular and cellular biochemistry 2003, 253(1–2):255-261.
22. McCarthy FM, Wang N, Magee GB, Nanduri B, Lawrence ML, Camon EB, Barrell DG, Hill DP, Dolan ME, Williams WP, et al.: AgBase: a functional genomics resource for agriculture. BMC genomics 2006, 7:229.
23. Dikic I: Mechanisms controlling EGF receptor endocytosis and degradation. Biochemical Society transactions 2003, 31(Pt 6):1178-1181.
24. Lalancette C, Faure RL, Leclerc P: Identification of the proteins present in the bull sperm cytosolic fraction enriched in tyrosine kinase activity: a proteomic approach. Proteomics 2006, 6(16):4523-4540.
25. Holmes-Davis R, Tanaka CK, Vensel WH, Hurkman WJ, McCormick S: Proteome mapping of mature pollen of Arabidopsis thaliana. Proteomics 2005, 5(18):4864-4884.
26. Hozumi A, Satouh Y, Ishibe D, Kaizu M, Konno A, Ushimaru Y, Toda T, Inaba K: Local database and the search program for proteomic analysis of sperm proteins in the ascidian Ciona intestinalis. Biochemical and biophysical research communications 2004, 319(4):1241-1246.
27. Martinez-Heredia J, Estanyol JM, Ballesca JL, Oliva R: Proteomic identification of human sperm proteins. Proteomics 2006, 6(15):4356-4369.
28. Tan Y, Fan L, Luo K, Zhu W, Lu G: [Establishment of the twodimensional gel electrophoretic protein map of the human sperm head]. Zhonghua nan ke xue = National journal of andrology 2004, 10(12):886-889.
29. Bridges SM, Bryce GB, Wang N, Williams WP, Burgess SC, Nanduri B: ProtQuant: a tool for the label-free quantification of mudPIT proteomics data. BMC Bioinformatics 2007, 8(Supple 7):S24.
30. Ferrandi B, Lange Consiglio A, Chiara F, Uber E, Marchini M, Baglioni A, Carnevali A, Cremonesi F, Porcelli F: Cytochemical study on human spermatozoa metabolism during in vitro capacitation. Andrologia 1987, 19(Spec No):278-283.

31. Pithukpakorn M: Disorders of pyruvate metabolism and the tricarboxylic acid cycle. Molecular genetics and metabolism 2005, 85(4):243-246.

32. Guthrie HD, Welch GR: Determination of intracellular reactive oxygen species and high mitochondrial membrane potential in Percoll-treated viable boar sperm using fluorescence-activated flow cytometry. Journal of animal science 2006, 84(8):2089-2100.

33. Peterson RN, Freund M: ATP synthesis and oxidative metabolism in human spermatozoa. Biology of reproduction 1970, 3(1):47-54.

34. Hunter T: When is a lipid kinase not a lipid kinase? When it is a protein kinase. Cell 1995, 83(1):1-4.

35. Payne DM, Rossomando AJ, Martino P, Erickson AK, Her JH, Shabanowitz J, Hunt DF, Weber MJ, Sturgill TW: Identification of the regulatory phosphorylation sites in pp42/mitogen-activated protein kinase (MAP kinase). The EMBO journal 1991, 10(4):885-892.

36. Breitbart H, Naor Z: Protein kinases in mammalian sperm capacitation and the acrosome reaction. Reviews of reproduction 1999, 4(3):151-159.

37. Walensky LD, Snyder SH: Inositol 1,4,5-trisphosphate receptors selectively localized to the acrosomes of mammalian sperm. The Journal of cell biology 1995, 130(4):857-869.

38. Choi D, Lee E, Hwang S, Jun K, Kim D, Yoon BK, Shin HS, Lee JH: The biological significance of phospholipase C beta 1 gene mutation in mouse sperm in the acrosome reaction, fertilization, and embryo development. Journal of assisted reproduction and genetics 2001, 18(5):305-310.

39. Mudgal P, Anand SR: Casein kinase II activity of buffalo sperm chromatin. Molecular reproduction and development 1998, 50(2):178-184.

40. Xu X, Toselli PA, Russell LD, Seldin DC: Globozoospermia in mice lacking the casein kinase II alpha' catalytic subunit. Nature genetics 1999, 23(1):118-121.

41. Breitbart H, Cohen G, Rubinstein S: Role of actin cytoskeleton in mammalian sperm capacitation and the acrosome reaction. Reproduction (Cambridge, England) 2005, 129(3):263-268.
42. Sanchez-Gutierrez M, Contreras RG, Mujica A: Cytochalasin-D retards sperm incorporation deep into the egg cytoplasm but not membrane fusion with the egg plasma membrane. Molecular reproduction and development 2002, 63(4):518-528.
43. Kumakiri J, Oda S, Kinoshita K, Miyazaki S: Involvement of Rho family G protein in the cell signaling for sperm incorporation during fertilization of mouse eggs: inhibition by Clostridium difficile toxin B. Developmental biology 2003, 260(2):522-535.
44. Giancotti FG, Ruoslahti E: Integrin signaling. Science (New York, NY) 1999, 285(5430):1028-1032.
45. Huang Z, Somanath PR, Chakrabarti R, Eddy EM, Vijayaraghavan S: Changes in intracellular distribution and activity of protein phosphatase PP1gamma2 and its regulating proteins in spermatozoa lacking AKAP4. Biology of reproduction 2005, 72(2):384-392.
46. Zwald NR, Weigel KA, Chang YM, Welper RD, Clay JS: Genetic selection for health traits using producer-recorded data. II. Genetic correlations, disease probabilities, and relationships with existing traits. Journal of dairy science 2004, 87(12):4295-4302.
47. Zwald NR, Weigel KA, Chang YM, Welper RD, Clay JS: Genetic selection for health traits using producer-recorded data. I. Incidence rates, heritability estimates, and sire breeding values. Journal of dairy science 2004, 87(12):4287-4294.
48. Chang YM, Gianola D, Heringstad B, Klemetsdal G: Effects of trait definition on genetic parameter estimates and sire evaluation for clinical mastitis with threshold models. Animal science 2004, 79:355-364.
49. Elias JE, Gygi SP: Target-decoy search strategy for increased confidence in large-scale protein identifications by mass spectrometry. Nature methods 2007, 4(3):207-214.
50. Elias JE, Gibbons FD, King OD, Roth FP, Gygi SP: Intensity-based protein identification by machine learning from a library of tandem mass spectra. Nature biotechnology 2004, 22(2):214-219.

51. Park GW, Kwon KH, Kim JY, Lee JH, Yun SH, Kim SI, Park YM, Cho SY, Paik YK, Yoo JS: Human plasma proteome analysis by reversed sequence database search and molecular weight correlation based on a bacterial proteome analysis. Proteomics 2006, 6(4):1121-1132.
52. Peng J, Elias JE, Thoreen CC, Licklider LJ, Gygi SP: Evaluation of multidimensional chromatography coupled with tandem mass spectrometry (LC/LC-MS/MS) for large-scale protein analysis: the yeast proteome. Journal of proteome research 2003, 2(1):43-50.
53. Qian WJ, Liu T, Monroe ME, Strittmatter EF, Jacobs JM, Kangas LJ, Petritis K, Camp DG 2nd, Smith RD: Probability-based evaluation of peptide and protein identifications from tandem mass spectrometry and SEQUEST analysis: the human proteome. Journal of proteome research 2005, 4(1):53-62.
54. Nesvizhskii AI, Keller A, Kolker E, Aebersold R: A statistical model for identifying proteins by tandem mass spectrometry. Analytical chemistry 2003, 75(17):4646-4658.
55. MacCoss MJ, Wu CC, Yates JR 3rd: Probability-based validation of protein identifications using a modified SEQUEST algorithm. Analytical chemistry 2002, 74(21):5593-5599.
56. Martens L, Hermjakob H, Jones P, Adamski M, Taylor C, States D, Gevaert K, Vandekerckhove J, Apweiler R: PRIDE: the proteomics identifications database. Proteomics 2005, 5(13):3537-3545.
57. McCarthy FM, Bridges SM, Wang N, Magee GB, Williams WP, Luthe DS, Burgess SC: AgBase: a unified resource for functional analysis in agriculture. Nucleic acids research 2007:D599-603.
58. Gerling IC, Singh S, Lenchik NI, Marshall DR, Wu J: New data analysis and mining approaches identify unique proteome and transcriptome markers of susceptibility to autoimmune diabetes. Mol Cell Proteomics 2006, 5(2):293-305.
59. Huang Y, Yan J, Lubet R, Kensler TW, Sutter TR: Identification of novel transcriptional networks in response to treatment with the anticarcinogen 3H-1,2-dithiole-3-thione. Physiological genomics 2006, 24(2):144-153.
60. Fazal MA, Palmer VR, Dovichi NJ: Analysis of differential detergent fractions of an AtT-20 cellular homogenate using oneand two-dimensional capillary electrophoresis. Journal of chromatography 2006, 1130(2):182-189.

Chapter 8

Histomorphological Studies on the Prostate Gland of Donkey Equus Asinus during Different Seasons

Alaa S. Abou-Elhamd, Ahmed O. Salem, and Aziza A. Selim

Department of Anatomy and Histology, Faculty of Veterinary Medicine, Assiut University, Assiut 71526, Egypt

ABSTRACT

The objective of this study is to describe the histological and histochemical structures of the prostate gland during different seasons of the year The experiment was carried out on the prostate gland of 24 sexually mature apparently healthy male donkeys (5 to 7 years)

distributed over the four seasons of the year. The prostate gland was enveloped externally by a thick fibromuscular capsule. Fibromuscular septa arose from the deep aspect of the capsule dividing the prostate into variable numbers of lobules of different sizes and shapes. Each prostatic lobe was made up of compound tubuloalveolar glands and duct system. The secretory end pieces were lined with principal secretory cells with occasional few basal ones. The principal cells varied from columnar to cuboidal in shape, depending upon the studied season. The principal cells showed PAS-positive reactivity. Seasonal variations were observed in the height of the principal cell lining the secretory end pieces, in the interstitial tissue/glandular tissue ratio, and in the PAS reactivity in the principal cells. In conclusion, the prostate gland of donkey appeared more active during spring. This reactivity decreased during other seasons of the year. Minimal reactivity was recorded during winter.

INTRODUCTION

The accessory genital glands were a series of glands situated between the vas deferens and the root of the penis. These glands are responsible for the secretion of the seminal plasma, which provides the substrate for conveying the sperm to the female and ensuring final maturation [1,2]. The accessory genital glands of donkey were made up of ampulla ductus deferentis, seminal vesicles, prostate gland, bulbourethral glands, and urethral glands [3].

The secretory portions of the prostate were tubuloalveolar in rabbits [4], dogs [5], boars [6], elephants [7], bulls [8], equines [9], men [10], camels [11], and buffalo bulls [12]. In rams, the prostate was compound tubular [13], while in red deer and goats [14–16], it was of branched tubular type.

The epithelial lining of the secretory end pieces varied from low cuboidal to high columnar cells as observed in rabbits, boars, elephants, bulls, common marmoset, camels, buffalo bulls, domestic animals, and men ([4, 6–8, 17–21], resp.). In dogs, the lining epithelium was simple, stratified, or pseudostratified [5, 22]. Frequently, flattened, large rounded, ovoid, wedged, or pyramidal-shaped cells were recorded between the lining cells of the secretory units of the prostate of dogs [22], shrew [23], camels [24], men [10], and buffalo bulls [17]. These basal cells possessed darkly stained cytoplasm and rounded nuclei with dense chromatin [18] in marmoset.

The glandular epithelium of the secretory end pieces of the prostate showed seasonal variations in red deer [14], bucks [15], rams [25], and camels [26].

The histological and histochemical studies on the prostate gland of equines especially those of donkeys are rare [9]. So the aim of the present work is to study the histological and histochemical structures of the prostate gland of donkey during different seasons of the year.

MATERIALS AND METHODS

As discussed in our previous work [3], the present study was performed on 24 sexually mature apparently healthy male donkeys (jacks) that were collected during four seasons of the year, six for each. Their age ranged between 5 and 7 years.

The animals were anesthetized and then thoroughly bled to death from the common carotid artery. The jacks were dissected, and their accessory genital glands were perfused in situ through the right and left internal pudendal arteries with the appreciate fixatives. They included neutral buffered formaldehyde, Bouin's fluid (for routine histological and morphometrical examination), and cold formol-calcium (for lipids).

The fixed specimens from the prostate gland were further processed for paraffin embedding. 5–7 μm thick paraffin sections were obtained and stained with the following stains. Routine histological examinations were performed by using Harris haematoxylin and eosin stain [27,28]. Collagenous fibers were detected by Crossmon's trichrome stain [29, 30]. For demonstration of elastic and reticular fibers, we used Verhoeff's methods [31, 32] and Gomori's reticulin stain [33], respectively. Periodic acid-schiff, PAS [34], alcian blue technique, pH 2.5 [35], and combined alcian blue-PAS technique [36] for detection of neutral and acid mucopolysaccharides. Glycogen was demonstrated by using Best's carmine method [37].

For demonstration of lipids, Sudan black staining as described by Bayliss and Adams [38]; we used the accessory genital glands of another 2 jacks each season.

The sections were examined and photographed on an Olympus microscope with DP72 camera and cell software.

For scanning electron microscopy, the specimens were fixed in 5% phosphate buffered glutaraldehyde for 24 hr at 4°C. Thereafter, the specimens were post-fixed in 1% buffered osmic acid and dehydrated in alcohol followed by amyl acetate. They were dried by the critical point drying using liquid CO_2 and mounted on specimen's tubes. The specimens were sputtercoated with gold, examined, and photographed at JEOL 5400 LV scanning electron microscope.

The morphometric studies were performed on the stained histological sections of the glands under investigation using Leica Q 500 MC image analyser. They were performed by two operators, in double blind, comparing the results obtained subsequently. The measurements were carried out on each gland of the 6 jacks in all seasons in the following manner. The height of the surface and the glandular epithelium, the nuclear/cell ratio of the principal cells of the surface, and glandular epithelium were calculated from fifteen random fields of the glands under investigation. The interstitial connective tissue/glandular tissue ratio of the studied glands was calculated from five random fields. All the data were presented as means ± SE, which were statistically analysed using SPSS (one way ANOVA and Scheffe tests).

RESULTS

The prostate gland (Glandula prostatica) of the donkey was represented only by the body or the external part of the gland (Pars externa, Corpus prostatica), which was retroperitoneal. It consisted of right and left somewhat prismatic-shaped lobes connected with isthmus. The prostate gland was located on the dorsolateral surface of the neck of the urinary bladder and the beginning of the urethra. Caudally, a muscular band originating from the urethralis muscle covered partially each prostatic lobe at its ventral surface. After incision of the ventral aspect of the pelvic urethra, 15–20 duct openings of the prostate were observed on both sides of the Colliculus seminalis (Figures 1(a)–1(d)).

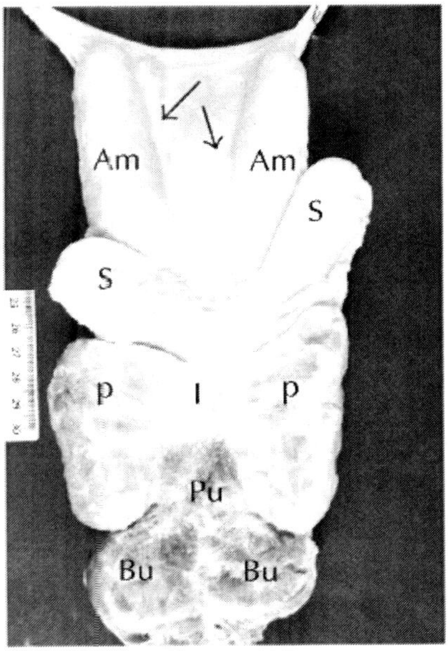

(a)

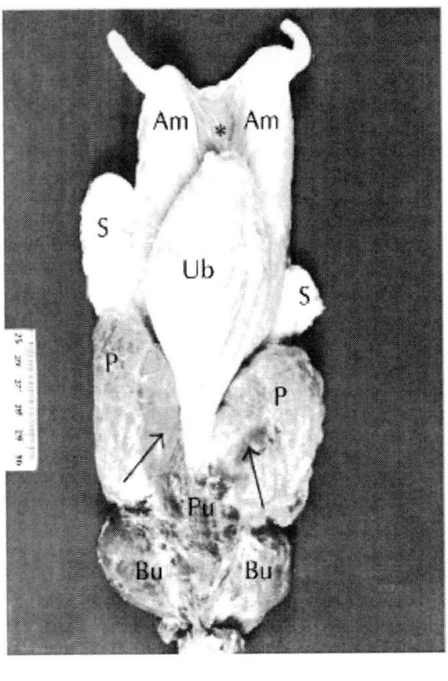

(b)

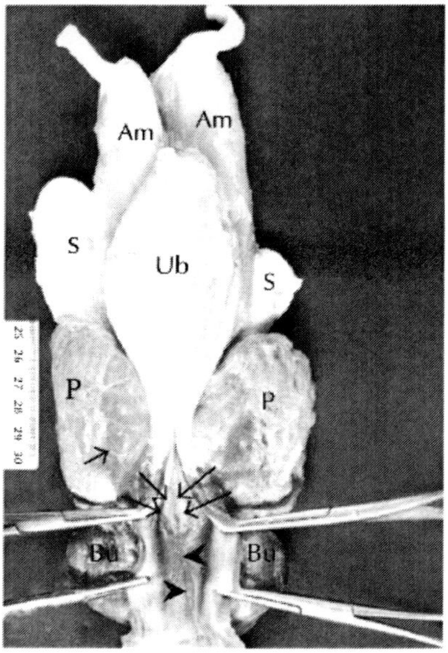

(c)

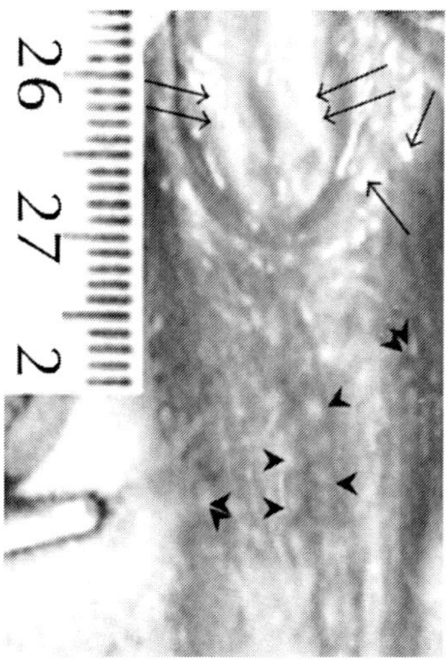

(d)

Figure 1: Photographs showing the accessory genital glands of the donkey during spring (dorsal view, (a); ventral view, (b)-(c)). Ductus deferens (arrowhead), ampulla of the deferent duct (Am), seminal vesicles (S), prostate gland (P) and its isthmus (I), band of urethralis muscle (arrow) covers the caudal pole of the prostate (P), bulbourethral glands (Bu), genital fold (asterisk), vestige Mullerian ducts (arrow), urinary bladder (Ub), and pelvic urethra (Pu). (d) High magnification photograph at the ventral aspect of an incised pelvic urethra of the donkey during spring showing opening of the ejaculatory ducts (double arrows), prostate gland openings (arrows), bulbourethral gland openings (arrowhead), and urethral gland duct openings (double arrowheads) adapted after Abou-Elhamd et al., [3].

Histological Observations

The prostate gland of the donkey consisted of stroma and parenchyma. The former was represented by capsule, septa, and interstitial connective tissue.

The prostate gland was enveloped externally by a thick capsule. The capsule was divided into outer fibrous and inner fibromuscular layers. The outer fibrous capsule was made up mainly of collagenous, reticular, and few fine elastic fibers (Figures 2(a)–2(c)). This layer contained small-sized arteries and veins, arterioles, venules, bundles of myelinated nerve fibers, and sympathetic ganglia (Figures 3(a) and 3(b)).

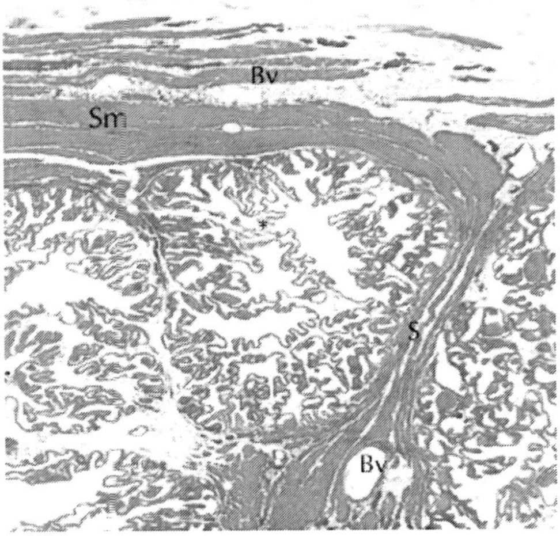

(a)

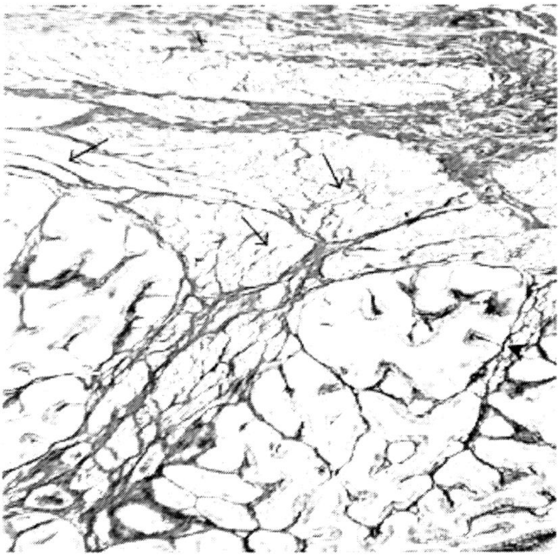

(b)

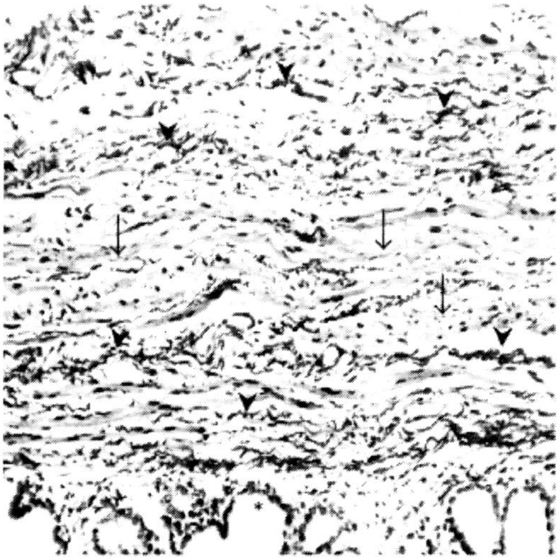

(c)

Figure 2: Photomicrographs of the fibromuscular capsule of the prostate of the donkey during winter by using of (a) Crossmon's trichrome stain showing the smooth muscle fiber bundles (Sm) and collagen fibers (green colour). Septa

(S), prostatic lobules (asterisk), blood vessels (Bv), and ×25. (b): Verhoff's stain showing the elastic (arrowhead) and smooth muscle fibers (arrow). Secretory end pieces (asterisk), ×200. (c): Gomori's stain showing the reticular fibers network (arrowhead) supporting the smooth muscle fibers. Collagen fibers (brown colour), prostatic lobules (asterisk), and×100

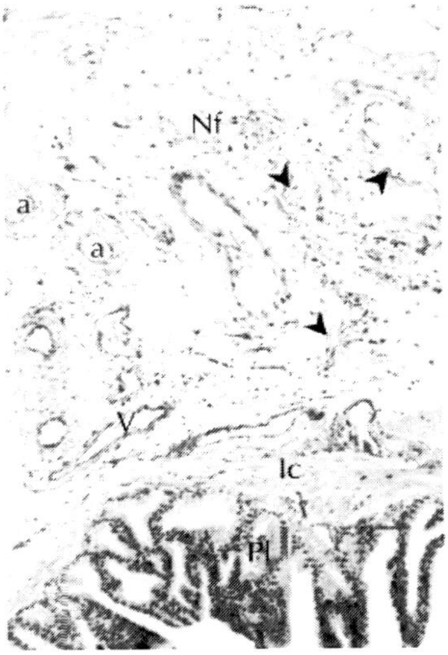

(a)

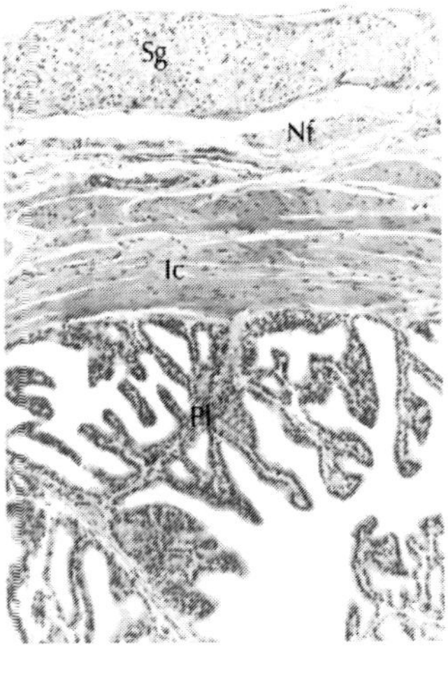

(b)

Figure 3: Photomicrographs of the prostatic capsule during winter showing fine elastic fibers (arrowhead), small-sized arteries (a), small-sized veins (V), bundles of myelinated nerve fibers (Nf), and sympathetic ganglion (Sg) within the outer fibrous layer. Inner fibromuscular capsule (Ic), and prostatic lobules (Pl). (a) Verhoff's stain. ×50. (b) Haematoxylin and eosin×100

The inner fibromuscular capsule consisted mainly of coarse collagenous fibers and thick bundles of smooth muscle ones (Figure 2(a)). The latter were concentrated mainly in the deep portion of the capsule with abundant elastic fibers. Moreover, fine elastic ones were seen elsewhere in the capsule in between the individual smooth muscle fibers (Figure 2(c)).

It was observed that the prostatic capsule is attached directly to the connective tissue adventitia of the seminal vesicle cranially at its dorsal aspect (Figure 4). In addition, bundles of skeletal muscle fibers of the urethralis muscle were also demonstrated, joining the prostatic capsule at its caudal pole ventrally (Figure 5(a)). Some of these skeletal muscle fibers penetrated the capsule and were demonstrated among the smooth muscle fiber bundles of the septa only in sections obtained from the caudal pole of the prostate (Figure 5(b)).

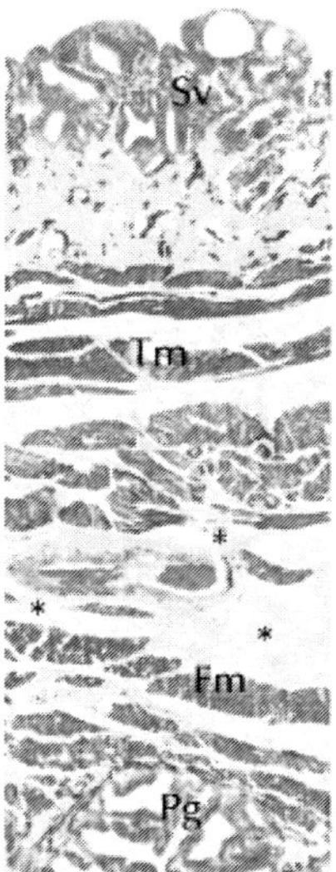

Figure 4: Photomicrograph showing the attachment (asterisk) of the seminal vesicle (Sv) with the capsule of the prostate gland (Pg) during winter. Colla-

gen fibers (green colour). Tunica muscularis of the seminal vesicle (Tm), and fibromuscular capsule of the prostate (Fm). Crossmon's trichrome stain×100

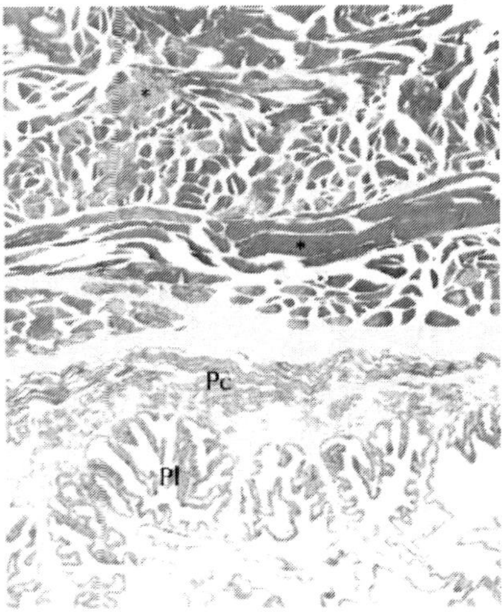

(a)

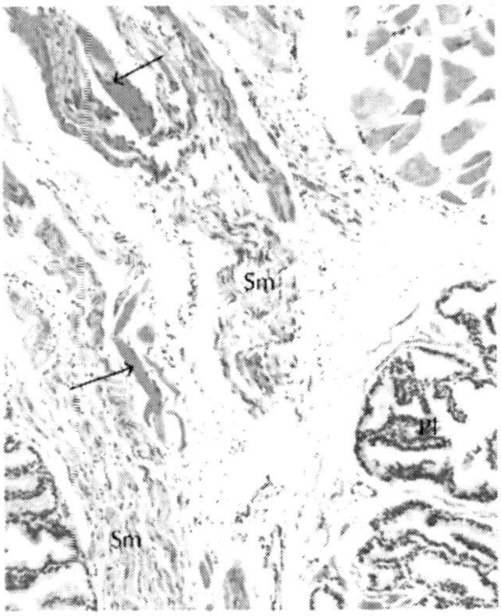

(b)

Figure 5: Photomicrographs showing the site of attachment of the skeletal muscle fibers (a) of the urethralis muscle (asterisk) to the prostatic capsule

(Pc) and the extension of some these fibers (arrow) within the fibromuscular septa (b). Collagen fibers (green colour), smooth muscle fibers (Sm), and prostatic lobules (Pl). (a) Crossmon's trichrome stain. ×50 . (b) Haematoxylin and eosin stain×100(asterisk).

Fibromuscular septa arose from the deep aspect of the capsule (Figures 2(a) and 2(b)) dividing the prostate into variable numbers of lobules of different sizes and shapes (Figure 6(a)). Structurally, the septa simulated nearly the capsule (Figure 6(b)), but the elastic fibers appeared more numerous and thicker (Figure 6(c)). It also contained small-sized blood vessels and bundles of myelinated nerve fibers.

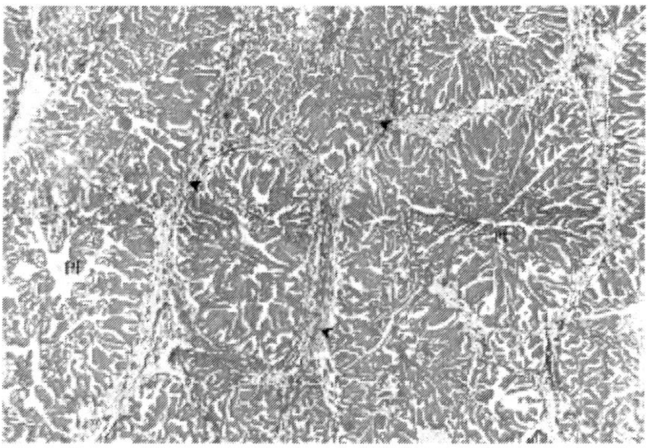

(a)

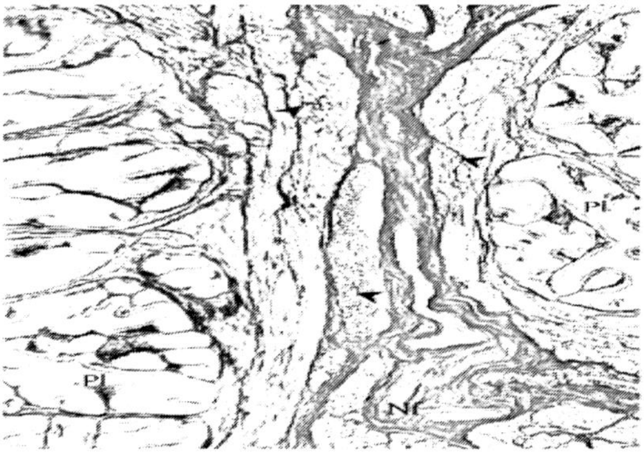

(b)

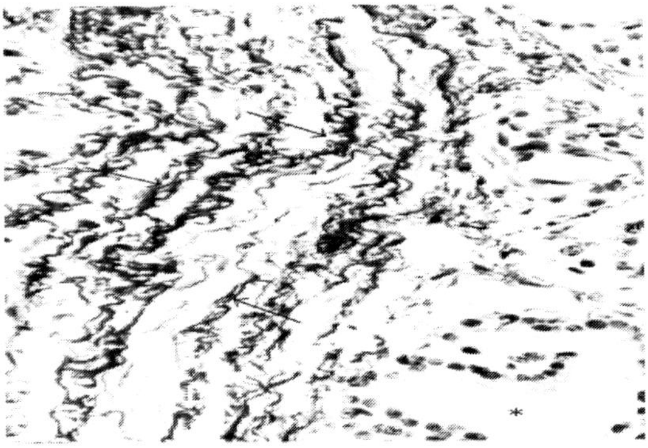

(c)

Figure 6: Photomicrographs of the fibromuscular capsule of the prostate of the donkey during winter after by using of (a) Crossmon's trichrome stain showing the smooth muscle fiber bundles (Sm) and collagen fibers (green colour). Septa (S), prostatic lobules (asterisk), and blood vessels (Bv). ×25. (b) Gomori's stain showing the reticular fibers network (arrowhead) supporting the smooth muscle fibers. Collagen fibers (brown colour), and prostatic lobules (asterisk). ×100. (c) Verhoff's stain showing the elastic (arrowhead) and smooth muscle fibers (arrow). Secretory end pieces (asterisk) ×200

The interstitial tissue of the prostate was made up mainly of a network of reticular fibers supporting the glandular end pieces (Figure 7(a)). In addition to the presence of fine elastic (Figure 7(b)) and collagenous fibers, singly distributed smooth muscle fibers were also demonstrated (Figures 8(a) and 8(d)).

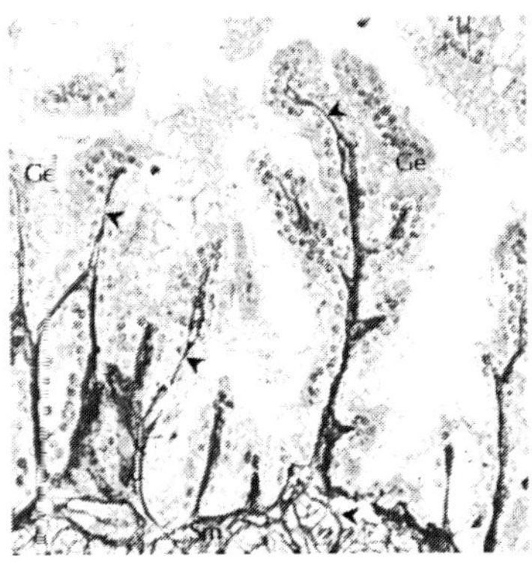

(a)

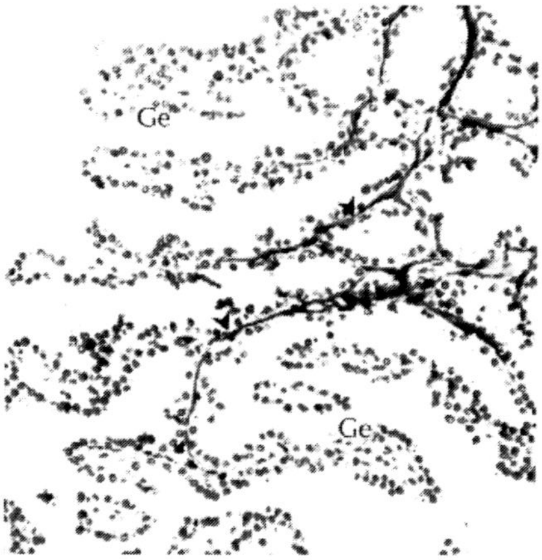

(b)

Figure 7: (a) Photomicrographs showing the reticular fibers network (arrowhead) supporting the muscle fibers of the septa (asterisk) during winter. Collagen fibers (brown colour), myelinated nerve fiber bundles (Nf), and prostatic lobules (Pl). Gomori's stain. ×100. (b) Photomicrograph showing the numerous elastic fibers (arrow) within the septa of the prostate of the donkey during winter. Secretory end pieces (asterisk). Verhoff's stain. ×400. (a)- (b), (a) Photomicrograph of the prostatic lobules during spring showing reticular fibers network (arrowhead) supporting the glandular epithelium (Ge) and smooth muscle fibers of the septa (Sm). Gomori's stain. ×200. (b) Photomicrograph showing fine elastic fibers (arrowhead) in the interstitial connective tissue of the prostate of the donkey during spring. Glandular epithelium (Ge). Verhoff's stain×200

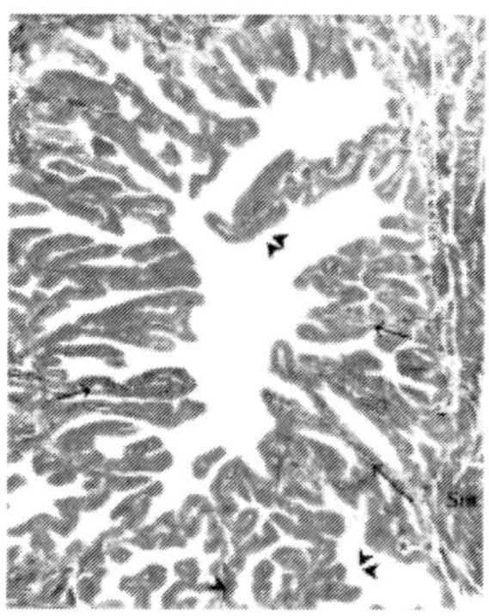

(a)

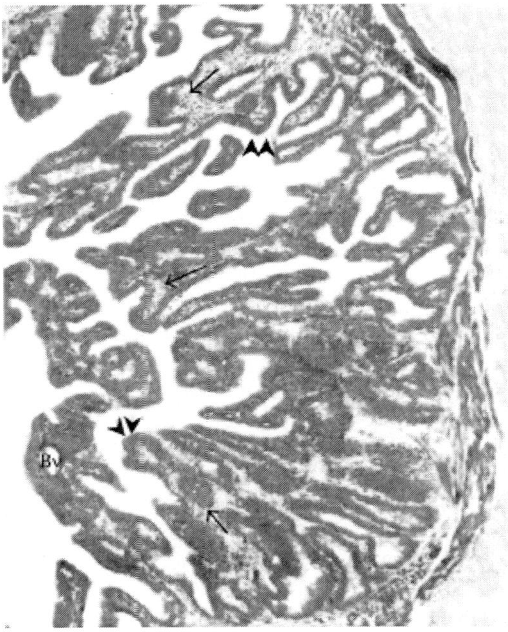

(b)

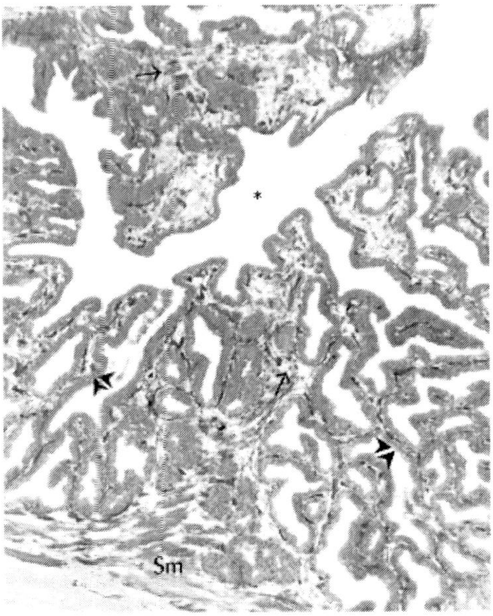

(c)

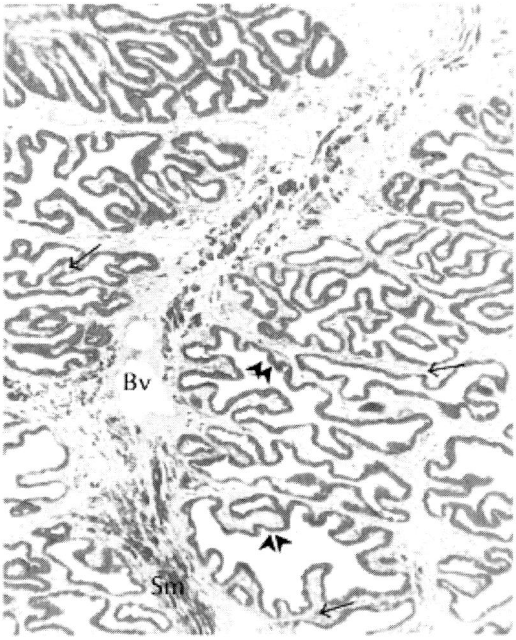

(d)

Figure 8: Photomicrographs showing the variation in the amount of the interstitial connective tissue (arrow) of the prostate gland of the donkey during spring (a), summer (b), autumn (c), and winter (d). Glandular epithelium (double arrowhead), collagen fibers (green colour), smooth muscle fiber bundles of the septa (Sm), singly distributed smooth muscle fibers (arrowhead), central collecting sinus (asterisk), and blood vessels (Bv). Crossmon's trichrome stain×100

The amount of the interstitial connective tissue supporting the prostatic parenchyma varied among the studied seasons, where highly significant () seasonal differences in the interstitial connective tissue/glandular tissue ratio were recorded. The lowest amount of the interstitial tissue was obtained in spring, where the interstitial connective tissue/glandular tissue ratio reached about 0.247 ± 0.015. This ratio increased gradually during summer (about 0.295 ± 0.019) and autumn (about 0.400 ± 0.025), while the highest ratio was observed during winter, where it measured about 0.480 ± 0.018 (Figures 8(a)–8(d) and Figure 9).

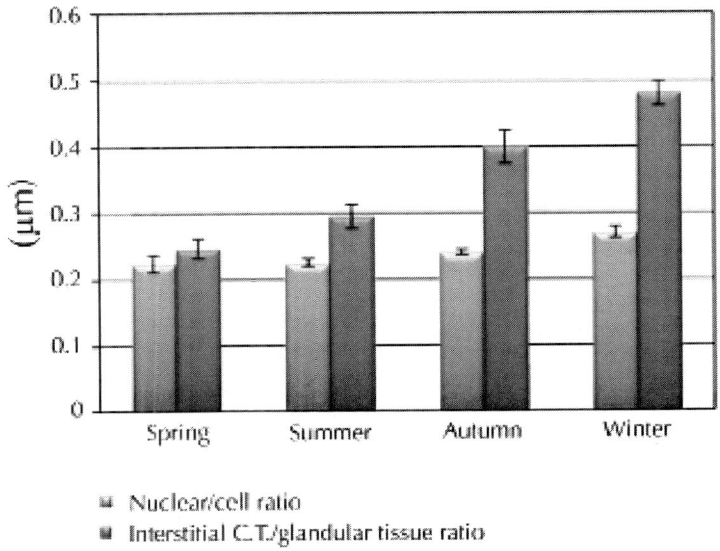

Figure 9: The nuclear/cell ratio of the principal cells of the glandular epithelium and the interstitial connective tissue/glandular tissue ratio of the prostate gland of the donkey showed significant seasonal variations.

The parenchyma of the prostatic lobes and isthmus is composed of compound tubuloalveolar glands and duct system (Figures 2(a), 5(a) and 8(a)–8(d)).

The compound tubuloalveolar glands were lined with principal secretory cells with, however, occasional few basal ones. The principal cells varied from columnar to cuboidal in shape, depending upon the studied season with somewhat distinct cell boundaries and fine granular acidophilic cytoplasm, which appeared more numerous during spring than the other seasons. Their deeply stained basely located nuclei were nearly round or ovoid in shape. Also, fine dark yellow to yellow brown granules were distributed within the cytoplasm of the glandular and ductal epithelial cells of the prostatic lobules. Large amount of these granules was clearly visible during winter. The basal cells appeared as small flat or triangular-shaped cells, wedged between the principal ones and the basement membrane. They were characterized by their somewhat small cytoplasm and large flattened or irregular-shaped nuclei (Figures 10(a)-10(b)).

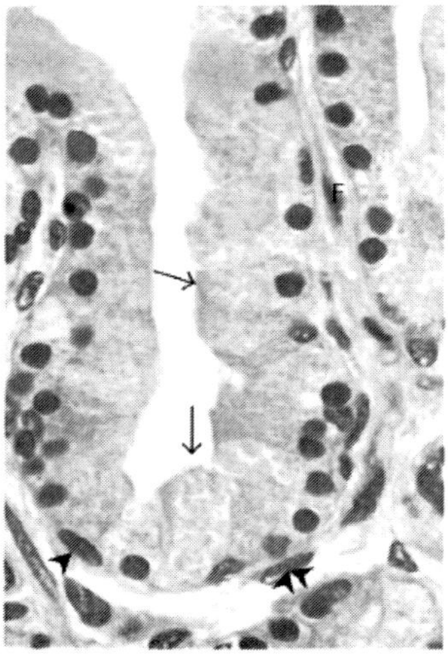

(a)

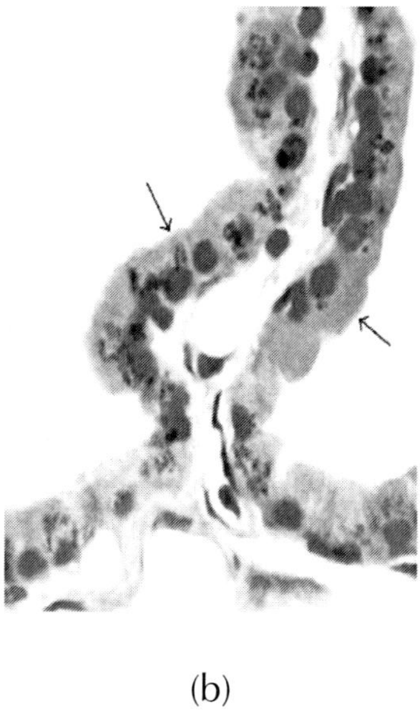

(b)

Figure 10: Photomicrographs of the glandular epithelium of the prostate during spring (a) and winter (b) showing the principal cells with fine acidophilic granular cytoplasm and rounded basely located nuclei (arrow). During winter, the principal cells contained large amount of lipofuscin pigments (brown colour). Basal cells with flattened (arrowhead) or irregular-shaped nuclei (double arrowhead), Fibroblasts (F). Haematoxylin and eosin stain. . ×1000

The height of the glandular epithelium revealed highly significant ($p < 0.01$) seasonal variations. During spring, the epithelial height reached its maximal value, where it measured about 14.67 μm ± 0.138. Then, it decreased gradually during summer (about 12.80 μm ± 0.397) and autumn (about 12.64 μm ± 0.279). The lowest value was obtained in winter, where it was about 11.31 μm ± 0.322 (Figures 11 and 12(a)–12(d)).

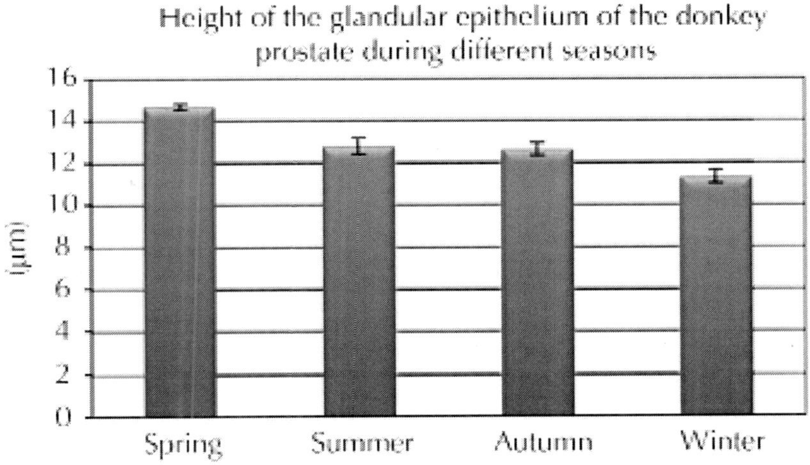

Figure 11: The height of the glandular epithelium of prostate gland of the donkey showed significant seasonal variations.

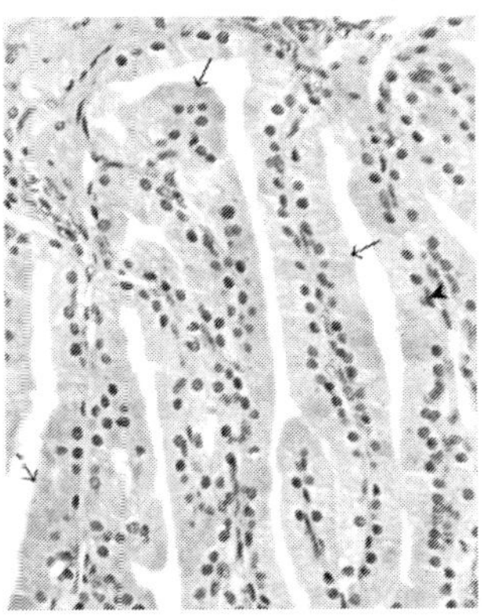

(a)

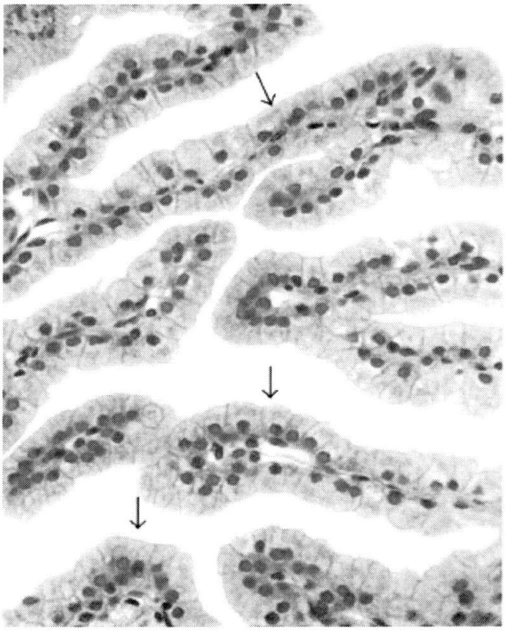

(b)

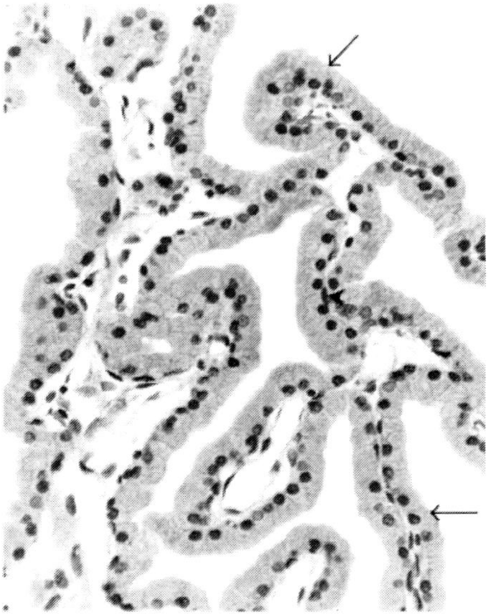

(c)

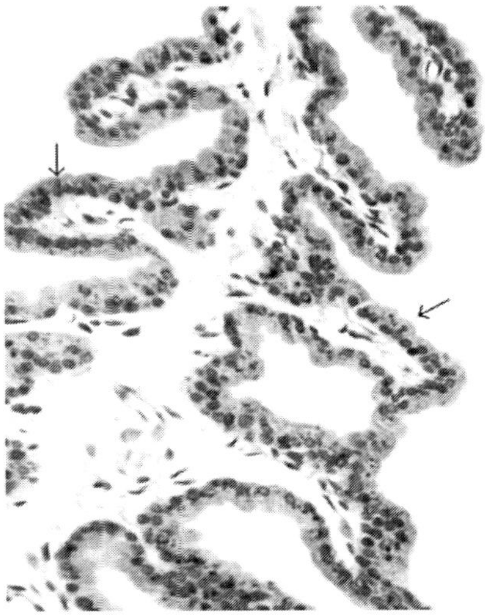

(d)

Figure 12: Photomicrographs showing the variation in the height of the glandular epithelium of the prostate during spring (a), summer (b), autumn (c), and winter (d). Principal cells (arrow), basal cells (arrowhead), and lipofuscin granules (brown colour in (d), fibroblasts (F). Haematoxylin and eosin stain×400.

The nuclear/cell ratio of the principal cells of the prostate varied among the studied seasons. This ratio showed highly significant () seasonal variations. The lowest ratio was recorded in spring, where it reached about 0.224 ± 0.013. This ratio increased gradually to about 0.225 ± 0.005 during summer, 0.241 ± 0.005 during autumn, and 0.270 ± 0.009 during winter (Figure 9).

The lumina of some secretory portions as well as that of the central collecting sinuses showed acidophilic secretory materials as well as concretes.

The duct system could be organized into tertiary, secondary, and primary ducts. The secretory portions were drained directly by a tertiary duct into a secondary duct or the central collecting sinus of the prostatic lobules (Figure 13(a)). The glandular epithelium of the secretory portions changed gradually into the ductal epithelium. Both the tertiary and secondary ducts and central collecting sinuses were lined with low cuboidal principal cells, with somewhat deeply stained acidophilic cytoplasm. Their spherical or ovoid nuclei appeared somewhat darkly stained occupying most of the cell (Figure 13(b)).

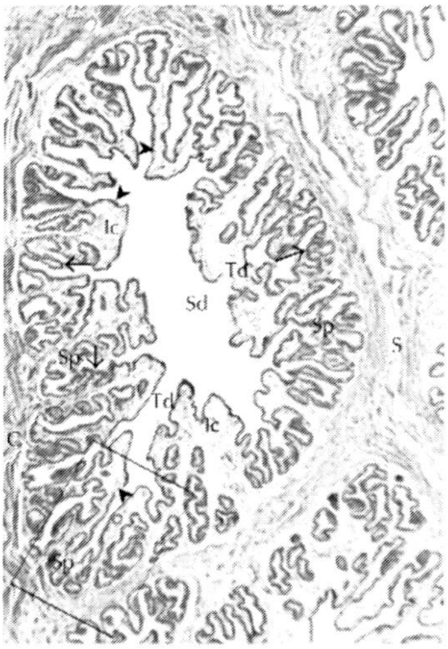

(a)

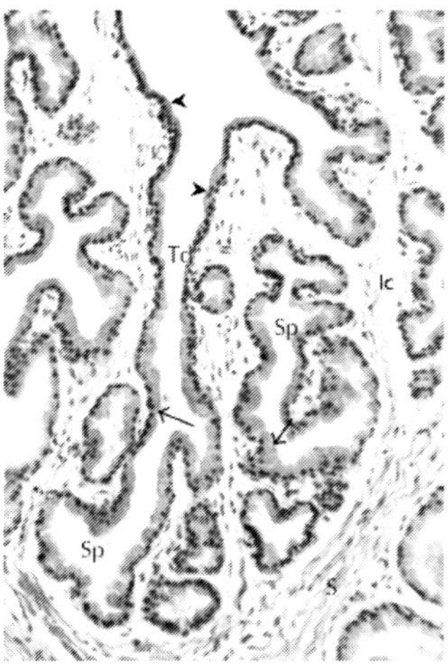

(b)

Figure 13: Photomicrographs of the prostatic lobules (a) and the higher magnification of the marked area (b) during winter. The secretory portions (Sp) drained by a tertiary duct (Td) into large secondary duct or collecting sinus (Sd), gradual change of the glandular epithelium (arrow) into ductal one (arrowhead). Fibromuscular capsule (C) connective tissue septa (S), interstitial connective tissue (Ic). Haematoxylin and eosin stain.(a):×50 (b):×100

The secondary ducts or central collecting sinuses of several prostatic lobules or even of a single lobule are drained directly into a long primary duct (Figure 14). These primary ducts were accompanied with few secretory end pieces, which opened directly into their lumina. The ducts were directed towards the cranial part of the pelvic urethra penetrating its muscle (Figures15(a) and 15(b)) to open on both sides of the Colliculus seminalis. These ducts were firstly lined with simple low cuboidal epithelial cells as those of the central collecting sinus, which changed gradually into a bilayered epithelium, consisting of superficial cuboidal cells and flat basal ones. Near its termination, the ductal lining epithelium changed into stratified cuboidal at its opening into the pelvic urethra (Figure 16(b)).

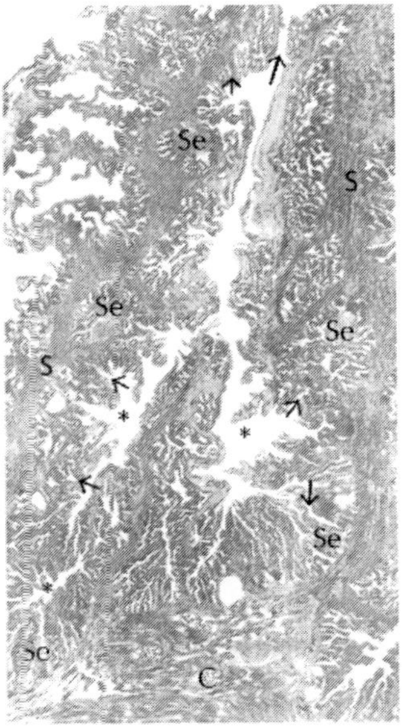

Figure 14: Photomicrograph of the prostate during spring showing the secretory end pieces (Se) drained directly by tertiary ducts (thin arrow) into collecting sinuses (asterisk), which are drained into long primary duct (thick arrow). Fibromuscular capsule (C), septa (S), and collagen fibers (green colour). Crossmon's trichrome stain×25.

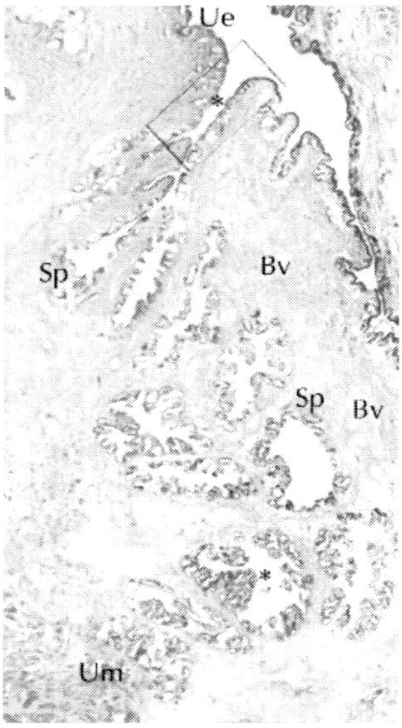

(a)

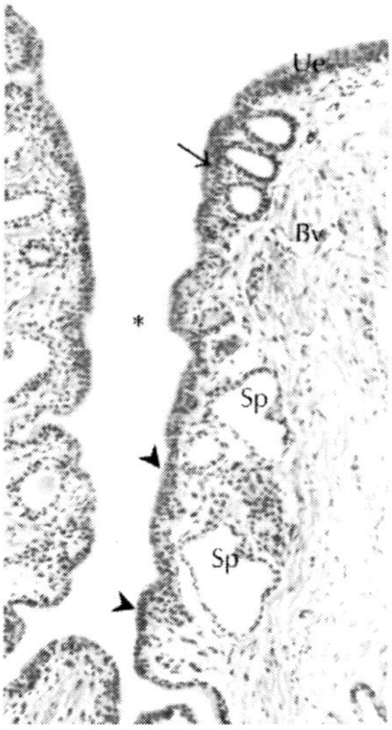

(b)

Figure 15: (a) Photomicrographs showing the penetration of the primary ducts (asterisk) to the urethral muscle (Um) during spring and high magnification of the marked area and (b) the change of the lining epithelium from bilayered epithelium (arrowhead) to stratified cuboidal (arrow) as that of the urethral epithelium (Ue). Secretory portions accompanied the duct (Sp), blood vessels (Bv). Haematoxylin and eosin stain. (a) ×25. (b):×200

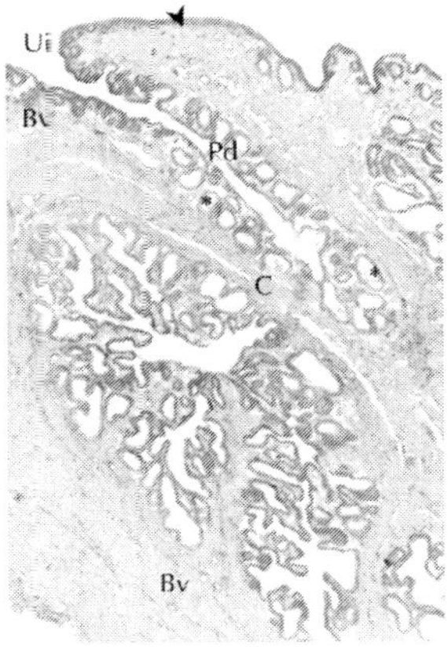

(a)

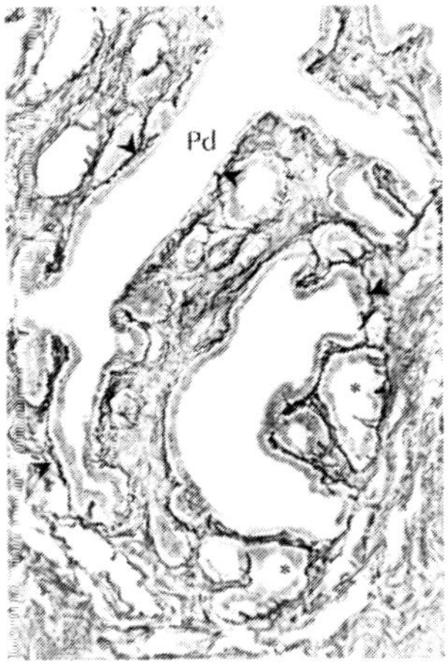

(b)

Figure 16: (a) Photomicrographs showing the presence of collagenous fibers (green colour) in the connective tissue layer supporting the primary duct (Pd) during autumn. Secretory end pieces accompanied the duct (asterisk). Urethral epithelium (arrowhead), urethral lumen (Ul), cavernous spaces (C), and blood vessels (Bv). Crossmon's trichrome stain. ×50. (b) Photomicrograph of the reticular fibers network (arrowhead) supporting the accompanied secretory end pieces (asterisk). Collagenous fibers (brown colour). Gomori's stain × 200.

The primary ducts were supported with highly vascular dense fibrous connective tissue layer made up mainly of collagenous (Figure 16(a)). Reticular fibers network was observed only under the epithelial lining of the duct and secretory portions (Figure 15(b)). Elastic fibers were demonstrated mainly parallel to the longitudinal axis of the duct (Figures 17(a) and 17(b)). This connective tissue layer contained also fibroblasts, fibrocytes, and blood vessels of variable calibers as well as cavernous spaces (Figures 15(a), 15(b), and 16(a)).

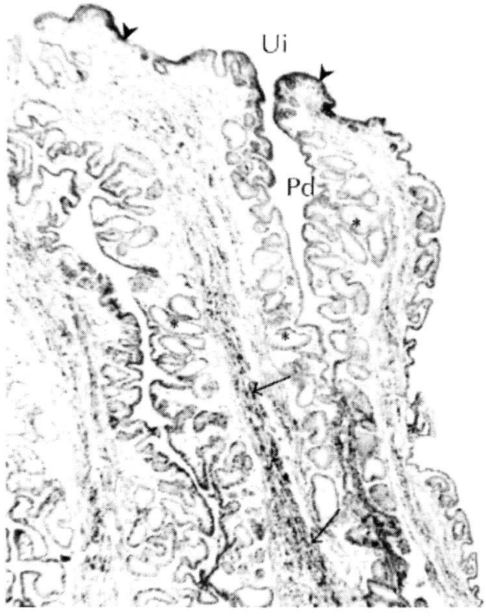

(a)

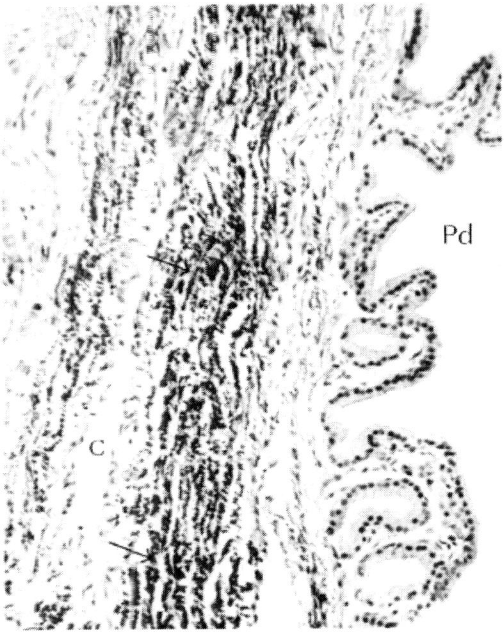

(b)

Figure 17: (a) Photomicrographs showing the parallelly arranged elastic fibers (thin arrow) to the longitudinal axis of the primary duct (Pd) during autumn. Secretory portions (asterisk) accompanying the duct, and urethral epithelium (arrowhead). Verhoff's stain×25. (b) High magnification photomicrograph of the elastic fibers (thin arrow) in the wall of the primary duct (Pd) during autumn. Cavernous spaces (C). Verhoff's stain×200

Scanning electron microscopy of the pelvic urethra during the studied seasons at the level of the Colliculus seminalis revealed numerous prostatic duct openings (Figure 18(a)), which are arranged into somewhat parallel rows on either side of the Colliculus seminalis. These openings appeared as elevated dome-shaped papillae upon the urethral membrane. At the tip of each papilla, the prostatic gland openings possessed irregular indentations and hexagonal-shaped cell luminal surface (Figures 18(b) and 18(c)). Variable numbers of spermatozoa could be observed within some prostatic duct openings (Figure 18(d)).

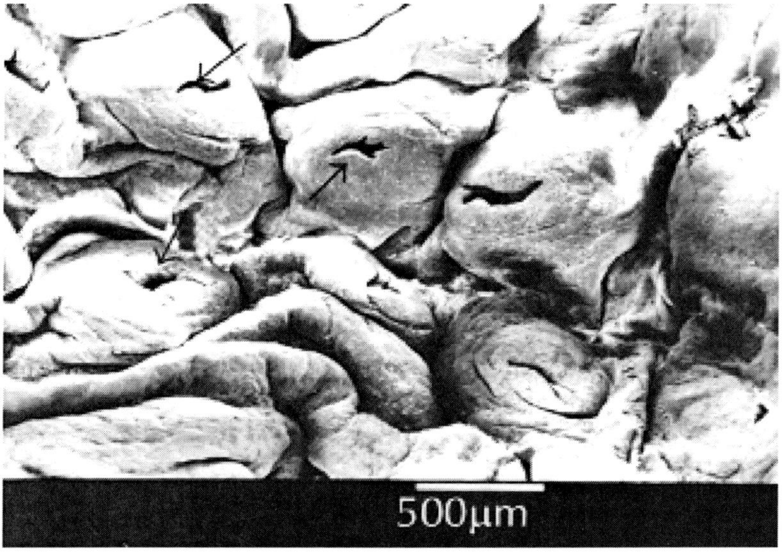

(a)

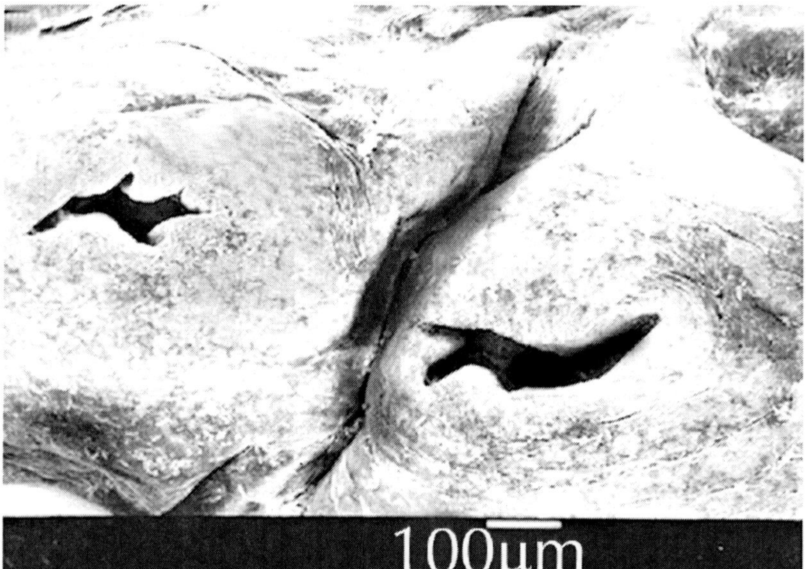

(b)

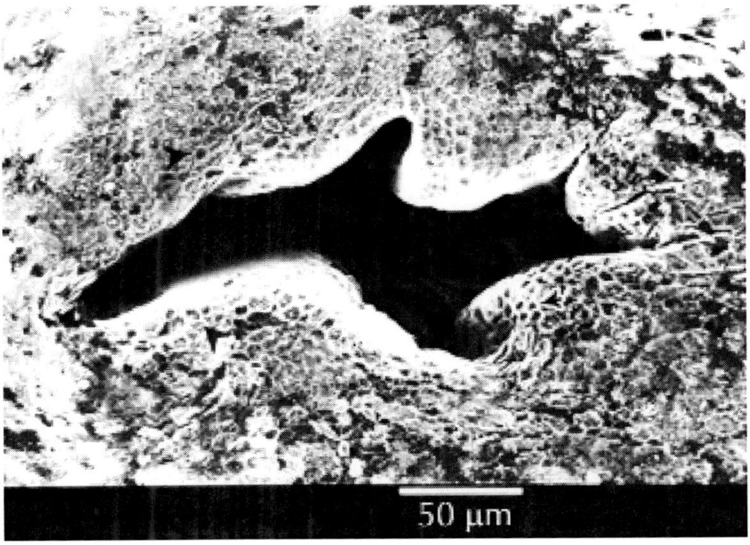

(c)

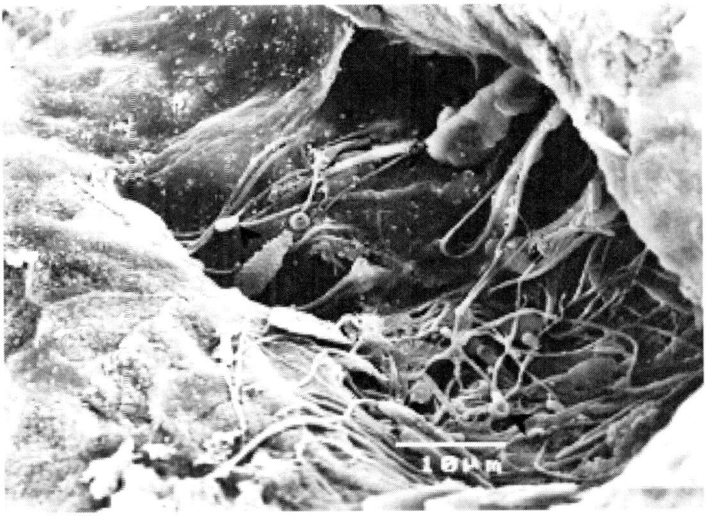

(d)

Figure 18: (a) Scanning electron micrograph of the luminal surface of the prostatic urethra at the level of the Colliculus seminalis during spring showing the arrangement of the prostate gland openings (arrow) into somewhat parallel rows. ((b)-(c)) High magnification scanning electron micrographs of

(a) showing the elevated dome-shaped like papillae of the duct openings with its irregular oval appearance and hexagonal-shaped cell surface (arrowhead). (d) High magnification scanning electron micrograph of the prostate duct opening containing variable numbers of spermatozoa (arrowhead). Scale bar was demonstrated on each figure.

HISTOCHEMICAL OBSERVATIONS

Carbohydrates

Neutral Mucopolysaccharides. During spring, the principal glandular epithelial cells lining the majority of the secretory end pieces of the prostatic lobules reacted very strongly to PAS in the form of diffuse homogenous substance filling the whole cytoplasm (Figure 19(a)). It was observed that in some glandular lobules or even in the same secretory portions, the intensity of the PAS-positive reactivity ranged from strong to moderate. But secretory portions that negatively reacted to PAS could not be demonstrated. The secretory materials observed within the lumina of some prostatic lobules showed very strong positive reaction. The epithelial lining of the duct had the same reactivity as that of the glandular one.

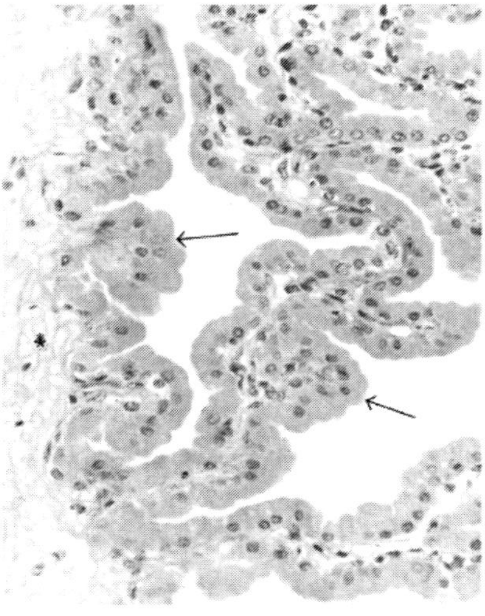

(a)

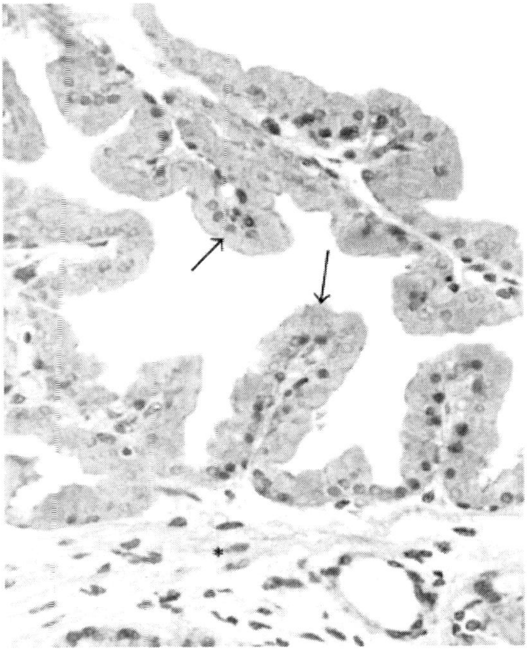

(b)

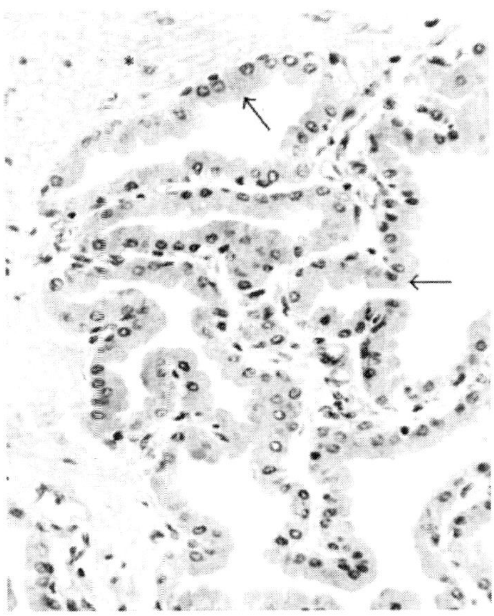

(c)

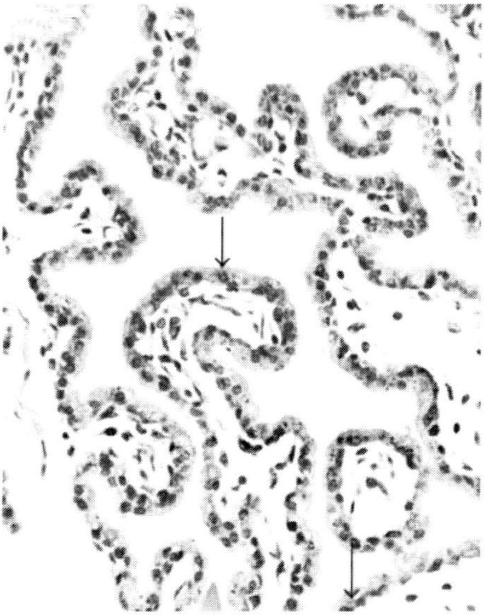

(d)

Figure 19: Photomicrographs showing the PAS reactivity within glandular epithelium (arrow) of the prostate gland of the donkey. Strong PAS positive reaction was observed during spring (a). This reaction decrease in intensity during summer (b) and becomes moderate during autumn (c). During winter (d), the majority of the secretory end pieces are weakly reacted, except the lipofuscin granules. Weakly reacted smooth muscle fiber bundles and connective tissue stroma (asterisk). Concretes (C). PAS/haematoxylin stain×400

During summer, the intensity of the PAS reaction was somewhat slightly lower than that during spring (Figure 19(b)). During autumn, a moderate PAS-positive reactivity was observed within the majority of the prostatic lobules, although some of them weakly reacted (Figure19(c)), while the secretory globules very strongly reacted. During winter, the majority of the secretory portions of the prostatic lobules weakly reacted to PAS, although few secretory portions showed moderate PAS reactivity. On the other hand, strong PAS-positive granules were detected within some glandular and ductal epithelial cells (Figure 19(d)).

In all studied seasons, the prostatic stroma weakly reacted to PAS while the reticular fibers supporting the smooth muscle fibers strongly reacted (Figures 19(a)–19(d)).

Glycogen

After Best's carmine staining, the prostate gland of the donkey did not reveal any positive glycogenic granules during the four seasons. Only the luminal content showed somewhat moderate reaction for Best's carmine stain (data not shown).

Acid Mucopolysaccharides

During the four studied seasons, the glandular and ductal epithelium of the prostatic lobules as well as the luminal contents, concretes, the capsule, septa, and the interstitial connective tissue were devoid of any alcianophilic positive reaction (Figures 20(a) and 20(b)).

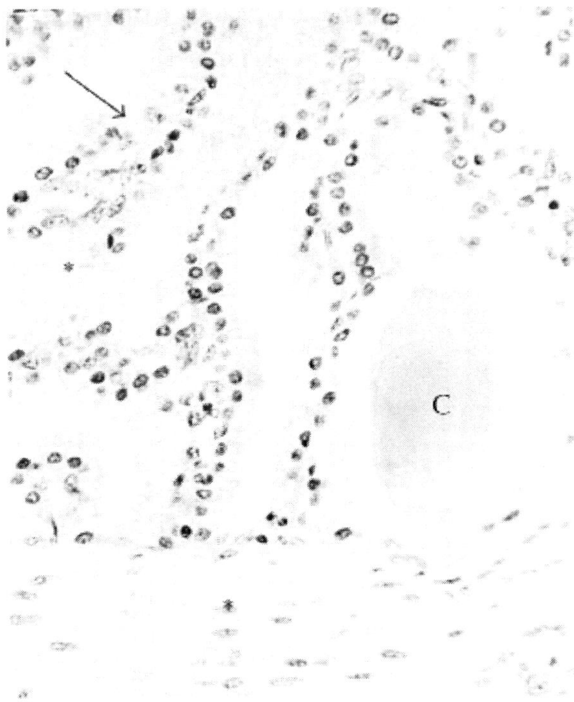

(a)

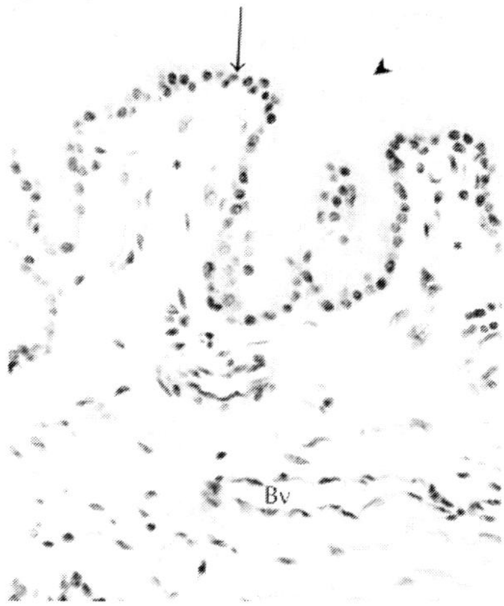

(b)

Figure 20: Photomicrographs of the prostate after alcian blue staining during spring (a) and winter (b) showing the negative reactivity of the glandular epithelium (arrow), stroma (asterisk), luminal contents (arrowhead), concretes (C), and blood vessels (Bv). Alcian blue/haematoxylin stain×400

With alcian blue-PAS staining technique, the histochemical picture of the prostate gland of the donkey concerning the pattern of distribution and the intensity of reaction was nearly the same as that observed with PAS technique during the all studied seasons (Figures 21(a) and 21(b)).

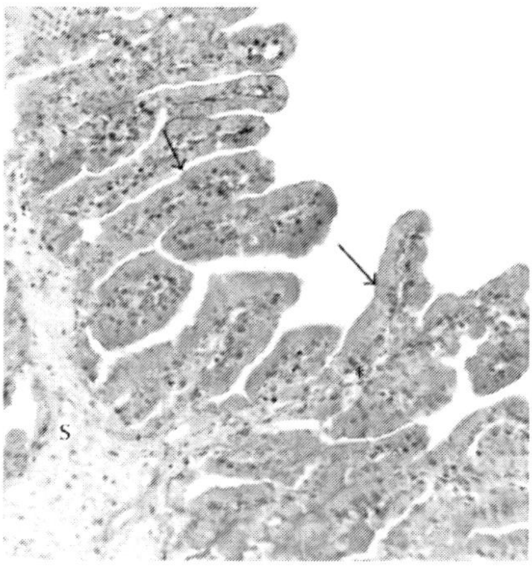

(a)

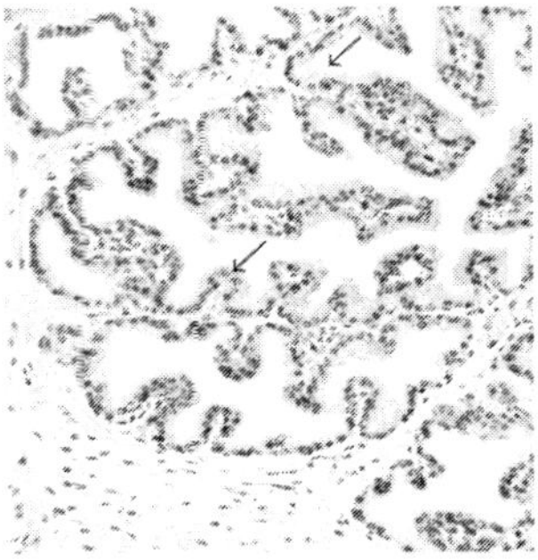

(b)

Figure 21: Photomicrographs of the prostate gland during spring (a) and winter (b) after alcian blue/PAS/haematoxylin staining showing nearly the same picture as PAS reactivity. Glandular epithelium (arrow), interstitial connective tissue (asterisk), and septa (S) ×200

Lipids

During spring, few sudanophilic granules were observed within the glandular and ductal epithelial cells of the prostate gland of the donkey. They were represented by small granules within the majority of these cells (Figure 22(a)). During the other seasons, the intensity and amount of sudanophilic granules increased than those observed during spring (Figure 22(b)). The components of the capsule, connective tissue septa and the secretory substances negatively reacted to Sudan black stain.

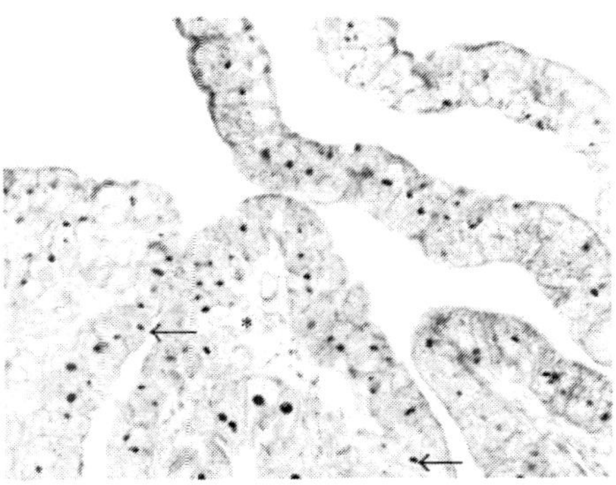

(a)

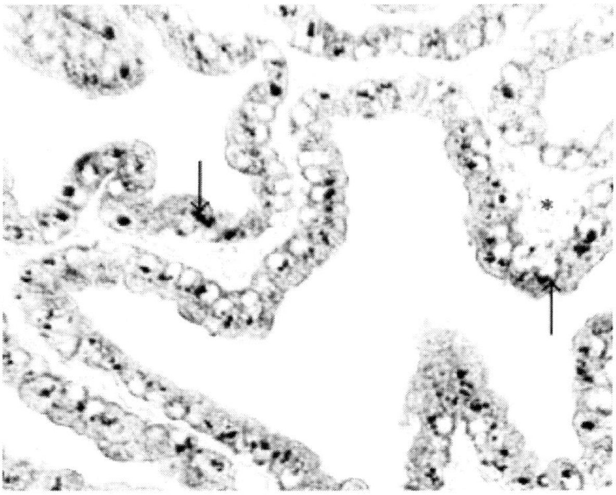

(b)

Figure 22: Photomicrographs showing few sudanophilic granules within the glandular and ductal epithelial cells (arrow) of the prostate of the donkey during spring (b). These granules increase in intensity and amount during winter (b). Negatively reacted interstitial connective tissue (asterisk). Sudan black stain. ×400.

Lipofuscins

After long Ziehl-Neelsen staining, few positive lipofuscin granules could be demonstrated during spring in some glandular and ductal epithelial cells of the prostatic lobules. These granules were nearly rounded ranging from bright red to magenta colour (Figure 23(a)). They increased slightly during summer (Figure 23(b)) while during autumn a further increment in their amount could be observed (Figure 23(c)). These lipofuscin pigments reached their maximal amount during winter (Figure 23(d)). In all studied seasons, lipofuscin pigments within the stroma of the prostatic glands of the donkey and the luminal contents could not be demonstrated.

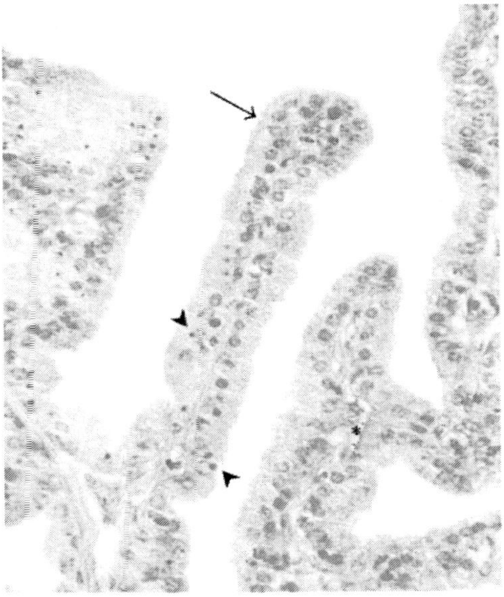

(a)

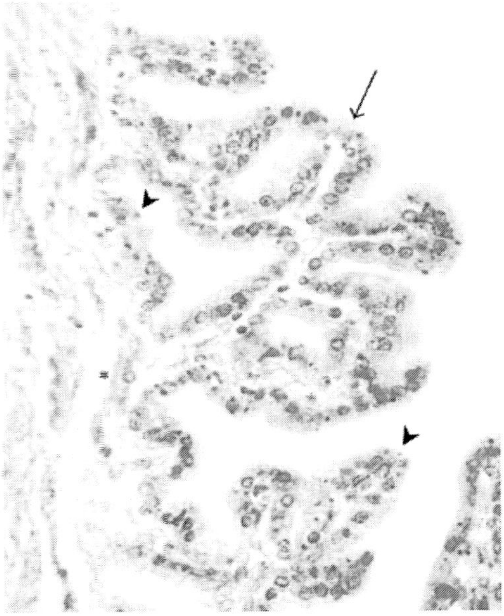

(b)

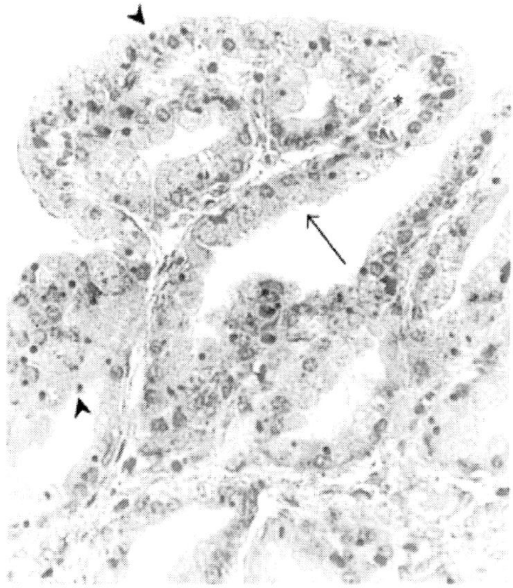

(c)

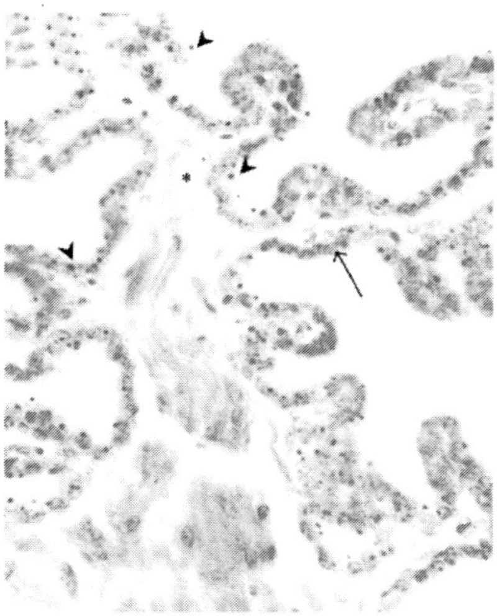

(d)

Figure 23: Photomicrographs showing the variation in the amount of lipofuscin granules (arrowhead) within the glandular epithelial cells (arrow) of the prostate of the donkey. Few granules are observed during spring (a), which increase in amount during summer (b) with further increase during autumn (c), where they reach their maximal amount during winter (d). Smooth muscle fibers (S), interstitial connective tissue (asterisk). Long Ziehl-Neelsen technique. ×400

DISCUSSION

The prostate gland of the donkey was made up only of Pars externa (Corpus prostatae), which consisted of right and left lobes, connected with isthmus and located on the dorsolateral surface of the neck of the urinary bladder and the beginning of the urethra. Similar results were reported in horses [19, 39–41] and equines [2, 9].

The prostate of the donkey was enveloped by thick capsule which had outer fibrous and inner fibromuscular layers. Simulated results were reported in bulls [8, 42, 43], common marmoset [18], horses [40], camels [11], and buffalo bulls [44].

The present study revealed that the capsule of the prostate is attached directly to the connective tissue adventitia of the seminal vesicles. This may be the cause of the difficulty to distinguish them on rectal palpation in horses [40].

The connective tissue septa of the prostate of the donkey were mainly fibromuscular in nature. Similar results were observed in bulls [8, 43] and buffalo bulls [17, 42, 45], while in camels, it was less fibrous and more muscular [11, 26, 46, 47].

The present study revealed that the interstitial tissue of the prostate gland of the donkey was made up of a network of reticular fibers supporting the glandular end pieces as that observed in the prostate of camels and buffalo bulls [26, 48]. In addition, fine elastic and collagenous fibers as well as single distributed smooth muscle fibers were also observed. A great amount of smooth muscle fibers were demonstrated in the interstitial connective tissue of the prostate gland of camels [46], stallions [19], and Mongolian gerbil [49]. The contraction of this muscle may be required to push the stored prostatic secretion into the lumen of the urethra [11, 50].

The parenchyma of the prostate gland of donkey was compound tubuloalveolar in type. However, it was of compound tubular type in red deer, horses, bucks, and domestic animals ([14, 15, 39, 40], resp.).

The present study revealed that the glandular epithelium of the prostate is made up of principal secretory cells with occasionally few basal ones. Similar description was observed in dogs [5], goats [51], common marmoset [18], camels [20, 46], goats [52] and domestic animals [19], while the glandular epithelium of the prostate of bucks [15], buffalo bulls [12, 48], gorilla [53], and camel [11] ranged from cuboidal to columnar.

The present study revealed that the principal glandular cells were columnar in shape with fine granular acidophilic cytoplasm. The basal cells appeared as small flat or triangular-shaped.

These cells were considered as a source of cellular regeneration and played a role in substrate transport [54]. This was supported by Chandler et al. [55] as after administration of cadmium to rats, the basal cells were found to replace epithelial cells in vivo.

Contrary to that observed in male opossum [56] and camels [11, 20, 26], the apical surface of the principal cells of the prostate of the donkey showed no apical protrusions, and this suggests that the mode of secretion of these cells may be a merocrine type. This finding was in agreement with that observed in dogs [57] as well as in bucks [58]. Both merocrine and apocrine modes of secretion were observed in the prostate gland of Mongolian gerbil [49].

Similar to that observed in the glandular epithelium of the prostate gland of baboons [59], dogs [60, 61], and house mice [62], fine dark yellow to yellow brown granules were distributed within the cytoplasm of the glandular and ductal epithelium of the prostate of the donkey. These granules were histochemically similar to lipofuscin pigments [21]. The prostatic stromal and glandular cells of the prostate gland of dogs underwent serial pathological changes of atrophy and apoptosis after castration. The atrophic cells were filled with numerous intracellular lipofuscin pigments. This indicates that the prostate was an androgen sensitive organ. Reference [62] added that there was an increase in apoptotic cells in ventral prostate of house mice on ageing related to the fall of testosterone level and increase of lipofuscin granules, which may be indicative stress in this tissue. In men prostatic tissue, the increase of lipofuscin might be secondary to cellular damage with a consequent catabolic process in the cells [63]. This confirmed the present results, in which lipofuscin pigments were observed during winter (in active season) and decreased during the rest of the seasons, where they reached their minimal amount during spring (active season).

The prostate gland of donkey reached its maximal activity during spring, where the glandular epithelium reached its maximal height (about 14.67 μm ± 0.138), and the nuclear/cell ratio of the principal cells reached the lowest value (about 0.224 ± 0.013). The connective tissue was sparse, where the interstitial connective tissue/glandular tissue ratio reached the lowest value (about 0.247 ± 0.015). The lowest activity was observed during winter, where the cell height reached the lowest value (about 11.31 μm ± 0.322), and the nuclear/cell ratio reached its maximal value (about 0.270 ± 0.009). The connective tissue was abundant and the interstitial connective tissue/glandular tissue ratio reached the maximal value (about 0.480 ± 0.018).

Seasonal variations were also observed in the prostate of bucks [15], rams [25], camels [26], and rats [64]. In addition, reducing androgen production by the Leydig cells causes involution of the prostatic epithelium and growth of stroma in adult animals [65, 66].

The duct system of the prostate of the donkey was organized into tertiary, secondary (central collecting sinuses), and primary ducts. The latter opened into dorsal aspect of the prostatic urethra. Contradictive speculations were mentioned concerning the duct system organization in prostate of the different animals. In stallions and bulls, the prostate has intercellular canaliculi in addition to the excretory ducts, which have the same glandular lining [39]. In camels, the prostate duct system was organized into connecting ducts, collecting sinuses, and interlobular ducts. The latter was lined with stratified epithelium, which changed near its termination into the transitional one [26]. In the present study, similar interlobular ducts were not absolutely seen where the interlobular connective tissue was free of them. In buffalo bulls, it was organized into intra- and interlobular ducts [12]. However, Wrobel and Dellmann [19] in the prostate of domestic animals mentioned only intraglandular ducts where their lining epithelium changed from simple columnar to transitional one at their terminal portions.

Our results showed that 15–20 prostatic duct openings are arranged on both sides of the Colliculus seminalis, representing the prostate gland ducts. Similar results were observed in equines [9], camels [46], buffalo bulls [12], and stallions [19]. Scanning electron microscope of the prostatic urethra showed that these openings appeared as elevated dome-shaped papillae upon the urethral surface (Figure 18).

The glandular epithelial cells of the prostate of the donkey reacted strongly to PAS, indicating the presence of neutral mucopolysaccharides. This reaction reached maximal intensity and amount during spring. During summer, the PAS reaction was nearly the same or somewhat slightly decreased more than that during spring. Then it reached its lowest reactivity during winter. In the epithelial cells of the prostate of rabbits, the neutral mucopolysaccharides were the precursors of fructose in the prostatic secretion [67].

Seasonal variations with PAS were also recorded in the secretory end pieces of the prostate of red deer and rams. In red deer, strong PAS-positive granules were observed in the epithelial lining of the prostatic tubules during the rut than in the pre-rut season [14]. In rams, during winter the PAS-positive granules were observed in the majority of the active cells, and these granules increased in amount during spring and summer and reached their maximum during autumn [25]. In camels, the total glandular reactivity to PAS is greater in spring and winter than in autumn and summer. This simply reflects the change in the amount of neutral mucopolysaccharides secreted by the prostate along the year being maximal in spring and minimal in summer [26].

In this work, the PAS-positive cells did not reveal any significant positive reaction to Best's carmine. Similar results were observed in dogs [5], buffalo bulls [48], and ferrets [68], where glycogen could not be observed in the prostate of these animals. These results were contrary to those observed in one-day-old poppy, opossum, shrew, camels, and young calves ([5, 11, 23,45, 56], resp.), where fine glycogenic granules were demonstrated in the prostatic glandular epithelium. These glycogen granules might be involved in the metabolic activity of the secretory units of camel's prostate [11].

Similar to that observed in the prostate of boars [6], dogs and cats [69], camels [24, 26], and Viscacha [70], the prostate of the donkey was devoid of any alcianophilic positive reaction. This result was in contrary that observed in the prostate of dogs [71], goats [16], buffalo bulls [12, 17, 48], and ferrets [68] in which the prostatic epithelium contained alcianophilic positive granules.

From the previous results, the secretory materials of the prostate gland of the donkey were neutral mucopolysaccharides and the prostate was suggested to be serous gland while in bulls [8, 72] and buffalo bulls [12, 17] two types of prostatic epithelial cells were recorded: serous and mucous cell types.

In a common agreement with Arcadi [5] Seaman and Winell [22] Brandes and Bourne [73], Miraglia et al. [18], Ali et al. [24], Nasr and Moustafa [11], Sudhakar et al. [45] in the prostate gland of dogs, men, common marmoset. camels, and buffalo bulls, respectively, the prostate of the donkey reacted positively to Sudan black stain. Few sudanophilic granules were distributed in the cytoplasm of the glandular and ductal epithelial cells during spring. During the other seasons, the intensity and amount of sudanophilic granules was increased.

Seasonal variations in the amount of lipid content were observed in the glandular epithelial cells of the prostate of bucks, in which the maximal sudanophilic materials were demonstrated in autumn (active season), while materials collected at the end of spring showed minimal lipid contents [15] This was on contrary to that observed in the prostate of goats [16] and buffalo bulls [48], which were free from sudanophilic materials.

The secretory materials of the prostate of domestic animals increased spermatozoal motility and contributed to vaginal plug formation. In bulls, the secretory fluids contain high quantities of fructose and citric acid; however, little else is known regarding its function [1]. In stallions, the prostatic secretion forms about 25–30% of the total volume of the ejaculate, and its function is to neutralize the seminal plasma, made acid by accumulation of metabolic carbon dioxide and lactate, and to initiate active movements of the ejaculated spermatozoa [19]. Also, Dym [74] reported that the prostatic secretion of men was colourless fluid that contained zinc, citric acid, and numerous proteolytic enzymes. The most potent one was fibrinolysin, which played a role in liquefaction of semen.

In conclusion, the prostate gland of donkey appeared more active during spring, which is manifested by increase in the epithelial height, decrease in the interstitial connective tissue glandular tissue ratio, and strong PAS reactivity in the epithelial lining of the secretory end pieces. This reactivity decreased during other seasons of the year. Minimal reactivity was recorded during winter.

ACKNOWLEDGMENTS

The authors would like to express deep thanks for Assiut University for funding of the project. Grateful thanks were extended for lab technicians in the Department of Anatomy and Histology, Assiut University for their grateful help.

REFERENCES

1. W. J. Banks, Male Reproductive System, Mosby Year Book, St. Louis, Lo, USA, 3rd edition, 1993.
2. M. C. G. Davies Morel, Equine Reproductive Physiology, Breeding and Stud Management, CABI Publishing, 2nd edition, 2003.
3. A. S. Abou-Elhamd, A. O. Salem, and A. A. Selim, "Histological and histochemical studies on the ampulla of the deferent duct of donkey (Equus asinus)," Journal of Advanced Veterinary Research, vol. 2, no. 4, pp. 261–270, 2012.
4. H. A. Bern, "The effects of sex steroids on the sex accessories of the male Dutch rabbit,"American Journal of Anatomy, vol. 84, no. 2, pp. 231–277, 1949.
5. J. A. Arcadi, "Some polysaccharide components of the prostate gland of the dog," The Anatomical Record, vol. 112, no. 3, pp. 593–607, 1952.
6. R. N. Aitken, "A histochemical study of the accessory genital glands of the boar," Journal of Anatomy, vol. 94, pp. 130–142, 1960.
7. R. V. Short, T. Mann, and M. F. Hay, "Male reproductive organs of the African elephant, Loxodonta africana," Journal of Reproduction and Fertility, vol. 13, no. 3, pp. 517–536, 1967.
8. R. A. Kainer, L. C. Faulkner, and M. Abdel-Raouf, "Glands associated with the urethra of the bull," American Journal of Veterinary Research, vol. 30, no. 6, pp. 963–974, 1969.
9. S. Sisson, The Anatomy of the Domestic Animals, vol. 1, W. B. Saunders, Philadelphia, Pa, USA, 1975.
10. D. H. Cormack, "The male reproductive system," in Ham's Histology, J. B. Lippincott, Philadelphia, Pa, USA, 9th edition, 1987.

11. M. T. Nasr and I. A. Moustafa, "Morphohistological and histochemical studies on the prostate gland of the camel (Camelus dromedarius) during different ages," Journal of the Egyptian Veterinary Medical Association, vol. 48, pp. 317–334, 1988.

12. Chandrapal and M. B. L. Bharadwaj, "Microanatomy of corpus prostate in buffalo (Bulbalus bulbalis) at different stages of maturity," Indian Veterinary Journal, vol. 70, pp. 1025–1029, 1993.

13. R. N. Aitken, "Observations on the development of the seminal vesicles, prostate and bulbourethral glands in the ram," Journal of Anatomy, vol. 93, no. 1, pp. 43–51, 1959.

14. E. Aughey, "Histology and histochemistry of the male accessory glands of the red deer,Cervus elaphus L," Journal of Reproduction and Fertility, vol. 18, no. 3, pp. 399–407, 1969.

15. A. Selim A, Histological and histochemical studies on the accessory genital glands of balady buck with special references to seasonal changes [M.S. thesis], Assiut University, Assiut, Egypt, 1974.

16. K. H. Wrobel, "Histochemical examinations of the prostatic parenchyma in the goat,"Zentralblatt für Veterinärmedizin C, vol. 1, pp. 64–72, 1972.

17. A. Abou-Elmagd and K. H. Wrobel, "The periurethral glandular complex in the water buffalo: an ultrastructural, histological and lectin-histochemical study," Archives of Histology and Cytology, vol. 52, no. 5, pp. 501–512, 1989.

18. T. Miraglia, M. Telles Filho, and A. L. Branco, "The male reproductive system of the common marmoset (Callithrix jacchus)," Acta Anatomica, vol. 76, no. 4, pp. 594–611, 1970.

19. K. H. Wrobel and H. D. Dellmann, "Male reproductive system," in Textbook of Veterinary Histology, H.-D. P. Dellmann, Ed., Lea & Febiger, Philadelphia, Pa, USA, 4th edition, 1993.

20. A. E. Aly and A. A. Khabir, "The ultrastructure of normal prostatic acini of the camel (Camelus dromedarius)," Zagazig Veterinary Journal, vol. 13, pp. 79–89, 1986.

21. M. B. Amin and D. G. Bostwick, "Pigment in prostatic epithelium and adenocarcinoma: a potential source of diagnostic confusion

with seminal vesicular epithelium," Modern Pathology, vol. 9, no. 7, pp. 791–795, 1996.

22. A. R. Seaman and M. Winell, "The ultrafine structure of the normal prostate gland of the dog," Acta Anatomica, vol. 51, pp. 1–28, 1962.
23. U. Kanwar and C. Sheikher, "Morphological and cytochemical studies on the shrew prostate gland," Acta Anatomica, vol. 98, no. 2, pp. 194–198, 1977.
24. H. A. Ali, K. A. Moniem, and M. D. Tingari, "Some histochemical studies on the prostate, urethral and bulbourethral glands of the one humped camel (Camelus dromedarius)," Histochemical Journal, vol. 8, no. 6, pp. 565–578, 1976.
25. A. A. Abbas, Histological and histochemical studies of the accessory genital glands of the balady ram with special reference to age and seasonal variations [M.S. thesis], Faculty of Veterinary Medicine, Zagazig University, 1976.
26. E.-S. M. Mosallam, Histological and histochemical studies of the male accessory glands of the adult camel (Camelus dromedarius) in the different seasons of the year [Ph.D. thesis], Cairo, Egypt, 1981.
27. H. F. Harris, "On the rapid conversion of haematoxylin into haematin in staining reactions," Journal of Applied Microscopy and Laboratory Methods, vol. 3, p. 777, 1900.
28. J. D. Bancroft and A. Steven, Theory and Practice of Histological Techniques, Churchill Livingstone, New York, NY, USA, 4th edition, 1996.
29. G. Crossmon, "A modification of Mallory's connective tissue with a discussion of principles involved," The Anatomical Record, vol. 69, pp. 33–38, 1937. View at Publisher· View at Google Scholar
30. P. Böck, Romeis Mikroskopishe Technik, vol. 17, Urban und Schwarzenberg, München, Germany, 1989.
31. F. H. Verhoeff, "Some new staining methods of wide applicability. Including a rapid differential stain for elastic tissue," The Journal of the American Medical Association, vol. 50, p. 876, 1908.
32. J. D. Bancroft and A. Steven, Theory and Practice of Histological Techniques, Churchill Livingstone, New York, NY, USA, 4th edition, 1996.

33. G. Gomori, "Silver impregnation of reticulum in paraffin sections," The American Journal of Pathology, vol. 13, no. 6, pp. 993–1002, 1937.
34. J. F. A. McManus, "Histological demonstration of mucin after periodic acid," Nature, vol. 158, no. 4006, p. 202, 1946.
35. H. F. Steedman, "Alcian blue 8GS; a new stain for mucin," The Quarterly Journal of Microscopical Science, vol. 91, pp. 477–479, 1950.
36. R. W. Mowry, "Observations on the use of sulphuric ether for the sulphation of hydroxyl groups in tissue sections," Journal of Histochemistry & Cytochemistry, vol. 4, p. 407, 1956.
37. F. Best, "Über karmin Färbung des Glykogens und der Kerne," Zeitsch. Wissenschaft. Microsk. & Mikrosk. Technick, vol. 23, pp. 319–322, 1906.
38. O. B. Bayliss and C. W. M. Adams, "Bromine-Sudan Black: a general stain for lipids including free cholesterol," The Histochemical Journal, vol. 4, no. 6, pp. 505–515, 1972.View at Publisher · View at Google Scholar ·
39. A. Trautmann and J. Fiebiger, "The male genital organs," in Fundamentals of the Histology of Domestic Animals, R. E. Habel and E. L. Biberstein, Eds., Comstock Publishing Associates Itheca, New York, NY, USA, 1957, translated and revised from 8th and 9th German.
40. R. Nickel, A. Schummer, and E. Seiferle, "Male genital organs," in The Viscera of the Domestic Mammals, Paul Parey, Berlin, Germany, 1st edition, 1973, translated and revised by Sack W. O.
41. K. M. Dyce, W. O. Sack, and C. J. G. Wensing, "The urogenital apparatus," in Textbook of Veterinary Anatomy, W. B. Saunders, Philadelphia, Pa, USA, 2nd edition, 1996.
42. M. F. A. Fahmy and A. M. H. Osman, "Certain morphological investigations on the male genital organs of water buffalo as guide for andrological diagnosis. IV. Accessory glands," Egyptian Journal of Veterinary Science, vol. 9, pp. 56–65, 1972.
43. G. Fehér and A. Haraszti, "Beiträge zur Morphologie und zu den altersbedingten Veranderungen der akzessorischen Geschlechtsdrüsen von Stieren," Acta Veterinaria Hungarica, vol. 14, pp. 141–145, 1964.

44. L. S. Sudhakar, L. D. Dhingra, and D. N. Sharma, "Histomorphological studies on the pars disseminata of the prostate gland of Murrah buffalo during postnatal development," Indian Journal of Animal Sciences, vol. 55, pp. 847–853, 1985.
45. L. S. Sudhakar, L. D. Dhingra, and D. N. Sharma, "Histochemical studies on the prostate gland of Murrah Buffalo during postnatal development," Indian Veterinary Journal, vol. 62, pp. 221–226, 1985.
46. H. A. Ali, M. D. Tingari, and K. A. Moniem, "On the morphology of the accessory male glands and histochemistry of the ampulla ductus deferentis of the camel (Camelus dromedarius)," Journal of Anatomy, vol. 125, no. 2, pp. 277–292, 1978.
47. A. B. A. Badawy, R. S. A. Ragab, and H. I. Youssef, "Histological and biochemical observations on the accessory reproductive glands of castrated camels," Journal of the Egyptian Veterinary Medical Association, vol. 42, pp. 113–120, 1982.
48. M. H. G. Moussa, A. B. A. Badawy, M. H. A. Kandil, and Y. M. Shahin, "Histological and histochemical studies of the accessory genital glands of buffalo-bull (Bubalis bubalis),"Anatomischer Anzeiger, vol. 153, no. 5, pp. 429–439, 1983.
49. S. S. Rochel, A. Bruni-Cardoso, S. R. Taboga, P. S. L. Vilamaior, and R. M. Góes, "Lobe identity in the Mongolian gerbil prostatic complex: a new rodent model for prostate study," Anatomical Record, vol. 290, no. 10, pp. 1233–1247, 2007. View at Publisher ·View at Google Scholar ·
50. D. H. Cormack, "The male reproductive system," in Essential Histology, Lippincott-Ravanen, Philadelphia, Pa, USA, 1st edition, 1997.
51. T. S. Yao and O. N. Eaton, "Postnatal growth and histological development of reproductive organs in male goats," The American Journal of Anatomy, vol. 95, no. 3, pp. 401–431, 1954.
52. A. Tsukise and K. Yamada, "Histochemistry of glycoconjugates in the secretory epithelium of the goat bulbourethral gland," Acta Anatomica, vol. 129, no. 4, pp. 344–352, 1987.
53. S. C. Jacobs, B. A. Beehler, and G. Boese, "The prostate of the gorilla," Prostate, vol. 5, no. 6, pp. 597–603, 1984.

54. A. Abou-Elmagd, "Morphologische Untersuchungen an Wandepithel und Anhangsdrüsen der Urethra des mannlichen Wasserbüffels (Bubalis bubalis)," inInaugural-Dissertation zur Erlangung der Tiermedizinischen Doktorwürde der Tierärztlichen, Fakultät der Ludwig-Maximilians-Universität, München, Germany, 1988.
55. J. A. Chandler, B. G. Timms, M. S. Morton, and G. V. Groom, "Proceedings: effect of cadmium administration in vivo on plasma testosterone and the ultrastructure of accessory sex organs of the rat," Journal of Endocrinology, vol. 69, no. 3, p. 21, 1976.
56. Z. Hruban, J. Martan, A. Slesers, D. F. Steiner, M. Lubran, and M. Rechcigl Jr., "Fine structure of the prostatic epithelium of the opossum (Didelphis virginiana Kerr),"Journal of Experimental Zoology, vol. 160, no. 1, pp. 81–105, 1965.
57. C. Hohbach and H. Ueberberg, "Ultrastructural and histochemical aspects of prostatic secretion in the dog," Pathology Research and Practice, vol. 173, no. 3, pp. 225–235, 1982.
58. H. E. S. Marei, H. A. El-Habback, and K. F. Abou-Esa, "Histology, fine structure and carbohydrate histochmistry of the epithelium of the accessory male genital glands of the Egyptian balady goat," Veterinary Medical Journal Giza, vol. 52, pp. 165–182, 2004.
59. J. Muntzing, H. Myhrberg, and J. Saroff, "Histochemical and ultrastructural study of prostatic tissue from baboons treated with antiprostatic drugs." Investigative Urology, vol. 14, no. 2, pp. 162–167, 1976.
60. J. B. Brennick, J. X. O›Connell, G. R. Dickersin, and R. H. Young, "Lipofuscin pigmentation (so-called "melanosis") of the prostate," American Journal of Surgical Pathology, vol. 18, no. 5, pp. 446–454, 1994.
61. Y.-J. Niu, T.-X. Ma, J. Zhang, Y. Xu, R.-F. Han, and G. Sun, "Androgen and prostatic stroma," Asian Journal of Andrology, vol. 5, no. 1, pp. 19–26, 2003.
62. M. Jara, R. Carballada, and P. Esponda, "Age-induced apoptosis in the male genital tract of the mouse," Reproduction, vol. 127, no. 3, pp. 359–366, 2004.
63. J. Muntzing and T. Nilsson, "Lipofuscin in malignant and non-malignant human prostatic tissue," Zeitschrift für Krebsforschung

und klinische Onkologie, vol. 77, no. 2, pp. 166–170, 1972. View at Publisher · View at Google Scholar

64. M. Garcia-Florez, C. A. Oliveira, and H. F. Carvalho, "Early effects of estrogen on the rat ventral prostate," Brazilian Journal of Medical and Biological Research, vol. 38, no. 4, pp. 487–497, 2005.
65. S. A. Thompson, D. R. Rowley, and P. M. Heidger Jr., "Effects of estrogen upon the fine structure of epithelium and stroma in the rat ventral prostate gland," Investigative Urology, vol. 17, no. 1, pp. 83–89, 1979.
66. Z. Weihua, M. Warner, and J.-Å. Gustafsson, "Estrogen receptor beta in the prostate,"Molecular and Cellular Endocrinology, vol. 193, no. 1-2, pp. 1–5, 2002. View at Publisher· View at Google Scholar ·
67. V. E. Filotto and P. Mongiardini, "Ricerche istochimiche sulle ghiandole annesse allápparato genitale maschile di (Lepus cuniculus)," Folia Clinica et Biologica, vol. 30, pp. 239–250, 1961.
68. S. Jacob and S. Poddar, "Morphology and histochemistry of the ferret prostate," Acta Anatomica, vol. 125, no. 4, pp. 268–273, 1986.
69. M. Wrobel, "Histochemical and electron microscopical examinations of the prostate gland in dog and cat," Zentralblatt für Veterinärmedizin C, vol. 1, pp. 93–116, 1972.
70. E. M. Chaves, C. Aguilera-Merlo, V. Filippa, F. Mohamed, S. Dominguez, and L. Scardapane, "Anatomical, histological and immunohistochemical study of the reproductive system accessory glands in male viscacha (Lagostomus maximusmaximus)," Journal of Veterinary Medicine Series C, vol. 40, no. 1, pp. 11–20, 2011. View at Publisher · View at Google Scholar ·
71. A. R. Seaman, "Cytological observation on the prostate gland of the dog," The Anatomical Record, vol. 118, p. 353, 1954.
72. J. Schencker, "Zur funktionellen Anatomie der Prostata des Rindes," Acta Anatomica, vol. 9, pp. 69–102, 1965.
73. D. Brandes and G. H. Bourne, "Histochemistry of the human prostate: normal and neoplastic," The Journal of Pathology and Bacteriology, vol. 71, no. 1, pp. 33–36, 1956.

74. M. Dym, "The male reproductive system," in Histology, Cell and Tissue Biology, L. Weiss, Ed., Macmillan Press, 5th edition, 1983.

Chapter 9

Role of Membrane Lipid Fatty Acids in Sperm Cryopreservation

Rajes Mandal, Damodar Badyakar, and Jitamanyu Chakrabarty

Department of Chemistry, National Institute of Technology, Durgapur, West Bengal 713209, India

ABSTRACT

Lipid is an important constituent of cell membrane. Membrane lipid composition of spermatozoa has been correlated to different function. Many researchers have related membrane lipid with survival success after cryopreservation or cold shock. Sperm maturation and acrosome reactions are natural phenomenon, but cryopreservation or cold shock is not. Therefore, sperm cells are not programmed for such change and undergo stress. So the change in membrane lipid composition due to cold shock or cryopreservation may be looked upon as response of spermatozoa to a certain stressed condition. A significant body of research worked on the relationship between membrane lipid and fatty acid composition and ability of cell to tolerate adverse change in temperature. However, as the approach of different research groups was different, it is very difficult to compare the changes. Studies have been done with different species, ejaculated/seminal or epididymal sperm. Lipid analyses have been done with whole cell membrane isolated by different methods. Fatty acids estimated were from whole cell, plasma membrane, head membrane, or phospholipids. The cryopreservation condition, media composition, and diluents/cryoprotectants were also different. At this onset a comprehensive review is needed to cover changes of sperm membrane lipid composition of different species under different cryopreservation conditions.

INTRODUCTION

Sperm cell is unique in many respects including structure and function. It is capable of fertilizing egg; it functions in a body different from its origin and gender. Its plasma membrane is also different from most other cell membranes in lipid composition. It contains high amount of polyunsaturated fatty acids (PUFA), especially diPUFA (phospholipids esterified with two PUFA), which is found only in sperm, retina, and certain brain areas [1, 2]. In particular, PUFA are known to contribute to membrane fluidity and flexibility [3–5]. Membrane lipid composition has been related to their specific functions, because it promotes the creation of microdomains with different fluidity, fusogenicity, and permeability characteristics [2], required for reaching and fusing with the oocyte.

Phospholipids are the most representative lipid fraction of the sperm cell membranes, of which phosphatidylcholine, phosphatidylethanolamine, and sphingomyelin are the major components [6]. Lipid and fatty acid composition of sperm cells differ not only for different animals [7, 8] but also for different species [9–12], even for fertile and subfertile population of same species [13–15].

The definite lipid pattern of ejaculated spermatozoa is reached only after epididymal maturation. Plasma membrane lipids of the goat [16], ram [17], and boar [18] spermatozoa have been shown to undergo marked changes during epididymal maturation. The lipid content of whole sperm decreases during epididymal maturation in boar, bull, ram, and rat [19–26], and the cholesterol content decreases in ram, rat, and hamster sperm [27–29]. The cholesterol : phospholipid ratio and concentration of phosphatidylserine, phosphatidylethanolamine, cardiolipin, and ethanolamine plasmalogen decrease in whole ram sperm [20, 27]. However, increases occur in the amount of the sulphoconjugated sterols in whole hamster and human sperm [28–30] and in unsaturated fatty acids in whole ram sperm [27]. Studies using plasma membrane isolated from boar spermatozoa confirm earlier results with whole sperm that the amount of lipid decreases during epididymal maturation [18]. Although there is a decrease in cholesterol, no significant change is seen in the cholesterol : phospholipid ratio. There are also decreases in phosphatidyl ethanolamine and phosphatidyl inositol as well as increases in dermosterol, cholesterol sulphate, phosphatidylcholine, and polyphosphoinositides. There is a decrease in the level of fatty acids and an increase in diacylglycerol but no change in the degree of saturation of fatty acids. Plasma membrane from the anterior head region of ram sperm is particularly rich in ethanolamine and choline phosphoglycerides [17]. The amount of dermosterol and ethanolamine in this region of the plasma membrane decreases whereas the cholesterol : phospholipid ratio increases, during epididymal maturation. The goat sperm plasma membrane is particularly rich in ether lipids phosphatidylcholine and phosphatidylethanolamine. Of all the membrane phospholipids, diacyl phosphatidylethanolamine decreases most strikingly (approx. 65%) during epididymal maturation of sperm [16].

Changes in the amount and composition of lipids in the plasma membrane of sperm during maturation are thought to explain why ejaculated sperm is more sensitive to cold shock than is testicular sperm [31, 32]. These changes may also account for the maturation-dependent decrease in charge density at the phospholipid-water interface of ram spermatozoa, detected by electron spin resonance [31] and the decrease in membrane fluidity of bull spermatozoa, seen by fluorescence polarization spectroscopy [33]. Analysis of testicular and ejaculated ram spermatozoa by fluorescence recovery after photobleaching (FRAP) indicates that there are regional differences in the decrease of plasma membrane fluidity [34]. During maturation, the diffusion rate of fluorescent lipid analogue increases in all regions of the sperm except the midpiece.

CHANGES IN LIPID ASSOCIATED WITH CRYOPRESERVATION

Cryopreservation affects sperm membrane integrity [35, 36]. Differences in fatty acid composition and lipid class ratios in spermatozoa among species are important factors in the freezability of the male gametes [37] (the different animals/species and cryopreservation methods are summarized in Table 1). According to Pettitt and Buhr [38] freezing and thawing results in lipid modifications and domains of sperm head plasma membrane react differently to cryopreservation. Furthermore, some studies [39, 40] investigated the ability of sperm cells to take up lipid components or fatty acids from the surrounding environment during incubation in vitro [41].

Table 1: Different animals/species and cryopreservation methods

Animal	Cryopreservation methods	Reference number
Human		
	Semen was diluted using human sperm preservation medium, TEST-Yolk buffer, or glycerol, subjected to slow manual cooling in liquid nitrogen (LN_2) vapour, and stored in LN_2.	[47]
	The procedure is based on the program of cooling speed doubling: from 20 to 5°C at 0.5°C/min; from 5 to 4°C at 1°C/min; from 4 to 3°C at 2°C/min; from 3 to 2°C at 4°C/min; from 2 to 1°C at 8°C/min; from 1 to −80°C at 10°C/min. After being held 10 minutes at the final temperature, −80°C then were transferred to LN_2.	[62]

	Normozoospermic, oligozoospermic, astheno-zoospermic, and oligoasthenozoospermic semen samples were frozen in pellets on the surface of dry ice using a glycerol-based cryoprotectant with egg yolk.	[65]
	Sperm cells were frozen or cold-shocked by lowering the temp. rapidly from 37 to 0°C on melting ice.	[66]
	Sperm cells were frozen using the programme: from 20 to −4°C at 5°C/min; from −4 to −30°C at 10°C/min; from −30 to −140°C at 20°C/min and then were transferred for storage to LN_2.	[67]
Ram and goat		
Merino rams	Ejaculates were obtained by electrical stimulation. Semen was also collected from the caput and cauda epididymis. Spermatozoa were cold-shocked by placing tubes containing the semen held at 37°C into a bath at 0°C for 10 min.	[20]
Zandi rams	The diluted semen was cooled at 4 to 5°C for 2 h. Then the samples were placed into the LN_2 vapor at a height of 4 cm above the liquid for 8 minutes, and then the straws were plunged into LN_2.	[80]
Goat	Epididymal sperms were cryopreserved using programmable freezer: from 30 ± 2° to 5°C at 0.25°C min, from 5 to −20°C at 5°C min, and from −20 to −100°C at 20°C min then transferred to LN_2.	[81]
Goat	Semen was frozen in pellet form on dry ice, and then plunged into LN_2.	[82]
Mahabadi bucks	Ejaculated semen samples were diluted and equilibrated at 5°C for 150 min. Samples were frozen in LN_2 vapor, 4 cm above the L, for 7 min; subsequently the straws were plunged into the LN_2 for storage.	[83]

Blanca-Celtiberica buck	Diluted semen was cooled to 5°C for 2 h, diluted further, and held at 5°C for 2 h; another sample was cooled to 5°C for 4 h; both samples were frozen over N_2 vapour for 10 min, 4 cm above N_2 level, plunged, and stored in LN_2.	[84]
San Clemente bucks and Tennessee Myotonic buck	Semen aliquots were cooled on ice for 1 h before transfer to a 5°C refrigerator and kept for total of 1-2 h; then extender was added. Fully extended semen was equilibrated at 5°C for 2 h. Semen was frozen by suspending straws in N_2 vapour for 10 min, then plunging into LN_2.	[85]
Saanen bucks	Semen samples were cryopreserved using programmable freezer using a fast freezing curve (from 25°C to 5°C at 0.25°C/min and from 5°C to −120°C at 20°C/min) that started at 28°C. After reaching a temperature of 5°C (~80 min), the straws were subjected to an equilibration time for 120 min. The freezing curve was implemented immediately after the equilibration time and was sustained until the temperature reached −120°C, then were placed in LN_2.	[87]
Spanish ibex (Capra pyrenaica)	The diluted sperm suspension was cooled to 13°C in a water bath, further cooled to 5°C over 1 h, kept for 2 more h, and frozen by placing in N_2 vapour 5 cm above the surface of LN_2 for 10 min before plunging into the LN_2 .	[102]
Bull		
Friesian bull	Semen was cooled to 5°C over 30 min, equilibrated for 6 h at 5°C, and frozen above the surface of LN_2 (a temperature of −120°C was attained in 7 min).	[73]
Holstein bulls	Semen was cooled to 5°C in 1 h; after 4 h it was pellet-frozen on solid CO_2.	[74]

Holstein, Jersey, and Guernsey	The semen was cooled immediately after collection to 15 to 20°C and held at this temperature for one-half to one hour; then diluted semen was cooled slowly to a storage temperature between 4 and 7°C.	[76]
Prim Holstein	Electroejaculated semen samples were cooled from 34 to 4°C in 1.5 h, held for 2 h, and then descended in LN_2. Rate: 4 to −10°C at 0. 7°C/10 s; −10 to −150°C at 7°C/10 s.	[77]
Holstein	Fresh sperm samples were cooled to 4°C and held for 1 h (addition of diluent). Cryostraws were placed ~5 cm above the LN_2 surface for 10 min and then put directly into the LN_2 for storage	[78]
Swiss brown bull	Diluted semen was cooled to 4-5°C over 2 h and then frozen by being placed into the LN_2 vapor at a height of 4 cm above the liquid for 8 min; after that, the straws were plunged into LN_2.	[79]
Boar		
	The semen was cooled to 22°C over 2 h and further cooled to 5°Cover 3 h by placing in a cold room. Samples were then frozen in LN_2 vapors at 30°C/min from 5°C a final temperature of −70°C. Then straws were plunged directly into LN_2.	[38]
Norwegian Landrace and Duroc	The diluted semen was cooled at 15°C over 3 h and then cooled to 4°C over 2 h period. Semen was frozen in a controlled rate freezer for 9 min. The freezing chamber was precooled to −100°C. Immediately after the straws were transferred to the chamber it was warmed at 10°C/min to −70°C and held for 1 min before lowering the temperature to −120°C at 50°C /min. The straws were held at −120°C for 4 min before transferring to LN_2.	[11]

Landrace, Large White, and commercial hybrids	Semen was cooled at 15°C for 3 h and was further cooled in a programmable freezer to 5°C over 90 min; samples were cryopreserved using programmable freezer. The freezing chamber was precooled to −110°C. Immediately after loading the straws it was warmed at 45°C/min to −60°C and held for 1 min before lowering the temperature to −130°C at 20°C/min. The straws were plunged into LN_2.	[41, 90]
Marsupial		
Eastern grey kangaroo (Macropus giganteus)	Epididymal sperms were subjected to cold shock by rapid cooling.	[91]
Koala (Phascolarctos cinereus)		
Common wombat (Vombatus ursinus)		
Canine samples		
Blue fox (Alopex lagopus)	Semen was cryopreserved in different extenders; FA and sterols of plasma membrane were analysed.	[10]
Red/silver fox (Vulpes vulpes)	Cooling at a moderate rate (2–5°C/min from 4-5°C to below the freezing point, i.e., from −7 to −15 or −20°C) and freezing at a rapid rate from −20 to −50 or −70°C.	[92, 94,95]

Dog	Cooling at a moderate rate (2–5°C/min from 4-5°C to below the freezing point, i.e., from −7 to −15 or −20°C) and freezing at a rapid rate from −20 to −50 or −70°C.	[94]
Beagle and Golden Retriever	The samples were maintained at a temperature of 4°C for total 1 h 30 min. Then the canine semen was frozen in LN_2 vapours (4 cm above the level of the LN_2) at −110°C for 10 min then immersed vertically in LN_2 for storage at −196°C.	[99]
Elephant		
African Elephant (Loxodonta Africana)	Ejaculated semen samples were stored at −70°C or cryopreserved in LN_2.	[9]
Asian Elephant (Elephas maximus)		
Stallion		
Andalusian stallions	The spermatozoa were slowly cooled to 4°C within 1 h and frozen horizontally in racks placed 4 cm above the surface of LN_2 for 10 min, after which they were directly plunged in LN_2.	[100, 101]
Bats/flying fox		

Indian flying-fox (Pteropus giganteus)	Electroejaculated semen samples were cooled at 50°C/min to 4°C.	[12]
Variable flying-fox (Pteropus hypomelanus)		
Grey-headed flying-fox (Pteropus poliocephalus)		
Rodrigues flying-fox (Pteropus rodricensis)		
Large flying-fox (Pteropus vampyrus)		

The major problem associated with cryopreservation of sperm cells is the loss of viability using freeze thaw process [36, 42–54]. Loss of viability is related to membrane leakiness which is induced by sperm phospholipids peroxidation [55, 56]. Different workers have assessed the effect of cryopreservation on sperm membrane fatty acid composition in different species including human.

Human System

Human sperm cryopreservation is considered to be an important therapeutic option with several practical applications [57, 58]. Analyses of the fatty acid pattern of membrane phospholipids and plasmalogen of human spermatozoa have demonstrated significant levels of PUFAs [59]. The major damage caused during cryopreservation is peroxidation of lipids especially phospholipid bound polyunsaturated fatty acids (PUFAs) [60, 61]. But it is also established that membrane stress rather than lipid peroxidation is related to sublethal cryodamage [62]. The lipid composition of whole spermatozoa is well documented [7, 59].

According to Schiller et al. [63], significant changes in lipid composition are associated with freezing/thawing. They suggested that matrix-assisted laser desorption and ionization time-of-flight (MALDI-TOF) mass spectra revealed clear differences between the spermatozoa and the seminal plasma as well as between the native and the cryopreserved spermatozoa. The concentration of 1-stearoyl and 1-palmitoyl-2-docosahexaenoyl-sn-glycero-3-phosphocholine shows rapid decrease following cryopreservation. Alvarez and Storey reported a reduction of some fatty acids in human spermatozoa after freezing, with a reduction in PUFA C18:2, C20:3, C20:4, and docosahexaenoic acid (C22:6 n-3; DHA) and an increase of the saturated fatty acid (SFA) C: 16 and SFA C: 18 after freezing [64]. Martínez-Soto et al. [65] confirmed a strong correlation between the fatty acid composition of the human spermatozoa or seminal plasma and the sperm parameters of the samples after thawing. They described a significant correlation between the fatty acid composition of the human spermatozoa or seminal plasma and the sperm parameters of the samples after thawing. PUFA, n-3, and specially DHA are directly correlated with sperm motility and viability after freezing/thawing, and monounsaturated fatty acids (MUFA) were inversely correlated. They also suggested that in the future the fatty acid composition could be used as a predictor of the capacity of cryopreservation of a seminal sample. The susceptibility of spermatozoa to rapid cold shock has been associated with a high ratio of membrane PUFA:SFA and with low levels of cholesterol within the sperm membrane [8]. Lipid diffusion which is reflected in the dynamics of the recovery of the lipid reporter probe ODAF [5-(N-octadecanoyl) aminofluorescein] during FRAP is significantly reduced after thawing in all regions of spermatozoa [66]. Correlation between fluidity and postthaw recoveries of motile and viable spermatozoa showed that there is marked variation between membrane anisotropy values, which were significantly high in cryopreserved samples compared to fresh samples. Furthermore, recovery of motile and viable spermatozoa is strongly correlated to anisotropy of fresh spermatozoa. The higher the membrane fluidity before freezing, the better the response of spermatozoa to cryopreservation [67] As PUFAs can influence membrane fluidity, it is not surprising to see that membrane fluidity is a predictor of cryogenic success in humans.

Other Systems

Apart from human spermatozoa other animal systems were also subjected to cryopreservation. The changes associated with lipid composition were studied thoroughly in animal spermatozoa like boar, bovine, marsupials, goat, ram, fowl, and so forth. The ability to cryopreserve spermatozoa from all of the domestic species is challenging. Even though all of the cells must endure similar physical stresses associated with the cryopreservation processes, sperm from the different species is very different in size, shape, and lipid composition, all of which affect cryosurvival. Thus, when a cryopreservation protocol has been optimized for sperm of one species, it may not be ideal for sperm of the other .

Cattle System

Increased concentrations of free cholesterol, free fatty acids, triacylglycerol, and cholesterol ester are associated with decreased sperm motility and fertility [69]. It is also elucidated from the works of bull semen that increased age of bulls has an inverse correlation with the fatty acid composition, especially PUFA and DHA. It is suggested by Argov-Argaman et al. [70] that such alterations might affect the semen's capacity to successfully undergo the cryopreservation procedures, which are widely used in intensive reproduction management.

Egg yolk is widely used and generally accepted as an essential ingredient in diluents employed for the freezing of bovine spermatozoa for use in artificial insemination (AI). It is known to be an efficient protectant of spermatozoa from cooling/thawing [71]. Different forms of lipid extracts confer cryoprotection to frozen spermatozoa [72]. Foulkes and Stewart [73] have demonstrated the maintenance of fertility in spermatozoa frozen in an egg yolk lipoprotein. Irreversible binding of egg yolk lipoprotein and its role in cryopreservation are well elucidated through immunological investigations [72]. Some authors are reluctant in using the whole egg yolk as an extender for cryopreservation as it diminishes the respiration and motility of spermatozoa [74–76]. Thus easy techniques for extraction of the essential part, low density lipoprotein (LDL), needed for cryopreservation have been suggested and it is also commented that LDL extenders have improved ability in retaining sperm viability and motility compared to the commercial extenders of egg yolk [77]. A comparative study of egg yolk from five avian species as cryoprotectant showed that pigeon egg yolk has the highest success after thawing in bull sperm [78]. Addition of bull semen extender with n-3 fatty acid and α-tocopherol enhanced postthaw sperm characteristics. Before semen freezing, percent DHA was higher in fatty acid treatment than that in the group without fatty acid and decreased significantly in both groups after thawing. A plausible reason for this decrease could be excessive lipid peroxidation during cryopreservation of sperm. This is due to excessive peroxidation as suggested earlier. But addition of α-tocopherol is effective and can reverse the effect [79]. Similar works in ram semen also showed similar result with FA and α-tocopherol [80]. According to Chakrabarty et al. [81], total lipid and its components, that is, neutral lipids, glycolipids, and phospholipids, decreased significantly after cryopreservation in case of goat semen. Among neutral lipids sterols, steryl esters and 1-O-alkyl-2,3-diacyl glycerol decreased appreciably, while, among phospholipids, major loss was observed for phosphatidylcholine and phosphatidylethanolamine. Unsaturated fatty acids bound to the phospholipids diminished while the percentage of saturated acids increased. Addition of egg yolk plays a major role during the freezing step of goat cryopreservation and the addition of trehalose significantly improved its cryoprotectant activity. Furthermore, neither glycerol nor egg yolk alone could reduce the intact acrosome percentage; however, combination of these two protectants significantly reduces the percentage of intact acrosome spermatozoa [82]. Salmani et al. [83] have suggested the use of soyabean-lecithin which is a suitable plant based cryoprotectant for caprine sperms. The beneficial effects of soyabean-lecithin as a substitute for egg yolk during cryopreservation of goat sperm are established in the works of Jiménez-Rabadán et al., Roof et al., Salmani et al., and Vidal et al. [84–87].

Boar System

The fatty acid composition of boar spermatozoa is interesting, since they contain some 25% docosapentaenoic acid (C22:5 n-6; DPA) and 30% DHA [88, 89]. Maldjian et al. [90] have reported a decrease in long chain PUFA and an increase in SFA taken up or passively bound to the spermatozoan membranes. Another distinct change in lipid content was that in the spermatozoan cholesterol level. A study on two different breeds (Norwegian Landrace and Duroc) of boar semen revealed no significant difference between breeds; however, there were significant male-to-male variations within breeds in postthaw percentages of live sperm. The most abundant fatty acids in the plasma membranes from both breeds were palmitic acid (C16:0), stearic acid (C18:0), oleic acid (C18:1 n-9), DPA, and DHA. The ratio of and all other membrane fatty acids was significantly related to survival rate (plasma membrane integrity) of sperm for both Norwegian Landrace and Duroc boars. Thus Waterhouse et al. [11] concluded that male-to-male differences in sperm survival rate after freezing and thawing may be partly related to the amount of long-chain PUFA in the sperm plasma membranes.

Marsupial System

Marsupial spermatozoa isolated from cauda epididymis had higher levels of long chain PUFA in membrane as compared to spermatozoa isolated from caput epididymis. A study conducted in Kangaroo, Koala, and Wombat confirmed the presence of high PUFA and a high ratio of unsaturated/saturated fatty acids, whereas cholesterol levels are found to be very low in all three species. According to White [8], cold shock resistance is related to high levels of membrane sterols and a low ratio of unsaturated/saturated membrane fatty acids. But the spermatozoa of the koala, common wombat, and Eastern grey kangaroo had very low levels of membrane sterols and very high ratios of unsaturated/ saturated membrane fatty acids, but are still resistant to cold shock injury [91].

Other Mammalian Systems

The wild blue or arctic fox (Alopex lagopus), is a canid species that has declining population densities within the northernmost regions of North America and Eurasia [92, 93]. The causes of the population decline of the wild blue fox within artic areas, particularly in Fennoscandia, have been attributed to urban expansion into the countryside and growing competition with the closely related and widely abundant red fox (Vulpes vulpes). Thus artificial insemination (AI) is an efficient tool for increasing the population. While spermatozoa collected from the silver fox can be frozen [94, 95], these same protocols and permutations of these protocols have failed to satisfactorily preserve blue fox spermatozoa [94, 95]. Miller et al. [10] carried out experiments in farmed blue fox and silver fox (a colour mutant of red fox) to study the lipid composition in the sperm membrane. It revealed higher ratio of unsaturated/saturated fatty acids and cholesterol in silver fox than blue fox. This may be considered as a key component for the difference in success rates of semen samples after thawing.

The continued loss of natural habitats and the limited ability of wildlife parks and zoos to manage and breed wildlife have created a need for new and improved management and breeding strategies [96]. In case of elephants cryogenic, protocols have successfully preserved spermatozoa from African Elephants (Loxodonta africana), but these protocols and their modified forms failed to preserve spermatozoa of Asian Elephants (Elephas maximus). During cryogenic attempts, the spermatozoa of Asian elephants experience extensive acrosomal damage and thereby become useless for future breeding attempts [97, 98]. In Asian and African elephants, the most abundant fatty acid in spermatozoa membranes was DHA, along with lauric acid (C12:0), myristic acid (C14:0), palmitic acid, stearic acid, and oleic acid [9]. It is been concluded that higher levels of DHA in postthaw samples of African elephants may be beneficial for cryopreservation in comparison to Asian elephant. The differences in fatty acid composition can also be due to nutritional difference and genetic difference in fatty acid metabolism between African and Asian elephants [9]. Similarly bull spermatozoa have been successfully cryopreserved and have high levels of DHA; meanwhile boar spermatozoa with low levels of DHA are difficult to freeze [7, 22].

When canine samples were preserved separately with LDL and egg yolk, recovery percentage of sperm motility was higher in samples incubated with LDL. LDL medium also resulted in an improved preservation of spermatozoa during the freezing process in terms of acrosomal integrity, flagellar plasma membrane integrity, and DNA integrity [99].

García et al. [100] also examined the fatty acid and plasmalogen of the phospholipids of the stallion spermatozoa to analyze its relationship with sperm quality after thawing. One of the major drawbacks for the use of frozen thawed semen in equine breeding is the large variation in freezability among stallions. This variability can be explained through susceptibility to lipid peroxidation [101]. As the antioxidant enzymes do not vary considerably among stallions, it is obvious that PUFA and plasmalogens may play a role in such variability.

A study of lipid profile of flying fox (Pteropus) also revealed that stearic acid (C18:0) was the predominant saturated fatty acid and oleic acid (C18:1 n-9) was the predominant unsaturated fatty acid in both acrosomal and plasma membranes. Higher levels of PUFA in the acrosome can attribute to cryogenic success [12]. Chicken egg yolk is the most widely used extender in sperm cryopreservation. But Santiago-Moreno et al. [102] have used Quail egg yolk as an alternative to chicken egg yolk for threatened wild ruminant species, the Spanish ibex. Results showed that this alternative is not a good extender for chicken egg yolk as it provided lower motility and viability.

SCOPE OF FUTURE WORK

Though a good amount of work has been done on the subject discussed above, lack of uniformity provides scope of lot more research work in this field. Change in phospholipids or cholesterol due to cryopreservation drew attention of many researchers as their addition in cryopreservation media provided beneficial effect. Number of works involving change in fatty acids is comparatively very small. Information is wanted with endangered species or animals under captive breeding.

ACKNOWLEDGMENTS

Fellowship of Rajes Mandal by NIT Durgapur is acknowledged.

REFERENCES

1. S. Ladha, "Lipid heterogeneity and membrane fluidity in a highly polarized cell, the mammalian spermatozoon," The Journal of Membrane Biology, vol. 165, no. 1, pp. 1–10, 1998.
2. S. R. Wassall and W. Stillwell, "Polyunsaturated fatty acid-cholesterol interactions: domain formation in membranes," Biochimica et Biophysica Acta: Biomembranes, vol. 1788, no. 1, pp. 24–32, 2009.
3. J. N. Israelachvili, S. Marcelja, and R. G. Horn, "Physical principles of membrane organization.,"Quarterly Reviews of Biophysics, vol. 13, no. 2, pp. 121–200, 1980.
4. A. D. Fleming and R. Yanagimachi, "Effects of various lipids on the acrosome reaction and fertilizing capacity of guinea pig spermatozoa with special reference to the possible involvement of lysophospholipids in the acrosome reaction," Gamete Research, vol. 4, no. 4, pp. 253–273, 1981.
5. S. Meizel and K. O. Turner, "Stimulation of an exocytotic event, the hamster sperm acrosome reaction, by cis-unsaturated fatty acids," FEBS Letters, vol. 161, no. 2, pp. 315–318, 1983.
6. T. Mann and C. Lutwak-Mann, Eds., Male Reproductive Function and Semen, Springer, Berlin, Germany, 1981.
7. A. Poulos, A. Darin Bennett, and I. G. White, "The phospholipid bound fatty acids and aldehydes of mammalian spermatozoa," Comparative Biochemistry and Physiology Part B: Comparative Biochemistry, vol. 46, no. 3, pp. 541–549, 1973.
8. I. G. White, "Lipids and calcium uptake of sperm in relation to cold shock and preservation: a review,"Reproduction, Fertility, and Development, vol. 5, no. 6, pp. 639–658, 1993.
9. J. E. Swain and R. R. Miller Jr., "A postcryogenic comparison of membrane fatty acids of elephant spermatozoa," Zoo Biology, vol. 19, no. 5, pp. 461–473, 2000.

10. R. R. Miller Jr., C. L. Cornett, K. E. Waterhouse, and W. Farstad, "Comparative aspects of sperm membrane fatty acid composition in silver (Vulpes vulpes) and blue (Alopex lagopus) foxes, and their relationship to cell cryopreservation," Cryobiology, vol. 51, no. 1, pp. 66–75, 2005.
11. K. E. Waterhouse, P. O. Hofmo, A. Tverdal, and R. R. Miller Jr., "Within and between breed differences in freezing tolerance and plasma membrane fatty acid composition of boar sperm," Reproduction, vol. 131, no. 5, pp. 887–894, 2006.
12. D. F. Melville, S. D. Johnston, and R. R. Miller Jr., "Flying-fox (Pteropus spp.) sperm membrane fatty acid composition, its relationship to cold shock injury and implications for cryopreservation success,"Cryobiology, vol. 65, no. 3, pp. 224–229, 2012.
13. Y. Aksoy, H. Aksoy, K. Altinkaynak, H. R. Aydin, and A. Özkan, "Sperm fatty acid composition in subfertile men," Prostaglandins Leukotrienes and Essential Fatty Acids, vol. 75, no. 2, pp. 75–79, 2006.
14. H. Tavilani, M. Doosti, I. Nourmohammadi et al., "Lipid composition of spermatozoa in normozoospermic and asthenozoospermic males," Prostaglandins Leukotrienes and Essential Fatty Acids, vol. 77, no. 1, pp. 45–50, 2007.
15. N. Am-in, R. N. Kirkwood, M. Techakumphu, and W. Tantasuparuk, "Lipid profiles of sperm and seminal plasma from boars having normal or low sperm motility," Theriogenology, vol. 75, no. 5, pp. 897–903, 2011.
16. A. P. S. Rana, G. C. Majumder, S. Misra, and A. Ghosh, "Lipid changes of goat sperm plasma membrane during epididymal maturation," Biochimica et Biophysica Acta—Biomembranes, vol. 1061, no. 2, pp. 185–196, 1991.
17. J. E. Parks and R. H. Hammerstedt, "Development changes occurring in the lipids of ram epididymal spermatozoa plasma membrane," Biology of Reproduction, vol. 32, no. 3, pp. 653–668, 1985.
18. M. Nikolopoulou, D. A. Soucek, and J. C. Vary, "Changes in the lipid content of boar sperm plasma membranes during epididymal

maturation," Biochimica et Biophysica Acta, vol. 815, no. 3, pp. 486–498, 1985.

19. R. M. C. Dawson and T. W. Scott, "Phospholipid composition of epididymal spermatozoa prepared by density gradient centrifugation," Nature, vol. 202, no. 4929, pp. 292–293, 1964.
20. P. J. Quinn and I. G. White, "Phospholipid and cholesterol content of epididymal and ejaculated ram spermatozoa and seminal plasma in relation to cold shock," Australian Journal of Biological Sciences, vol. 20, no. 6, pp. 1205–1215, 1967.
21. D. E. Grogan, D. T. Mayer, and J. D. Sikes, "Quantitative differences in phospholipids of ejaculated spermatozoa and spermatozoa from three levels of the epididymis of the boar," Journal of Reproduction and Fertility, vol. 12, no. 3, pp. 431–436, 1966.
22. A. Poulos, J. K. Voglmayr, and I. G. White, "Phospholipid changes in spermatozoa during passage through the genital tract of the bull," Biochimica et Biophysica Acta, vol. 306, no. 2, pp. 194–202, 1973.
23. A. Poulos, P. D. C. Brown-Woodman, I. G. White, and R. I. Cox, "Changes in phospholipids of ram spermatozoa during migration through the epididymis and possible origin of prostaglandin $F_{2\alpha}$ in testicular and epididymal fluid," Biochimica et Biophysica Acta: Lipids and Lipid Metabolism, vol. 388, no. 1, pp. 12–18, 1975.
24. C. Terner, J. MacLaughlin, and B. R. Smith, "Changes in lipase and phosphatase activities of rat spermatozoa in transit from the caput to the cauda epididymidis," Journal of Reproduction and Fertility, vol. 45, no. 1, pp. 1–8, 1975.
25. R. W. Evans and B. P. Setchell, "Lipid changes in boar spermatozoa during epididymal maturation with some observations on the flow and composition of boar rete testis fluid.," Journal of Reproduction and Fertility, vol. 57, no. 1, pp. 189–196, 1979.
26. M. I. Aveldaño, N. P. Rotstein, and N. T. Vermouth, "Lipid remodelling during epididymal maturation of rat spermatozoa. Enrichment in plasmenylcholines containing long-chain polyenoic fatty acids of the n-9 series," Biochemical Journal, vol. 283, no. 1, pp. 235–241, 1992.

27. T. W. Scott, J. K. Voglmayr, and B. P. Setchell, "Lipid composition and metabolism in testicular and ejaculated ram spermatozoa.," Biochemical Journal, vol. 102, no. 2, pp. 456–461, 1967.

28. G. Bleau and W. J. A. VandenHeuvel, "Desmosteryl sulfate and desmosterol in hamster epididymal spermatozoa," Steroids, vol. 24, no. 4, pp. 549–556, 1974.

29. Y. Legault, M. Bouthillier, G. Bleau, A. Chapdelaine, and K. D. Roberts, "The sterol and sterol sulfate content of the male hamster reproductive tract," Biology of Reproduction, vol. 20, no. 5, pp. 1213–1219, 1979.

30. G. Lalumiere, G. Bleau, A. Chapdelaine, and K. D. Roberts, "Cholesteryl sulfate and sterol sulfatase in the human reproductive tract," Steroids, vol. 27, no. 2, pp. 247–260, 1976.

31. R. H. Hammerstedt, A. D. Keith, S. Hay, N. Deluca, and R. P. Amann, "Changes in ram sperm membranes during epididymal transit," Archives of Biochemistry and Biophysics, vol. 196, no. 1, pp. 7–12, 1979. · ·

32. J. K. Voglmayr, T. W. Scott, B. P. Setchell, and G. M. Waites, "Metabolism of testicular spermatozoa and characteristics of testicular fluid collected from conscious rams.," Journal of Reproduction and Fertility, vol. 14, no. 1, pp. 87–99, 1967. · ·

33. S. Vijayasarathy and P. Balaram, "Regional differentiation in bull sperm plasma membranes,"Biochemical and Biophysical Research Communications, vol. 108, no. 2, pp. 760–769, 1982. · ·

34. D. E. Wolf and J. K. Voglmayr, "Diffusion and regionalization in membranes of maturing ram spermatozoa," Journal of Cell Biology, vol. 98, no. 5, pp. 1678–1684, 1984. · ·

35. C. O. Bwanga, "Cryopreservation of boar semen. I: a literature review," Acta Veterinaria Scandinavica, vol. 32, no. 4, pp. 431–453, 1991.

36. P. F. Watson, E. Kunze, P. Cramer, and R. H. Hammerstedt, "A comparison of critical osmolality and hydraulic conductivity and its activation energy in fowl and bull spermatozoa," Journal of Andrology, vol. 13, no. 2, pp. 131–138, 1992.

37. J. E. Parks and D. V. Lynch, "Lipid composition and thermotropic phase behavior of boar, bull, stallion, and rooster sperm membranes," Cryobiology, vol. 29, no. 2, pp. 255–266, 1992. · ·

38. M. J. Pettitt and M. M. Buhr, "Extender components and surfactants affect boar sperm function and membrane behavior during cryopreservation," Journal of Andrology, vol. 19, no. 6, pp. 736–746, 1998.

39. A. R. Neill and C. J. Masters, "Metabolism of fatty acids by bovine spermatozoa," Biochemical Journal, vol. 34, pp. 279–287, 1972.

40. A. R. Neill and C. J. Masters, "Metabolism of fatty acids by ovine spermatozoa," Journal of Reproduction and Fertility, vol. 34, no. 2, pp. 279–287, 1973. · ·

41. S. Cerolini, A. Maldjian, F. Pizzi, and T. M. Gliozzi, "Changes in sperm quality and lipid composition during cryopreservation of boar semen," Reproduction, vol. 121, no. 3, pp. 395–401, 2001. · ·

42. E. F. Graham and B. O. Crabo, "Some methods of freezing and evaluating human spermatozoa," in The Integrity of Frozen Spermatozoa, pp. 274–304, National Academy of Sciences, Washington, DC, USA, 1976.

43. K. D. Smith, L. J. Rodriguez-Rigau, and E. Steinberger, "The influence of ovulatory dysfunction and timing of insemination on the success of artificial insemination donor (AID) with fresh or cryopreserved semen," Fertility and Sterility, vol. 36, no. 4, pp. 496–502, 1981.

44. M. A. Richter, R. V. Haning Jr., and S. S. Shapiro, "Artificial donor insemination: fresh versus frozen semen: the patient as her own control," Fertility and Sterility, vol. 41, no. 2, pp. 277–280, 1984.

45. F. W. Hanson, J. W. Overstreet, and D. F. Katz, "A study of the relationship of motile sperm numbers in cervical mucus 48 hours after artificial insemination with subsequent fertility," American Journal of Obstetrics and Gynecology, vol. 143, no. 1, pp. 85–90, 1982.

46. G. M. Centola, "Effect of cryopreservation on human sperm motility," Molecular Andrology, vol. 1, no. 4, pp. 399–412, 1989.

47. G. M. Centola, R. F. Raubertas, and J. H. Mattox, "Cryopreservation of human semen: comparison of cryopreservatives, sources of variability, and prediction of post-thaw survival," Journal of Andrology, vol. 13, no. 3, pp. 283–288, 1992.

48. J. K. Critser, B. W. Arneson, D. V. Aaker, A. R. Huse-Benda, and G. D. Ball, "Cryopreservation of human spermatozoa. II. Postthaw chronology of motility and of zona-free hamster ova penetration,"Fertility and Sterility, vol. 47, no. 6, pp. 980–984, 1987.

49. J. K. Critser, A. R. Huse-Benda, D. V. Aaker, B. W. Arneson, and G. D. Ball, "Cryopreservation of human spermatozoa. I. Effects of holding procedure and seeding on motility, fertilizability, and acrosome reaction," Fertility and Sterility, vol. 47, no. 4, pp. 656–663, 1987.

50. J. K. Critser, A. R. Huse-Benda, D. V. Aaker, B. W. Arneson, and G. D. Ball, "Cryopreservation of human spermatozoa. III. The effect of cryoprotectants on motility," Fertility and Sterility, vol. 50, no. 2, pp. 314–320, 1988.

51. E. Z. Drobnis, C. Q. Zhong, and J. W. Overstreet, "Separation of cryopreserved human semen using sephadex columns, washing, or Percoll gradients," Journal of Andrology, vol. 12, no. 3, pp. 201–208, 1991.

52. R. H. Hammerstedt, J. K. Graham, and J. P. Nolan, "Cryopreservation of mammalian sperm: what we ask them to survive," Journal of Andrology, vol. 11, no. 1, pp. 73–88, 1990.

53. L. Weidel and G. S. Prins, "Cryosurvival of human spermatozoa frozen in eight different buffer systems," Journal of Andrology, vol. 8, no. 1, pp. 41–47, 1987.

54. J. W. Overstreet and E. Z. Drobnis, "Sperm transport in the female tract," in Advances in Donor Insemination, C. L. R. Barratt and I. D. Cooke, Eds., Cambridge University Press, Cambridge, UK, 1993.

55. J. G. Alvarez and B. T. Storey, "Assessment of cell damage caused by spontaneous lipid peroxidation in rabbit spermatozoa," Biology of Reproduction, vol. 30, no. 2, pp. 323–331, 1984. · ·

56. J. G. Alvarez, J. C. Touchstone, L. Blasco, and B. T. Storey, "Spontaneous lipid peroxidation and production of hydrogen peroxide and superoxide in human spermatozoa. Superoxide dismutase as major enzyme protectant against oxygen toxicity," Journal of Andrology, vol. 8, no. 5, pp. 338–348, 1987.

57. J. T. Anger, B. R. Gilbert, and M. Goldstein, "Cryopreservation of sperm: indications, methods and results," Journal of Urology, vol. 170, no. 4 I, pp. 1079–1084, 2003. · ·

58. P. Holoch and M. Wald, "Current options for preservation of fertility in the male," Fertility and Sterility, vol. 96, no. 2, pp. 286–290, 2011. · ·

59. A. Lenzi, M. Picardo, L. Gandini, and F. Dondero, "Lipids of the sperm plasma membrane: From polyunsaturated fatty acids considered as markers of sperm function to possible scavenger therapy,"Human Reproduction Update, vol. 2, no. 3, pp. 246–256, 1996. · ·

60. R. J. Aitken, "The role of free oxygen radicals and sperm function," International Journal of Andrology, vol. 12, no. 2, pp. 95–97, 1989. · ·

61. A. Agarwal, K. Makker, and R. Sharma, "Clinical relevance of oxidative stress in male factor infertility: an update," American Journal of Reproductive Immunology, vol. 59, no. 1, pp. 2–11, 2008. · ·

62. J. G. Alvarez and B. T. Storey, "Evidence that membrane stress contributes more than lipid peroxidation to sublethal cryodamage in cryopreserved human sperm: glycerol and other polyols as sole cryoprotectant," Journal of Andrology, vol. 14, no. 3, pp. 199–209, 1993.

63. J. Schiller, J. Arnhold, H. J. Glander, and K. Arnold, "Lipid analysis of human spermatozoa and seminal plasma by MALDI-TOF mass spectrometry and NMR spectroscopy—effects of freezing and thawing,"Chemistry and Physics of Lipids, vol. 106, no. 2, pp. 145–156, 2000. · ·

64. J. G. Alvarez and B. T. Storey, "Evidence for increased lipid peroxidative damage and loss of superoxide dismutase activity as a mode of sublethal cryodamage to human sperm during cryopreservation,"Journal of Andrology, vol. 13, no. 3, pp. 232–241, 1992.

65. J. C. Martínez-Soto, J. Landeras, and J. Gadea, "Spermatozoa and seminal plasma fatty acids as predictors of cryopreservation success," Andrology, vol. 1, no. 3, pp. 365–375, 2013. ··

66. C. A. James, A. Wolfe, S. Mackie, A. Ladha, and R. Prentice, "Lipid dynamics in the plasma membrane of fresh and cryopreserved human spermatozoa," Human Reproduction, vol. 14, no. 7, pp. 1827–1832, 1999. · ·

67. M. N. Giraud, C. Motta, D. Boucher, and G. Grizard, "Membrane fluidity predicts the outcome of cryopreservation of human spermatozoa," Human Reproduction, vol. 15, no. 10, pp. 2160–2164, 2000.· ·

68. P. H. Purdy, "A review on goat sperm cryopreservation," Small Ruminant Research, vol. 63, no. 3, pp. 215–225, 2006. · ·

69. S. Cerolini, K. A. Kelso, R. C. Noble, B. K. Speake, F. Pizzi, and L. G. Cavalchini, "Relationship between spermatozoan lipid composition and fertility during aging of chickens," Biology of Reproduction, vol. 57, no. 5, pp. 976–980, 1997. · ·

70. N. Argov-Argaman, K. Mahgrefthe, Y. Zeron, and Z. Roth, "Variation in lipid profiles within semen compartments-the bovine model of aging," Theriogenology, vol. 80, no. 7, pp. 712–721, 2013. · ·

71. P. H. Phillips, "Preservation of bull semen," The Journal of Biological Chemistry, vol. 130, article 415, Abstract, 1939.

72. A. D. Cookson, A. N. Thomas, and J. A. Foulkes, "Immunochemical investigation of the interaction of egg-yolk lipoproteins with bovine spermatozoa," Journal of Reproduction and Fertility, vol. 70, no. 2, pp. 599–604, 1984. · ·

73. J. A. Foulkes and D. L. Stewart, "Fertility of dairy cattle after artificial insemination with semen frozen in a lipoprotein diluent," Journal of Reproduction and Fertility, vol. 51, no. 1, pp. 175–177, 1977. · ·

74. M. M. Pace and E. F. Graham, "Components in egg yolk which protect bovine spermatozoa during freezing," Journal of Animal Science, vol. 39, no. 6, pp. 1144–1149, 1974.

75. P. F. Watson, "The interaction of egg yolk and ram spermatozoa studied with a fluorescent probe,"Journal of Reproduction and Fertility, vol. 42, no. 1, pp. 105–111, 1975. · ·

76. R. F. Kampschmidt, D. T. Mayer, and H. A. Herman, "Lipid and lipoprotein constituents of egg yolk in the resistance and storage

of bull spermatozoa," Journal of Dairy Science, vol. 36, pp. 733–742, 1953.·

77. M. Moussa, V. Martinet, A. Trimeche, D. Tainturier, and M. Anton, "Low density lipoproteins extracted from hen egg yolk by an easy method: cryoprotective effect on frozen-thawed bull semen,"Theriogenology, vol. 57, no. 6, pp. 1695–1706, 2002. · ·
78. L. Su, X. Li, J. Quan et al., "A comparison of the protective action of added egg yolks from five avian species to the cryopreservation of bull sperm." Animal Reproduction Science, vol. 104, no. 2–4, pp. 212–219, 2008. · ·
79. A. Towhidi and J. E. Parks, "Effect of n-3 fatty acids and α-tocopherol on post-thaw parameters and fatty acid composition of bovine sperm," Journal of Assisted Reproduction and Genetics, vol. 29, no. 10, pp. 1051–1056, 2012. · ·
80. A. Towhidi, S. Zeinoaldini, R. Ardebili, N. Dadashpour Davachi, and A. H. Nasiri, "Combined n-3 fatty acids and α-tocopherol supplementation improved the ovine sperm cryosurvival," Iranian Journal of Biotechnology, vol. 11, no. 4, pp. 238–243, 2013. · ·
81. J. Chakrabarty, D. Banerjee, D. Pal, J. De, A. Ghosh, and G. C. Majumder, "Shedding off specific lipid constituents from sperm cell membrane during cryopreservation," Cryobiology, vol. 54, no. 1, pp. 27–35, 2007. · ·
82. E. M.-E. Aboagla and T. Terada, "Effects of egg yolk during the freezing step of cryopreservation on the viability of goat spermatozoa," Theriogenology, vol. 62, no. 6, pp. 1160–1172, 2004. ··
83. H. Salmani, A. Towhidi, M. Zhandi, M. Bahreini, and M. Sharafi, "In vitro assessment of soybean lecithin and egg yolk based diluents for cryopreservation of goat semen," Cryobiology, vol. 68, no. 2, pp. 276–280, 2014. · ·
84. P. Jiménez-Rabadán, M. Ramón, O. García-Álvarez, et al., "Effect of semen collection method (artificial vagina vs. electroejaculation), extender and centrifugation on post-thaw sperm quality of Blanca-Celtibérica buck ejaculates," Animal Reproduction Science, vol. 132, no. 1-2, pp. 88–95, 2012. · ·
85. D. J. Roof, S. Bowley, L. L. Price, and D. J. Matsas, "Comparison of two commercial extenders for cryopreservation of goat semen

without sperm washing," Theriogenology, vol. 77, no. 2, pp. 412–420, 2012. · ·

86. H. Salmani, M. M. Nabi, H. Vaseghi-Dodaran et al., "Effect of glutathione in soybean lecithin-based semen extender on goat semen quality after freeze-thawing," Small Ruminant Research, vol. 112, no. 1–3, pp. 123–127, 2013. · ·
87. A. H. Vidal, A. M. Batista, E. C. B. da Silva et al., "Soybean lecithin-based extender as an alternative for goat sperm cryopreservation," Small Ruminant Research, vol. 109, no. 1, pp. 47–51, 2013. · ·
88. P. C. Penny, R. C. Noble, A. Maldjian, and S. Cerolini, "Potential role of lipids for the enhancement of boar fertility and fecundity," Pig News and Information, vol. 25, pp. 119–126, 2000.
89. J. A. Rooke, C.-C. Shao, and B. K. Speake, "Effects of feeding tuna oil on the lipid composition of pig spermatozoa and in vitro characteristics of semen," Reproduction, vol. 121, no. 2, pp. 315–322, 2001.· ·
90. A. Maldjian, F. Pizzi, T. Gliozzi, S. Cerolini, P. Penny, and R. Noble, "Changes in sperm quality and lipid composition during cryopreservation of boar semen," Theriogenology, vol. 63, no. 2, pp. 411–421, 2005.· ·
91. R. R. Miller Jr., C. J. Sheffer, C. L. Cornett, R. McClean, C. MacCallum, and S. D. Johnston, "Sperm membrane fatty acid composition in the Eastern grey kangaroo (Macropus giganteus), koala (Phascolarctos cinereus), and common wombat (Vombatus ursinus) and its relationship to cold shock injury and cryopreservation success," Cryobiology, vol. 49, no. 2, pp. 137–148, 2004. ··
92. W. Farstad, A. Krogenæs, E. Nagyova, A. L. Hafne, and P. Hyttel, "In vitro techniques in fox reproduction," Livestock Production Science, vol. 36, no. 1, pp. 23–27, 1993.
93. W. Farstad, "Reproduction in foxes: current research and future challenges," Animal Reproduction Science, vol. 53, no. 1–4, pp. 35–42, 1998. · ·
94. W. Farstad, "Semen cryopreservation in dogs and foxes," Animal Reproduction Science, vol. 42, no. 1–4, pp. 251–260, 1996.
95. W. Farstad, J. A. Fougner, and C. G. Torres, "The effect of sperm number on fertility in blue fox vixens (Alopex lagopus) artificially

inseminated with frozen silver fox (Vulpes vulpes) semen," Theriogenology, vol. 37, no. 3, pp. 699–711, 1992.

96. B. L. Lasley, N. M. Loskutoff, and G. B. Anderson, "The limitation of conventional breeding programs and the need and promise of assisted reproduction in nondomestic species," Theriogenology, vol. 41, no. 1, pp. 119–132, 1994.

97. R. Buice, D. Maloy, C. Wraath, and N. M. Loskutoff, "Effects of various cryoprotectants on epididymal sperm from African elephants (Loxodonta africana)," in Proceedings of the Association of Zoo Veterinary Technicians, Baltimore, Md, USA, 1995.

98. E. O'Brien, S. Hoffman, T. Schawang et al., "Effects of different cryoprotectants and the short and long term storage of semen from the African elephant," in Proceedings of the 2nd International Elephant Research Symposium, Springfield, Mo, USA, 1997.

99. D. Bencharif, L. Amirat, M. Anton et al., "The advantages of LDL (Low Density Lipoproteins) in the cryopreservation of canine semen," Theriogenology, vol. 70, no. 9, pp. 1478–1488, 2008.

100. B. M. García, L. G. Fernández, C. O. Ferrusola et al., "Fatty acids and plasmalogens of the phospholipids of the sperm membranes and their relation with the post-thaw quality of stallion spermatozoa,"Theriogenology, vol. 75, no. 5, pp. 811–818, 2011.

101. C. Ortega Ferrusola, L. González Fernández, J. M. Morrell et al., "Lipid peroxidation, assessed with BODIPY-C 11, increases after cryopreservation of stallion spermatozoa, is stallion-dependent and is related to apoptotic-like changes," Reproduction, vol. 138, no. 1, pp. 55–63, 2009.

102. J. Santiago-Moreno, M. A. Coloma, A. Toledano-Díaz et al., "A comparison of the protective action of chicken and quail egg yolk in the cryopreservation of Spanish ibex epididymal spermatozoa,"Cryobiology, vol. 57, no. 1, pp. 25–29, 2008.

Chapter 10

Practical Applications Of Sperm Selection Techniques As A Tool For Improving Reproductive Efficiency

J. M. Morrell[1], and H. Rodriguez-Martinez[2]

[1]Division of Reproduction, Department of Clinical Sciences, Swedish University of Agricultural Sciences-SLU, Box 7054, 75007 Uppsala, Sweden

[2]Department of Clinical and Experimental Medicine, Faculty of Health Sciences, Linköping University, 581 85 Linköping, Sweden

ABSTRACT

Modern biotechnologies are used extensively in the animal breeding industry today. Therefore, it is essential that sperm handling procedures do not modulate the normal physiological mechanisms occurring in the female reproductive tract. In this paper, the different selection mechanisms occurring in vivo are described briefly, together with their relevance to artificial insemination, followed by a detailed description of the different selection processes used in reproductive biotechnologies. These selection methods included fractionated semen collection, cryopreservation, biomimetic sperm selection, selection based on hyaluronic acid binding, and last, but not least, sperm sex selection. Biomimetic sperm selection for AI or for cryopreservation could improve pregnancy rates and help to reverse the decline in fertility seen in several domestic species over the recent decades. Similarly, selection for hyaluronic acid binding sites may enable the most mature spermatozoa to be selected for IVF or ICSI.

INTRODUCTION

Modern biotechnologies such as artificial insemination (AI) and sperm cryopreservation have revolutionized the animal breeding industry. However, to unleash the full potential of these undoubtedly powerful technologies, the events that take place in the female reproductive tract between AI and fertilization should be considered, so that we do not inadvertently hinder, or even counteract, normal physiological processes [1, 2]. Moreover, in recent years there may have been a decline in fertility in some species, associated with an increase in the use of AI, for example in dairy cattle [3]. The aim of this paper is to examine the ways in which spermatozoa are "selected" during preparation for AI and how these processes may impact sperm fertility. First, the different selection mechanisms in the female reproductive tract will be examined briefly, followed by a discussion of the relevance of these mechanisms to AI. Sperm selection with regard to cryopreservation will be considered followed by a critique of different methods for sperm selection, with particular focus on Single Layer Centrifugation (SLC). The effectiveness of selecting spermatozoa for in vitro fertilization (IVF) and intra cytoplasmic sperm injection (ICSI) according to possession of hyaluronic acid binding sites will be discussed. Lastly, sperm selection for assisted reproduction (ART) according to content of sex chromosomes will be evaluated.

SELECTION MECHANISMS WITHIN THE FEMALE REPRODUCTIVE TRACT

At ejaculation, billions of spermatozoa are released into the female reproductive tract and start to make their way to the site of fertilization. However, only a few thousand spermatozoa are present in the oviducts at any one time, and only one spermatozoon will eventually fertilize each oocyte. As spermatozoa pass along the female reproductive tract they are subjected to several selection mechanisms responsible for filtering out immature or damaged spermatozoa [1], at the same time as they are acquiring fertilizing ability. Thus, only spermatozoa that are functionally normal should reach the potential site of fertilization in the oviducts, the isthmic-ampullary junction.

(i) The cervix: semen deposition takes place in the vagina, close to the posterior cervix, in human beings and some other species, for example, ruminants and rodents. In other species, for example, horses and dogs, where semen deposition takes place directly into the uterus, the uterotubal junction acts as the only filter. In species with vaginal deposition of semen, the cervix acts as a sperm reservoir where the spermatozoa may reside for up to 24 h, and it also serves as a filtration system. Immotile or morphologically abnormal spermatozoa become trapped by the viscous mucous in the cervical lumen [4] whereas normal motile spermatozoa are thought to orientate along the long axis of mucosal threads, aligning themselves along the longitudinal mucosal folds of the cervix (where the mucus is basically composed of sialic acid) for antegrade movement [5]. Damaged spermatozoa and microorganisms are trapped in the highly viscous central mucous which propels them in a retrograde direction for subsequent expulsion. During the stages of the oestrus cycle under progesterone dominance, cervical mucous is viscous and nearly impenetrable to spermatozoa.

(ii) The uterus: although sperm-uterine interaction has been studied mostly in the pig, it is believed that many of the observations in this species are pertinent to other species too. It has been shown that some spermatozoa attach to the uterine epithelium whereas others remain in the uterine lumen, the latter tending to have damaged plasma membranes [6]. Moreover, using uterine explants, spermatozoa attached to uterine epithelial cells (UEC) were shown to have normal ultrastructure and mitochondrial membrane potential [7, 8]. Thus, it has been suggested that the uterus, like the cervix, may act as a sperm reservoir and filtration mechanism, although the latter is based on direct interactions between the spermatozoa and the uterine epithelial cells (UECs) rather than on a physical barrier.

(iii) The uterotubal junction (UTJ) and distal isthmus may constitute a third sperm reservoir and filtering system. When biopsies were taken from this region at various times after mating, Mburu et al. [9] identified bound and nonbound sperm populations. In a later study the bound spermatozoa were found to have better membrane viability than the unbound group [10]. Further work with explants revealed that bound spermatozoa have both a prolonged lifespan [11] and better chromatin integrity [12] compared to those that do not bind. It is thought that spermatozoa that have temporarily bound to UEC or the epithelial cells of the UTJ subsequently become free to pass along the oviducts in an antegrade direction.

(iv) oviductal selection: oviductal proteins modify the zona pellucida (ZP) of freshly ovulated oocytes, thus affecting the ability of spermatozoa to interact with them. Incubation of human spermatozoa in the presence of oviductal proteins apparently reduces their affinity for the ZP [13], enabling the oviduct to actively select sperm subpopulations with specific ligands for fertilization.

(v) Selection for a functional acrosome and binding sites. sperm penetration of the cumulus matrix surrounding the oocyte in the cumulus oophorus complex is facilitated by sperm membrane-bound hyaluronidase [14] and by their hyperactivated motility pattern. Zona binding involves a wide range of sperm surface components and at least one of the three glycoproteins of which the ZP is composed. Zona binding acts as a trigger for the acrosome reaction (AR). The spermatozoon then enters the perivitelline space between the ZP and the oolemma, and the tip of the sperm makes contact with the oolemma, followed by lateral attachment of the spermatozoa [14]. The site of fusion is at the central region of the spermatozoa near to, or at, the equatorial region, and involves an integrin on the oocyte and an integrin ligand on the sperm plasma membrane.

RELEVANCE OF PHYSIOLOGICAL SELECTION TO ARTIFICIAL INSEMINATION

In AI, semen doses containing lower sperm numbers than are normally present in the ejaculate are deposited in the uterus or cervix during oestrus [1]. This site of semen deposition is non physiological for ruminants, bypassing the cervical sperm reservoir in these species. This means, in effect, that the person preparing the semen doses is acting as a partial substitute for the cervix, diluting the seminal plasma and selecting only those ejaculates with low proportions of immotile or morphologically abnormal spermatozoa to be used in AI. However, the presence of some seminal plasma in the uterus is nonphysiological in ruminants and may have a negative effect on fertility. Furthermore, the spermatozoa remain in contact with seminal plasma (SP) for much longer in the extended semen than they would under physiological conditions. SP contains decapacitating factors to prevent the spermatozoa capacitating too soon relative to the potential time of fertilization. Prolonged contact with SP may, therefore, impact negatively on sperm functionality. However, the type of semen extender used may also affect the ability of the spermatozoa to interact with the female reproductive tract [7].

The prolonged contact between stallion spermatozoa and seminal plasma during cooled storage may partially account for the lower pregnancy rates achieved in mares inseminated on the day following semen collection compared with AI using freshly ejaculated semen. Although semen extenders are used to dilute the seminal plasma, the formulations currently in use for stallion semen may not be sufficiently effective in maintaining the spermatozoa in an optimal condition for fertilization.

Conversely, SP also contains components that are considered beneficial to sperm survival [15]. Proteins in SP have various effects promoting or inhibiting sperm functions including motility, oviduct binding, zona binding/penetration, and ultimately fertilization [16]. Spermadhesins, for example, bind to the sperm surface on ejaculation and prevent capacitation [16]. It is speculated that removal of these proteins during preparation techniques such as flow cytometric sperm sexing, may destabilize the membrane and precapacitate the spermatozoa, thus shortening their functional life [15, 17].

Once the spermatozoa have been deposited in the uterus, they are subjected to the previously described selection mechanisms and interactions with the female reproductive tract. Therefore, it is essential that the sperm handling techniques prior to sperm deposition do not compromise sperm membranes, sperm motility or sperm longevity, since this will impair their ability to progress up the female reproductive tract.

SPERM SELECTION FOR FREEZING

Some individuals produce ejaculates that are better able to withstand cryopreservation than others, that is, with higher cryosurvival. In the semen industry, it is usual to select animals that are "good" freezers as breeding sires, since the market for straws of frozen semen with poor viability is nonexistent. However, this selection of sires inevitably impacts on the gene pool, since only spermatozoa surviving cryopreservation contribute their DNA to the next generation. Thus, by actively selecting for cryogenic spermatozoa, there may have been inadvertent selection for undesirable traits, such as reduced fertility.

Cryopreservation can have a profound effect on sperm viability and function, both because of the physical changes occurring during ice crystal formation and dissolution, and due to the effects of the cryopreservation medium on sperm membrane composition. Furthermore, cryopreservation may severely reduce or block binding proteins on the sperm surface that are necessary for binding to oviductal epithelium [1]. Frozen-thawed spermatozoa exhibit "capacitation-like" membrane changes, which may be evidence of membrane damage as well as actual capacitation. Reactive oxygen species, such as the superoxide anion (), are produced during capacitation in all species, and possibly also $ONOO^-$ in bovines [18], accompanied by increased activity of the mitochondrial respiratory chain. The additional sperm energy requirements needed to support these activities must be supplied by oxidative substrates in the surroundings, namely, the semen extender in stored semen doses. Thus the composition of the cryopreservation medium is important for supporting capacitation.

Whether cryosurvival ("freezability") is a function of the spermatozoa themselves or of the composition of the seminal plasma is the subject of much discussion. The boar ejaculate is produced in several fractions, each containing a different proportion of spermatozoa and SP, the latter being of different composition in the various fractions depending on the relative contributions of the accessory glands [19]. Spermatozoa present in the first 10 mL of the sperm-rich fraction of boar ejaculates (known as portion 1 or P1) were found to survive cryopreservation better than spermatozoa in the rest of the ejaculate (portion 2, P2) [20]. Moreover, when spermatozoa in the different fractions were separated from SP and subsequently mixed with SP from the other fraction in a crossover experiment, the kinematics of P2 spermatozoa were improved whereas those of P1 spermatozoa deteriorated [21]. In contrast, boar spermatozoa collected from the whole of the sperm-rich fraction were found to have better motility than those in P1, P2, or P1 subsequently mixed with P2 (P1+P2) [22]. Moreover, the sperm-rich fractions of stallion ejaculate were found to contain spermatozoa with lower %DFI (DNA fragm entation index) than those from the subsequent (sperm-poor) fractions [23]. Taken together, these observations suggest that spermatozoa are affected by the composition of SP, and at least boar and stallion spermatozoa may require exposure to SP in the correct ratio (or relative amounts of specific constituents) to achieve their optimum motility and membrane integrity.

This finding could have implications for enhancing sperm survival in species such as the stallion, where there are marked differences between individuals in sperm survival during cryopreservation or even during cooled storage. Removal of some [24], or all, of the SP [25, 26], prolongs stallion sperm survival during cooled storage. In contrast to possible negative effects of SP on sperm survival, SP may play a role in the postmating clearance of spermatozoa from the uterus, at least in mares [27]. Ejaculation in most other species is not differentiated into clear fractions, as it is in the boar and stallion, but even so there may be individual variation in the composition of SP that modulate cryosurvival. Identification of the components of SP that enhance fertility, either by their action on spermatozoa or on the female reproductive tract, would be of considerable benefit to the animal AI industry.

An alternative method for enhancing sperm survival during storage, either cooled or by cryopreservation, would be to select subpopulations of good quality spermatozoa prior to storage. Preliminary results suggest that sperm fertility is not adversely affected by such selection methods and may be improved, for example stallion spermatozoa [28]. The selection of the best quality spermatozoa is reviewed in the next section. However, it is pertinent to note here that stallion spermatozoa selected by SLC through Androcoll-E on the basis of sperm quality show increased progressive motility after thawing than unselected spermatozoa, which (it is speculated) could result in better pregnancy rates after AI with frozen thawed sperm doses.

BIOMIMETIC SPERM SELECTION

Biomimetics is the use of technologies and/or processes that mimic a naturally occurring event. Several mechanisms have been suggested that mimic the selection taking place in the female reproductive tract [29]. These methods either separate the spermatozoa from SP or, in addition, permit selection of the better quality spermatozoa from the rest of the ejaculate. There have been several extensive reviews recently on the merits and demerits of various sperm selection techniques used to improve sperm quality for assisted reproduction, for example, for human spermatozoa [30], and for animal spermatozoa [29].

Basically, the methods can be divided into those that result in removal of seminal plasma only (sperm washing), and methods that select spermatozoa on the basis of certain characteristics, such as sperm migration (based on sperm motility), filtration (based on membrane integrity), and colloid centrifugation (based on sperm motility, morphology, viability and chromatin integrity). Colloid centrifugation can be subdivided into density gradient centrifugation (DGC) and Single Layer Centrifugation (SLC) [31]. A brief description of each of these techniques follows.

Sperm Washing

The extended ejaculate is centrifuged, the supernatant (consisting of seminal plasma and extender) removed and the sperm pellet resuspended in a suitable volume of the extender. The spermatozoa are thus separated from most of the seminal plasma [32]. However, there is no selection of the spermatozoa and dead, moribund, and abnormal cells [33] as well as sources of reactive oxygen species (ROS), may remain, which are detrimental to sperm viability. There have been reports of chromatin damage in human spermatozoa due to this technique [34], although this may be due to centrifuging human semen without extender rather the technique itself. Extenders for animal semen, particularly milk- or egg yolk-based extenders, typically contain antioxidants which may counteract ROS released during centrifugation.

Migration

There are several variations, all relying on the ability of motile spermatozoa to move from one suspension to another [34]. The original sperm population is either underneath, on top of, or to one side of the migration medium [34]. The spermatozoa move away from the SP; thus selection is based on sperm motility and does not provide any selection based on morphology, chromatin integrity, viability, or acrosome integrity [35]. Spermatozoa with tail abnormalities are prevented from migrating into the swim-up medium. Some studies show significantly better midpiece- and tail-morphology after swim-up than after washing [33]. Adding hyaluronic acid to the migration medium may also select for spermatozoa with intact membranes [36]. The main disadvantage of any migration method is the low-recovery rate, for example, 10%–20% [33], which renders them impractical for preparing spermatozoa for AI in most animal species.

Filtration

The spermatozoa interact with the filter substance, for example, glass fibres, Sephadex beads, or membrane pores, but are also selected on the basis of being ability to move [37]. Nonviable spermatozoa adhere to the matrix more than motile, functional spermatozoa [38], although the mechanism of action is uncertain [39]. Immotile and dead spermatozoa may agglomerate because of changes in surface charges [40], or protein changes on the sperm surface after capacitation may allow sperm binding to sephadex particles [41]. Filtration of canine spermatozoa through Sephadex G-15 increased the proportion of viable spermatozoa and decreased the proportion of altered acrosomes compared to the unfiltered sample [37]. Filtered bovine spermatozoa showed improved post-thaw viability compared to unfiltered spermatozoa [42].

There are claims that filtration methods are not only useful for eliminating leukocytes (sources of ROS) and selecting motile spermatozoa, but may also aid selection for morphologically normal [43] and possibly acrosome-intact spermatozoa [39]. In contrast, Januskauskas et al. [42] found no effect on the proportion of spermatozoa with intact acrosomes. The filtrate is not considered to be as clean as for other sperm separation methods [30], presumably because some SP and cellular debris remain in the sample. However, fewer spermatozoa are lost than with other methods, with approximately 63% recovery rate being reported [42].

Colloid Centrifugation

In this method, extended semen is centrifuged through a colloid, separating spermatozoa from SP and selecting the spermatozoa that are motile, viable, and have good chromatin integrity. During DGC or SLC, cells move to a point in the gradient that matches their own density—the isopycnic point [44]. By altering the centrifugation force and time, and the physical properties of the colloid, the good quality spermatozoa are allowed to pellet in the bottom of the tube. Until recently, colloid centrifugation was confined solely to DGC, which involved using several layers of colloid of different density (hence "density gradient"), but recently a new method, SLC through a species-specific colloid (Androcoll) was developed by the current authors at the Swedish University for Agricultural Sciences [31], which uses only one layer of Androcoll. Thus, time is saved during preparation and the method can be scaled-up successfully to allow large volumes of ejaculate to be centrifuged [45]. Species-specific formulations of Androcoll (with a suffix to denote the species) have been developed for stallion [31], boar [22], bull [46], dog [47], and cat [48].

Sperm washing is used frequently in the equine breeding industry, either to remove most of the SP prior to extending and cooling the sample, or prior to freezing. However, it should be noted that sperm washing does not improve the quality of the sperm samples since the majority of the spermatozoa are retained during processing. In fact, some of the most motile spermatozoa may be removed with the supernatant [26]. Most of the true selection methods have been tested by researchers at one time or another with the semen of various species but are rarely considered practical for use in the field, mainly because of the large volume of ejaculate or high-sperm concentration involved in preparing sperm doses for animal AI.

In a comparison of SLC and sperm washing for stallion spermatozoa, it was found that sperm washing did not confer any beneficial effect on the sperm samples and, in fact, had a negative effect on sperm motility and chromatin integrity [26]. The SLC-selected samples from the same ejaculates showed both better sperm motility and chromatin integrity, which were maintained over the duration of the experiment (72 h).

However, the situation for animal AI is rather different to human ART, since much larger numbers of spermatozoa are required in animal breeding. Thus, with the exception of SLC, the sperm selection methods described above are impractical for incorporating into processing protocols for AI doses in animal breeding. Not only does SLC select good quality spermatozoa, as does DGC [31], but also SLC is user friendly and can be scaled up to produce sufficient numbers of spermatozoa even for boar and stallion AI doses [45]. Attempts to scale up DGC have not achieved the same yields as small-scale preparations, although the sperm quality is reported to be good [49]. SLC-selected sperm samples have been shown to be functionally normal in ICSI and AI studies in the horse [28, 50], and in bovine IVF [46]. Furthermore, there was an indication that SLC may have advantages over DGC for preparing spermatozoa for ICSI from sperm samples of very poor quality [50].

The major applications for SLC-selection are as follows:(i)improving sperm quality in AI doses (e.g., stallion [28]);(ii)increasing the "shelf-life" of in vitro stored sperm samples (stallion [25] and boar [22]);(iii) removal of pathogens [51, 52];(iv)to improve cryosurvival by removing dead and dying spermatozoa prior to cryopreservation, or used post-thawing to select the live spermatozoa [53, 54];(v)to select spermatozoa that are morphologically normal and have good chromatin integrity for AI [55], ICSI [50], or IVF [46], thus increasing the yield of zygotes developing to the blastocyst stage;(vi)in combination with other methods of sperm sexing, to speed up the process [56].

HBA: RELEVANCE FOR IVF, ICSI, AND AI

During epididymal maturation, spermatozoa acquire hyaluronic acid binding sites which are necessary for the acquisition of motility and for binding to the ZP/oocyte [57]. Spermatozoa not possessing these binding sites are unable to fertilize oocytes even in IVF. Therefore, detection of the proportion of spermatozoa with these binding sites may indicate the potential fertility of the sperm sample. Since ICSI circumvents all natural barriers to fertilization, the success rate of the technique is dependent on the quality of the spermatozoa selected for injection [58]. Using normal morphology as the sole criterion for selection increases the possibility of using spermatozoa with abnormal chromosomes [59]. Therefore, it was hypothesized that an effective test for selecting normal spermatozoa would increase the success rate of embryo production by ICSI, particularly in pigs [60]. Park et al. [58] reported an increase in ICSI efficiency when boar spermatozoa adhering to droplets of hyaluronic acid (HA) were selected for ICSI, compared to controls using motile spermatozoa that had been slowed down by passage through a solution of poly vinyl pyrrolidone (PVP). Although the blastocyst development was the same in the two groups, the frequency of normal diploidy in the group treated with HA was significantly higher (75.5%) than in the PVP-group (68.2%). The authors concluded that using the HA-binding spermatozoa was superior to morphological sperm selection alone in producing chromosomally normal embryos by ICSI [58]. Similar results were seen for human ART, where a higher fertilization rate was obtained using HA-selected spermatozoa for ICSI [61]. The latter authors also found a significant inverse correlation between percentage of HA binding and protamine deficiency, DNA fragmentation, and abnormal sperm morphology ().

Recently an assay was developed for determining the ability of human spermatozoa to bind to hyaluronan. A kit (HBA—the hyaluronan binding assay, Medicult, Denmark) is commercially available for use with human semen samples for IVF, consisting of glass slides coated with hyaluronan. A drop of the sperm sample in phosphate buffered saline is applied to the coated slide and, after a short incubation at ambient temperature (22°C), the number of spermatozoa bound to the hyaluronan coating is counted. A variant for selecting spermatozoa for

ICSI made by the same company consists of hyaluronan-coated dishes (PICSI dishes) from which bound spermatozoa can be selected one by one for use in ICSI.

Although originally developed for human spermatozoa, both the HBA and PICSI dishes have been evaluated for use with stallion spermatozoa destined for AI and ICSI, respectively. When the HBA was used with stallion spermatozoa subjected to cool storage, binding varied between stallions (11%–24% [62]) but was less than indicated for human spermatozoa (28%–89%; [63]). However, the ejaculates used in this trial had been extended in a commercial extender (INRA96; IMV) and stored in the refrigerator overnight, which may have blocked or inactivated some of the binding sites.

Use of the PICSI dishes when selecting spermatozoa for ICSI produced variable results, with lower cleavage rates but a higher proportion of cleaved oocytes developing to the blastocyst stage than for spermatozoa selected by the operator on the basis of apparent "normal" morphology alone [50]. Since previous studies have shown that bovine oocytes can cleave when fertilized with chromosomally abnormal bull spermatozoa, but development is subsequently blocked [64], it would appear that the spermatozoa binding in the PICSI dishes did have a better chance of being chromosomally normal than those selected on the basis of subjective morphology assessment by a skilled operator.

SEX SELECTION

For many centuries, animal breeders and researchers have endeavoured to control the sex of the offspring born, for various reasons. Initially male offspring were preferred, for example, for beef production, because of the better feed conversion efficiency and lean-to-fat ratio of males whereas females were preferred for dairy purposes, except that some males of high-genetic merit were still required as sires. Current husbandry practices in the pig industry favour same-sex groups on welfare grounds (to prevent fighting) and because of a more even live-weight gain, with all members of the group reaching slaughter weight within a specified time. However, if male pigs are left entire, the meat develops "boar taint" as the animal reaches sexual maturity, which is considered undesirable by the consumer. Therefore, young males must be castrated, which has welfare considerations. One mechanism for avoiding castration would be to produce only female piglets in litters destined for intensive meat production, obtained by using sexed sperm doses for AI.

Many methods have been proposed for separating X- and Y-chromosome bearing spermatozoa, based on physical properties, for example, size of the sperm head, or functional properties, for example, swimming speed. However, the only method which has been shown to work reliably is that of selection and separation of spermatozoa whose DNA is stained vitally with a bis-benzimidazole dye, H33342 [65], and separated into X- and Y-chromosome bearing groups using the sorting capacity of a flow cytometer [66, 67]. This method functions because the X chromosome is larger than the Y and therefore takes up more of the DNA-specific stain. In cattle, for example, the difference in DNA content between the X and Y chromosome is approximately 4.2%, whereas for pigs it is approximately 3.8%. However, the process of sorting sufficient numbers for an insemination dose in the flow cytometer is long since the stained spermatozoa must pass one at a time through a laser beam for detection of their DNA content. Although a commercial enterprise exists for sexing bull spermatozoa, the method is considered too expensive for commercial application in pig breeding, where much larger numbers of spermatozoa are needed per AI dose than for cattle. Therefore, flow cytometric sperm sexing for AI has been confined largely to the cattle breeding industry, and for ICSI in the equine breeding industry.

Even in the bovine breeding industry, flow cytometric sperm sexing has not fulfilled its original promise: sexed sperm doses are too expensive for widespread application, the fertility of sexed sperm doses is lower than unsexed sperm doses [68], which is not merely a reflection of the lower sperm numbers used but may be attributed to impaired sperm function caused by the sexing process [69]. It is worth noting that the first method [65, 66] developed for sperm sexing used a lower concentration of the vital dye, Hoechst 33342 than the method described later [67]. The higher dye concentration was linked to chromosomal abnormalities in rabbits, particularly in conjunction with laser illumination [70] whereas the lower concentration was used to produce 5 successive generations of rabbits without any evidence of fertility problems [71]. Since food dye is added to sperm samples stained with the higher concentration of dye to quench the excessive fluorescence [72], it would seem to be better to use lower concentrations of Hoechst 33342 initially to reduce the possibility of negative effects.

Furthermore, the flow cytometric technique is not applicable to all bulls; there appears to be a difference in "sortability" between individuals [69]. A similar variation between males was observed for stallions [73]; the latter authors attributed the variation in "sortability" to differences in the number of dead spermatozoa present in the sample. Therefore, there is still a need in the animal breeding industry to develop a technique for sperm sexing that would provide sufficient spermatozoa for AI doses, does not compromise sperm fertility, and is widely applicable to a range of individuals and species.

One possible alternative to flow cytometric separation is colloid centrifugation, either density gradient centrifugation (DGC) or the recently developed technique of single layer centrifugation (SLC). Since the X chromosome is larger than the Y, while no difference has been detected in the volume of the sperm head, there is a theoretical difference in density between the two sperm types. Thus, if there is no other factor contributing to sperm density, it should be possible to separate the two types using colloid centrifugation. However, spermatozoa change in density as they mature due to changes in the composition of their membranes, and the distribution in density due to the maturity of the spermatozoa overlaps that of the sex chromosome. Therefore, it is not certain that it would be possible to sex spermatozoa in sufficient numbers with colloid centrifugation to be useful for AI doses. To date, attempts have been made to sex small numbers of bull spermatozoa with DGC for subsequent IVF [74, 75]. The authors of the first paper claimed a shift in the sex ratio of embryos produced whereas the authors of the second found no change in the sex ratio.

Another possibility for sperm sexing is that sperm surface proteins may be sex linked [76]. Recent research has identified proteins on either X- or Y-chromosome bearing spermatozoa. The use of antibodies to these sperm surface proteins may enable the two subpopulations of spermatozoa to be separated.

A combination of techniques would also be relevant for sperm sexing. Thus, the speed of flow sorting can be increased by first removing the dead and dying spermatozoa from the population, for example by DGC or SLC [77]. Such a combination may increase the "sortability" of sperm samples. Since SCL with Androcoll appears to be better at removing spermatozoa with damaged chromatin, at least from stallion ejaculates [50], and is a simpler technique to use than DGC, it would appear to be advantageous to combine SLC with Androcoll and flow cytometry for producing sexed sperm doses for AI.

CONCLUSIONS

There are many mechanisms by which spermatozoa may be "selected" for use in ART, varying from a relatively crude fractionation of boar semen as it is being ejaculated to a highly refined process based on the possession/expression of certain cell surface molecules. Any selection mechanisms taking place in vitro must not harm the spermatozoa or modulate their interaction with the female reproductive tract if fertility is to be maintained. Biomimetic selection of the best quality spermatozoa for AI or for cryopreservation could improve pregnancy rates and may help to reverse the decline in fertility seen in several domestic species over the recent decades, for example in dairy cattle [78] and horses [79]. Similarly, selection for hyaluronic acid binding sites may enable the most mature spermatozoa to be selected for IVF or ICSI, resulting in a more efficient production of blastocysts than at present, or even help to identify the best males to be selected as breeding sires. Finally, as previously discussed in this paper, the animal breeding industry is still waiting for an effective, practical method of sexing spermatozoa, which is applicable to the semen of all males. Perhaps this achievement will become the most notable contribution to the animal breeding industry of the 21st century, as AI and sperm cryopreservation were to the 20th century.

ACKNOWLEDGMENTS

J. Morrell is funded by the Swedish Farmers' Foundation, Stockholm (V0750239), and the Swedish Ministry of Agriculture, Jönköping (31-3389/09).

REFERENCES

1. S. S. Suarez, "Interactions of spermatozoa with the female reproductive tract: inspiration for assisted reproduction," Reproduction, Fertility and Development, vol. 19, no. 1, pp. 103–110, 2007.
2. D. Rath, H. J. Schuberth, P. Coy, and U. Taylor, "Sperm interactions from insemination to fertilization,"Reproduction in Domestic Animals, vol. 43, no. 5, pp. 2–11, 2008.
3. H. Rodriguez-Martinez, J. Hultgren, R. Båge, et al., "Reproductive performance in high-producing dairy cows: can we sustain it under current practice?" in IVIS Reviews in Veterinary Medicine, I.V.I.S, Ed., International Veterinary Information Service, Ithaca, NY, USA, 2008,
4. C. Barros, P. Vigil, E. Herrera, B. Arguello, and R. Walker, "Selection of morphologically abnormal sperm by human cervical mucus," Archives of Andrology, vol. 12, pp. 95–107, 1984.
5. K. J. Mullins and R. G. Saacke, "Study of the functional anatomy of bovine cervical mucosa with special reference to mucus secretion and sperm transport," Anatomical Record, vol. 225, no. 2, pp. 106–117, 1989.
6. H. Rodriguez-Martinez, L. Nicander, S. Viring, S. Einarsson, and K. Larsson, "Ultrastructure of the uterotubal junction in preovulatory pigs," Anatomia, Histologia, Embryologia, vol. 19, no. 1, pp. 16–36, 1990.
7. U. Taylor, D. Rath, H. Zerbe, and H.-J. Schuberth, "Interaction of intact porcine spermatozoa with epithelial cells and neutrophilic granulocytes during uterine passage," Reproduction in Domestic Animals, vol. 43, no. 2, pp. 166–175, 2008.
8. U. Taylor, H. J. Schuberth, D. Rath, H. W. Michelmann, C. Sauter-Louis, and H. Zerbe, "Influence of inseminate components on porcine leucocyte migration in vitro and in vivo after pre- and post-ovulatory insemination," Reproduction in Domestic Animals, vol. 44, no. 2, pp. 180–188, 2009.
9. J. N. Mburu, H. Rodriguez-Martinez, and S. Einarsson, "Changes in sperm ultrastructure and localisation in the porcine oviduct around ovulation," Animal Reproduction Science, vol. 47, no. 1-2, pp. 137–148, 1997.

10. J. N. Mburu, S. Einarsson, N. Lundeheim, and H. Rodriguez-Martinez, "Distribution, number and membrane integrity of spermatozoa in the pig oviduct in relation to spontaneous ovulation," Animal Reproduction Science, vol. 45, no. 1-2, pp. 109–121, 1996.
11. E. Töpfer-Petersen, A. Wagner, J. Friedrich et al., "Function of the mammalian oviductal sperm reservoir," Journal of Experimental Zoology, vol. 292, no. 2, pp. 210–215, 2002.
12. F. Ardón, D. Helms, E. Sahin, H. Bollwein, E. Töpfer-Petersen, and D. Waberski, "Chromatin-unstable boar spermatozoa have little chance of reaching oocytes in vivo," Reproduction, vol. 135, no. 4, pp. 461–470, 2008.
13. M. J. Munuce, A. Serravalle, A. M. Caille et al., "Human tubal secretion can modify the affinity of human spermatozoa for the zona pellucida," Fertility and Sterility, vol. 91, no. 2, pp. 407–413, 2009.
14. P. Talbot, B. D. Shur, and D. G. Myles, "Cell adhesion and fertilization: steps in oocyte transport, sperm-zona pellucida interactions, and sperm-egg fusion," Biology of Reproduction, vol. 68, no. 1, pp. 1–9, 2003.
15. W. M. Maxwell, S. P. de Graaf, R. H. Ghaoui, and G. Evans, "Seminal plasma effects on sperm handling and female fertility," Society of Reproduction and Fertility, vol. 64, pp. 13–38, 2007.
16. I. Caballero, J. M. Vazquez, E. M. García et al., "Major proteins of boar seminal plasma as a tool for biotechnological preservation of spermatozoa," Theriogenology, vol. 70, no. 8, pp. 1352–1355, 2008.
17. J. M. Vazquez, I. Parrilla, M. A. Gil et al., "Improving the efficiency of insemination with sex-sorted spermatozoa," Reproduction in Domestic Animals, vol. 43, no. 4, pp. 1–8, 2008.
18. P. C. Rodriguez, L. B. Valdez, T. Zaobornyj, A. Boveris, and M. T. Beconi, "Nitric oxide and superoxide anion production during heparin-induced capacitation in cryopreserved bovine spermatozoa,"Reproduction in Domestic Animals. In press.
19. U. Lavon and J. C. Boursnell, "The split ejaculate of the boar: contributions of the epididymides and seminal vesicles," Journal of Reproduction and Fertility, vol. 42, no. 3, pp. 541–552, 1975.

20. F. Saravia, M. Wallgren, and H. Rodríguez-Martínez, "Freezing of boar semen can be simplified by handling a specific portion of the ejaculate with a shorter procedure and MiniFlatPack packaging,"Animal Reproduction Science, vol. 117, no. 3-4, pp. 279–287, 2010.
21. F. Saravia, M. Wallgren, A. Johannisson et al., "Exposure to the seminal plasma of different portions of the boar ejaculate modulates the survival of spermatozoa cryopreserved in MiniFlatPacks,"Theriogenology, vol. 71, no. 4, pp. 662–675, 2009.
22. J. M. Morrell, F. Saravia, M. van Wienen, H. Rodriguez-Martinez, and M. Wallgren, "Sperm survival following colloid centrifugation varies according to the part of the sperm-rich fraction used," Society of Reproduction and Fertility, vol. 66, pp. 85–86, 2009.
23. M. Kareskoski and T. Katila, "Components of stallion seminal plasma and the effects of seminal plasma on sperm longevity," Animal Reproduction Science, vol. 107, no. 3-4, pp. 249–256, 2008.
24. C. Aurich, "Factors affecting the plasma membrane function of cooled-stored stallion spermatozoa,"Animal Reproduction Science, vol. 89, no. 1–4, pp. 65–75, 2005.
25. J. M. Morrell, A.-M. Dalin, and H. Rodriguez-Martinez, "Comparison of density gradient and single layer centrifugation of stallion spermatozoa: yield, motility and survival," Equine Veterinary Journal, vol. 41, no. 1, pp. 53–58, 2009.
26. J. M. Morrell, H. Rodriguez-Martinez, and A. Johannisson, "Single layer centrifugation of stallion spermatozoa improves sperm quality compared with sperm washing," Reproductive Biomedicine. In press.
27. M. H. T. Troedsson, A. Desvousges, A. S. Alghamdi et al., "Components in seminal plasma regulating sperm transport and elimination," Animal Reproduction Science, vol. 89, no. 1–4, pp. 171–186, 2005.
28. G. Mari, E. Iacono, G. Kutvölgyi, B. Mislei, H. Rodriguez-Martinez, and J. M. Morrell, "Stallion spermatozoa prepared by Single Layer Centrifugation with Androcoll-E are capable of fertilisation in vivo," Reproduction in Domestic Animals. In press.

29. J. M. Morrell and H. Rodriguez-Martinez, "Biomimetic techniques for improving sperm quality in animal breeding: a review," Open Andrology Journal, vol. 1, pp. 1–9, 2009.
30. R. R. Henkel and W.-B. Schill, "Sperm preparation for ART," Reproductive Biology and Endocrinology, vol. 1, article 108, 2003
31. J. M. Morrell, A.-M. Dalin, and H. Rodriguez-Martinez, "Prolongation of stallion sperm survival by centrifugation through coated silica colloids: a preliminary study," Animal Reproduction, vol. 5, pp. 121–126, 2008.
32. L. Björndahl, M. Mohammadieh, M. Pourian, I. Söderlund, and U. Kvist, "Contamination by seminal plasma andrology lab corner factors during sperm selection," Journal of Andrology, vol. 26, no. 2, pp. 170–173, 2005.
33. T. Hallap, M. Håård, U. Jaakma, B. Larsson, and H. Rodriguez-Martinez, "Does cleansing of frozen-thawed bull semen before assessment provide samples that relate better to potential fertility?"Theriogenology, vol. 62, no. 3-4, pp. 702–713, 2004.
34. D. Mortimer, "Sperm preparation methods," Journal of Andrology, vol. 21, no. 3, pp. 357–366, 2000.
35. T. Somfai, S. Bodó, S. Nagy et al., "Effect of swim up and Percoll treatment on viability and acrosome integrity of frozen-thawed bull spermatozoa," Reproduction in Domestic Animals, vol. 37, no. 5, pp. 285–290, 2002.
36. M. Shamsuddin and H. Rodriguez-Martinez, "A simple, non-traumatic swim-up method for the selection of spermatozoa for in vitro fertilization in the bovine," Animal Reproduction Science, vol. 36, no. 1-2, pp. 61–75, 1994.
37. T. Mogas, T. Rigau, J. Piedrafita, S. Bonet, and J. E. Rodriguez-Gil, "Effect of column filtration upon the quality parameters of fresh dog semen," Theriogenology, vol. 50, no. 8, pp. 1171–1189, 1998.
38. E. Bussalleu, E. Pinart, M. M. Rivera et al., "Effects of filtration of semen doses from subfertile boars through neuter Sephadex columns," Reproduction in Domestic Animals, vol. 43, no. 1, pp. 48–52, 2008.

39. M. Anzar, E. F. Graham, and N. Iqbal, "Post-thaw plasma membrane integrity of bull spermatozoa separated with a sephadex ion-exchange column," Theriogenology, vol. 47, no. 4, pp. 845–856, 1997.
40. Z. Ahmad, M. Anzar, M. Shahab, N. Ahmad, and S. M. H. Andrabi, "Sephadex and sephadex ion-exchange filtration improves the quality and freezability of low-grade buffalo semen ejaculates,"Theriogenology, vol. 59, no. 5-6, pp. 1189–1202, 2003.
41. J. C. Samper, D. W. Hamilton, J. L. Pryor, K. J. Loseth, M. H. T. Troedsson, and B. G. Crabo, "Mechanism of sephadex trapping of capacitated stallion spermatozoa," Biology of Reproduction, pp. 729–737, 1995.
42. A. Januskauskas, K. Lukoseviciute, S. Nagy, A. Johannisson, and H. Rodriguez-Martinez, "Assessment of the efficacy of Sephadex G-15 filtration of bovine spermatozoa for cryopreservation," Theriogenology, vol. 63, no. 1, pp. 160–178, 2005.
43. N. M. Ibrahim, D. N. Foster, and B. G. Crabo, "Localization of clusterin on freeze-preserved bull spermatozoa before and after glass wool-sephadex filtration," Journal of Andrology, vol. 22, no. 5, pp. 891–902, 2001.
44. H. Pertoft, "Fractionation of cells and subcellular particles with Percoll," Journal of Biochemical and Biophysical Methods, vol. 44, no. 1-2, pp. 1–30, 2000.
45. J. M. Morrell, A. Johannisson, A.-M. Dalin, and H. Rodriguez-Martinez, "Single-layer centrifugation with Androcoll™-E can be scaled up to allow large volumes of stallion ejaculate to be processed easily,"Theriogenology, vol. 72, no. 6, pp. 879–884, 2009.
46. M. Thys, L. Vandaele, J. Morrell et al., "In vitro fertilizing capacity of frozen-thawed bull spermatozoa selected by single-layer (Glycidoxypropyltrimethoxysilane) silane-coated silica colloidal centrifugation,"Reproduction in Domestic Animals, vol. 44, no. 3, pp. 390–394, 2009
47. J. M. Morrell, H. Rodriguez-Martinez, and C. Linde Forsberg, "Single layer centrifugation on a colloid selects motile and morphologically normal spermatozoa from dog semen:

preliminary results,"Reproduction in Domestic Animals, vol. 43, article 61, 2008, abstract P29.

48. K. Chatdarong, P. Thuwanut, and J. M. Morrell, "Single-layer centrifugation through colloid selects improved quality of epididymal cat sperm," Theriogenology, vol. 73, no. 9, pp. 1284–1292, 2010.

49. A. J. Edmond, A. R. Teague, S. P. Brinsko, et al., "Effect of density gradient centrifugation on quality and recovery of equine spermatozoa," Animal Reproduction Science, vol. 107, article 318, 2008, abstract 16.

50. J. M. Morrell, S. Colleoni, I. Lagutina, H. Rodriguez-Martinez, G. Lazzari, and C. Galli, "Stallion spermatozoa selected by Single Layer Centrifugation with Androcoll™-E have normal functionality after ICSI," Animal Reproduction Science, vol. 121S, pp. S196–S197, 2010.

51. M. Wallgren, H. Rodriguez-Martinez, and J. M. Morrell, "Single Layer Centrifugation with Androcoll™-P removes, or substantially reduces, bacterial contamination in boar sperm samples," inProceedings of the 11th International Symposium on Spermatology, Okinawa, Japan, June 2010.

52. J. M. Morrell, "Prevention of pathogen transmission through breeding in horses," Reproduction in Domestic Animals, vol. 44, supplement 3, 2009, abstract 15.3.

53. B. Macías García, J. M. Morrell, C. Ortega-Ferrusola et al., "Centrifugation on a single layer of colloid selects improved quality spermatozoa from frozen-thawed stallion semen," Animal Reproduction Science, vol. 114, no. 1–3, pp. 193–202, 2009.

54. B. M. García, L. G. Fernández, J. Morrell et al., "Single-layer centrifugation through colloid positively modifies the sperm subpopulation structure of frozen-thawed stallion spermatozoa," Reproduction in Domestic Animals, vol. 44, no. 3, pp. 523–526, 2009.

55. J. Morrell, A. Johannisson, A.-M. Dalin, and H. Rodriguez-Martinez, "Morphology and chromatin integrity of stallion spermatozoa prepared by density gradient and single layer centrifugation through silica colloids," Reproduction in Domestic Animals, vol. 44, no. 3, pp. 512–517, 2009.

56. W. M. C. Maxwell, I. Parrilla, I. Caballero et al., "Retained functional integrity of bull spermatozoa after double freezing and thawing using PureSperm® density gradient centrifugation," Reproduction in Domestic Animals, vol. 42, no. 5, pp. 489–494, 2007.

57. G. Huszar, C. C. Ozenci, S. Cayli, Z. Zavaczki, E. Hansch, and L. Vigue, "Hyaluronic acid binding by human sperm indicates cellular maturity, viability, and unreacted acrosomal status," Fertility and Sterility, vol. 79, no. 3, pp. 1616–1624, 2003.

58. C. Y. Park, S. J. Uhm, S. J. Song, et al., "Increase of ICSI efficiency with hyaluronic acid binding sperm for low aneuploidy frequency in pig," Theriogenology, vol. 64, no. 5, pp. 1158–1169, 2005.

59. W. Rohini Edirisinghe, A. Murch, S. Junk, and J. L. Yovich, "Cytogenetic abnormalities of unfertilized oocytes generated from in-vitro fertilization and intracytoplasmic sperm injection: a double-blind study," Human Reproduction, vol. 12, no. 12, pp. 2784–2791, 1997.

60. M. Nakai, N. Kashiwazaski, A. Takizawa et al., "Viable piglets generated from porcine oocytes matured in vitro and fertilized by intracytoplasmic sperm head injection," Biology of Reproduction, vol. 68, no. 3, pp. 1003–1008, 2003.

61. M. H. Nasr-Esfahani, S. Razavi, A. A. Vahdati, F. Fathi, and M. Tavalaee, "Evaluation of sperm selection procedure based on hyaluronic acid binding ability on ICSI outcome," Journal of Assisted Reproduction and Genetics, vol. 25, no. 5, pp. 197–203, 2008.

62. J. M. Morrell, S. Meurling, and H. Rodriguez-Martinez, "Can the HBA be used predictively for stallion spermatozoa," in Proceedings of the 11th International Symposium on Spermatology, Okinawa, Japan, June 2010.

63. H. Ye, G.-N. Huang, Y. Gao, and D. Y. Liu, "Relationship between human sperm-hyaluronan binding assay and fertilization rate in conventional in vitro fertilization," Human Reproduction, vol. 21, no. 6, pp. 1545–1550, 2006.

64. A. N. Fatehi, M. M. Bevers, E. Schoevers, B. A. J. Roelen, B. Colenbrander, and B. M. Gadella, "DNA damage in bovine sperm does not block fertilization and early embryonic development but

induces apoptosis after the first cleavages," Journal of Andrology, vol. 27, no. 2, pp. 176–188, 2006.

65. K. D. Keeler, N. M. Mackenzie, and D. W. Dresser, "Flow microfluorometric analysis of living spermatozoa stained with Hoechst 33342," Journal of Reproduction and Fertility, vol. 68, no. 1, pp. 205–212, 1983.
66. J. M. Morrell, K. D. Keeler, D. E. Noakes, N. M. Mackenzie, and D. W. Dresser, "Sexing of sperm by flow cytometry," Veterinary Record, vol. 122, no. 14, pp. 322–324, 1988.
67. L. A. Johnson, J. P. Flook, and H. W. Hawk, "Sex preselection in rabbits: live births from X and Y sperm separated by DNA and cell sorting," Biology of Reproduction, vol. 41, no. 2, pp. 199–203, 1989.
68. G. E. Seidel Jr., "Overview of sexing sperm," Theriogenology, vol. 68, no. 3, pp. 443–446, 2007.
69. S. L. Underwood, R. Bathgate, M. Ebsworth, W. M. C. Maxwell, and G. Evans, "Pregnancy loss in heifers after artificial insemination with frozen-thawed, sex-sorted, re-frozen-thawed dairy bull sperm," Animal Reproduction Science, vol. 118, no. 1, pp. 7–12, 2010.
70. B. L. Libbus, S. D. Perreault, L. A. Johnson, and D. Pinkel, "Incidence of chromosome aberrations in mammalian sperm stained with Hoechst 33342 and UV-laser irradiated during flow sorting," Mutation Research, vol. 182, no. 5, pp. 265–274, 1987.
71. J. M. Morrell and D. W. Dresser, "Offspring from inseminations with mammalian sperm stained with Hoechst 33342, either with or without flow cytometry," Mutation Research, vol. 224, no. 2, pp. 177–183, 1989.
72. L. A. Johnson and G. R. Welch, "Sex preselection: high-speed flow cytometric sorting of X and Y sperm for maximum efficiency," Theriogenology, vol. 52, no. 8, pp. 1323–1341, 1999.
73. J. R. Clulow, G. Evans, L. H. A. Morris, and W. M. C. Maxwell, "Factors influencing the «sortability» of stallion spermatozoa into X- and Y-chromosome bearing populations," Animal Reproduction Science, vol. 113, no. 1–4, pp. 220–228, 2009.
74. C. A. Wolf, K. E. Brass, M. I. B. Rubin, S. E. Pozzobon, F. D. Mozzaquatro, and F. D. de la Corte, "The effect of sperm selection

by Percoll or swim up on the sex ratio of in vitro produced bovine embryos,"Animal Reproduction, vol. 5, pp. 110–115, 2008.

75. G. M. Machado, J. O. Carvalho, E. S. Filho et al., "Effect of Percoll volume, duration and force of centrifugation, on in vitro production and sex ratio of bovine embryos," Theriogenology, vol. 71, no. 8, pp. 1289–1297, 2009.

76. S. R. Blecher, R. Howie, S. Li, J. Detmar, and L. M. Blahut, "A new approach to immunological sexing of sperm," Theriogenology, vol. 52, no. 8, pp. 1309–1321, 1999.

77. F. K. Hollinshead, J. K. O›Brien, W. M. C. Maxwell, and G. Evans, "Assessment of in vitro sperm characteristics after flow cytometric sorting of frozen-thawed bull spermatozoa," Theriogenology, vol. 62, no. 5, pp. 958–968, 2004.

78. H. Dobson, R. F. Smith, M. D. Royal, C. H. Knight, and I. M. Sheldon, "The high-producing dairy cow and its reproductive performance," Reproduction in Domestic Animals, vol. 42, no. 2, pp. 17–23, 2007.

79. T. Katila, T. Reilas, K. Nivola, T. Peltonen, and A.-M. Virtala, "A 15-year survey of reproductive efficiency of Standardbred and Finnhorse trotters in Finland—descriptive results," Acta Veterinaria Scandinavica. In press.

Chapter 11

Recent Advances in Application of Male Germ Cell Transplantation in Farm Animals

Ali Honaramooz*, and Yanfei Yang

Department of Veterinary Biomedical Sciences, Western College of Veterinary Medicine, University of Saskatchewan, 52 Campus Drive, Saskatoon, Saskatchewan, Canada S7N 5B4

ABSTRACT

Transplantation of isolated germ cells from a fertile donor male into the seminiferous tubules of infertile recipients can result in donor-derived sperm production. Therefore, this system represents a major development in the study of spermatogenesis and a unique functional assay to determine the developmental potential and relative abundance of spermatogonial stem cells in a given population of testis cells. The application of this method in farm animals has been the subject of an increasing number of studies, mostly because of its potential as an alternative strategy in producing transgenic livestock with higher efficiency and less time and capital requirement than the current methods. This paper highlights the salient recent research on germ cell transplantation in farm animals. The emphasis is placed on the current status of the technique and examination of ways to increase its efficiency through improved preparation of the recipient animals as well as isolation, purification, preservation, and transgenesis of the donor germ cells.

DEVELOPMENT OF MALE GERM CELL TRANSPLANTATION TECHNIQUE IN RODENTS

Germ cell transplantation (GCT), also referred to as spermatogonial stem cell (SSC) transplantation, is a powerful technology first introduced in 1994 by Brinster and colleagues. Although initially developed using a mouse model, GCT has important applications in the study and manipulation of spermatogenesis in many species. In this method, testis cells obtained from a fertile donor male are transferred into the seminiferous tubules of infertile recipient testes where donor-derived sperm production can occur, allowing the recipient to sire progeny [1, 2] (Figure 1). In essence, donor SSCs deposited in the lumen of the recipient seminiferous tubules are allowed by the Sertoli cells to migrate to the basolateral compartment of the tubule, to proliferate, form new colonies and initiate donor-derived spermatogenesis [3, 4]. Following the original introduction of GCT in mice [1, 2], the technique was also successful among rats [5, 6]. In laboratory rodents, GCT not only provides a unique opportunity for gaining new insight into spermatogenesis and the biology of the stem cell niche, but also presents a unique functional bioassay to test the competence of putative SSCs. Furthermore, GCT also offers a new strategy for preservation of male fertility and an alternative approach for generation of transgenic animals [7, 8].

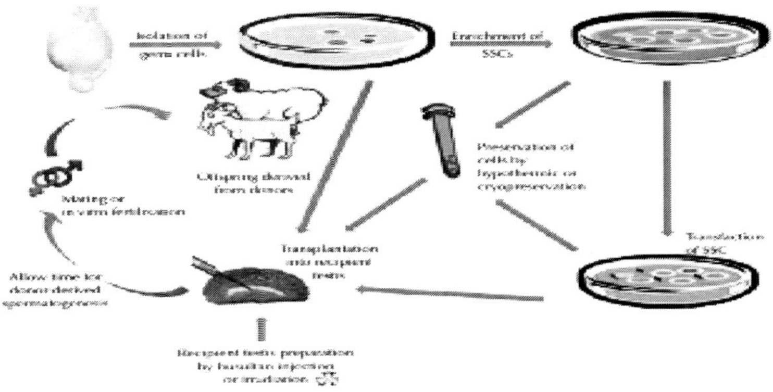

Figure 1: A schematic representation of procedures involved in germ cell transplantation in farm animals. A single-cell suspension of germ cells is prepared after enzymatic digestion of the donor testis for transplantation into recipient testes. Alternatively, the number of spermatogonial stem cells (SSCs) can be enriched in the donor cells and the resultant cells can be used fresh or preserved (for short term through hypothermic preservation or long-term by cryopreservation) and/or transfected with genes of interest before transplantation. The recipient animal can be treated with busulfan or undergo local irradiation of the testes to reduce the number of endogenous SSCs, in preparation for germ cell transplantation. Transplanted SSCs can form colonies of donor-derived spermatogenesis and produce sperm to allow the recipient to sire progeny carrying the donor haplotype.

CROSS-SPECIES APPLICATION OF MALE GERM CELL TRANSPLANTATION

Rather surprisingly, cross-species (xenogeneic/heterologous) transplantation of testis cells from donor rats into recipient mice resulted in complete rat spermatogenesis [9]. This development sparked an interest in the idea of using the laboratory mouse as a universal recipient model for testis cells from different donor species. However, while hamster testis cells transferred into recipient mouse testes also developed complete donor-derived spermatogenesis [10], GCT from genetically more distant donor species, including farm animals, into mice only resulted in colonization or proliferation of SSCs but not in complete spermatogenesis [11–15] (Table 1). This block in differentiation of donor germ cells is believed to be due to the incompatibility of donor germ cells and mouse Sertoli cells [16]. Although GCT from nonrodent species into the mouse testis did not result in complete spermatogenesis, it still is the only available bioassay for detecting the colonization potential of SSCs in a given population of donor testis cells from any species [11, 13, 17]. Interestingly, when (rather than transferring isolated testis cells into the seminiferous tubules) small fragments of testis tissue were transplanted under the back skin of recipient mice, complete donor-derived spermatogenesis was observed from a wide range of donor species, including farm animal species [18–26].

Table 1: Summary of germ cell transplantation in different donor and recipient species

			Donor-derived			
Donor	**Recipient**	**Colonization of SSCs**	**Spermatocytes**	**Spermatozoa**	**Offspring**	**Transgenic progeny**
Mouse	Mouse	+	+	+ [2]	+	+ [1, 27, 28]
Rat	Rat	+	+	+	+	+ [29, 30]
Rat	Mouse	+	+	+ [9, 31]	—	—
Hamster	Mouse	+	+	+ [10]	—	—
Rabbit	Mouse	+	[11]	—	—	—
Dog	Mouse	+	[11]	—	—	—
Pig	Mouse	+	[13]	—	—	—
Cattle	Mouse	+	[13]	—	—	—
Horse	Mouse	+	[13]	—	—	—
Baboon	Mouse	+	[14]	—	—	—
Mouse	Pig	– [32]	–	—	—	—
Goat	Goat	+ [33]	+	+	+	+ [34]
Cattle	Cattle	+ [35]	+	+ [36]	—	—
Cat	Mouse	+	[12]	—	—	—
Pig	Pig	+ [32]	+	+ [37]	—	—
Dog	Dog	+	+	+ [38]	—	—
Sheep	Sheep	+	+	+ [39, 40]	+ [40]	—

+: positive results; negative results.

CELL TRANSFER TECHNIQUES

The original procedures described for the transfer of donor male germ cells into the seminiferous tubules of recipient mice could not be directly applied in farm animals. Therefore, we used ultrasound-guided cannulation of the centrally located rete testis [41] to infuse donor germ cells by gravity flow which was successful in vivo for pigs and goats [32, 33]. The procedure could be completed in 15–30 min and resulted in filling of about half of the recipient seminiferous tubules with donor cells. This methodology has been successfully adapted for use in rams and bulls in vivo [36, 40, and 42]. Injection into the extratesticular rete testis using ultrasound guidance or surgical dissection was also reported to be applicable for use in rams [39, 43]. The success of the rete testis injection approach was further shown through donor-derived sperm production by the recipients [34, 44] and birth of progeny carrying the donor characteristics [34, 40].

PREPARATION OF RECIPIENT ANIMALS

The success of GCT between unrelated laboratory rodents appears to depend on the availability of recipients of strain that are genetically compatible with the donor animals, are inherently immunodeficient, or have undergone immunosuppressive treatments [1, 45, and 46]. Surprisingly, however, recipient pigs, goats, sheep, and bulls with fully functional immune systems did not reject germ cells from unrelated donors, making the practical application of the approach more feasible in farm animals [32–34, 39, 40].

Studies show that donor-derived spermatogenesis could be significantly improved when the recipient's endogenous germ cells are suppressed or depleted [6, 47]. Unlike in laboratory rodents, mutant animals with genetically impaired spermatogenesis are not readily available for use in work with farm animals. The azoospermic Klinefelter bull used in a study was determined not to be a useful recipient model for GCT [42], while limited donor-derived spermatogenesis was observed after GCT into two boars affected by the immotile short-tail sperm defect [37]. An alternative to the use of recipient animal models with congenital germ cell deficiency is removal of endogenous germ cells by cytoablative methods to facilitate further access to, and the availability of, the stem cell niche. We and others have achieved partial ablation of endogenous germ cells using busulfan (a chemotherapy agent) treatment of postnatal pigs [37, 48] and also during the in utero development of piglets [48]. This latter approach is particularly useful for preparation of piglets because treating a pregnant sow will result in producing multiple potential recipients at higher efficiency, but without the harmful health effects observed after treating postnatal piglets [48]. Where the facilities are available, local irradiation of testes can also be very effective in reducing the number of endogenous germ cells in recipient goats, rams and bulls [36, 48, and 49].

For practical reasons, most researchers have used immature recipients for GCT in farm animals, while recipients for GCT in laboratory rodents are typically adults. The use of immature recipient testis not only facilitates access of the transplanted donor germ cells to the tubular basolateral compartment (because it lacks the hindering multiple layers of germ cells), it also provides a more favorable environment than adult testes for engraftment and expansion of donor germ cells [50]. In our previous studies, we used immature pig and goat recipients with no pretreatment [32–34], resulting in ~7% donor-derived progeny in goats [34], while after preparation of immature recipients with testis irradiation, the progeny rate averaged ~8% or 10% in sheep and goats, respectively, [27, 40]. These results may indicate that while gradual progress in the efficiency of GCT in farm animals is being achieved, recipient preparation of immature recipients may not be as critical as that for adult recipients [6, 50]. It may also be concluded that recipient preparation is only part of the requirements for a successful GCT, and that other aspects of the system also need to be optimized before a higher efficiency is expected.

PREPARATION OF THE DONOR GERM CELLS

The efficiency of GCT is also highly dependent on the relative abundance of SSCs transplanted [3, 51–53]. In the adult testis, SSCs are a rare population, making up only ~0.02% to 0.2% of testis cells in mice and rats [54–56]. The efficiency of colony establishment is also low, and only 1% [53] or 7–20% of the transplanted SSCs will actually colonize the recipient testis [3, 52, and 53]. Naturally, increasing the number of SSCs in the donor population of cells prior to GCT will have a direct effect on the number of expected spermatogenic colonies in recipients [51, 52, and 57].

Choice of Donors

For GCT in rodents, several strategies including the use of cryptorchid, vitamin-A deficient or Steel (Sl) mutant mice can be used to increase the proportion of nondifferentiated spermatogonia in the population of donor cells [58–61]. Surgical induction of cryptorchidism in the donor, 2-3 months prior to use in GCT, is a common strategy resulting in elimination of a large number of differentiated germ cells, and thereby up to 23-fold increase in the relative number of SSCs [51]. These strategies have not been well pursued for use in farm animal GCT, partly to avoid the added complication of the procedure. On the other hand, testes from immature donors have been a frequent source of cells for use in farm animal GCT, because they provide a population of cells with a naturally higher proportion of germline stem cells than those of adults. In the neonatal testis, gonocytes are the only type of germ cells present, comprising 1-2% of total number of isolated testis cells in rodents [62, 63] or ~7% of intratubular cells in piglets [48]. Gonocytes have germline stem cell potential and upon transplantation into recipient testes are able to establish complete spermatogenesis [62]. Therefore, the neonatal/immature testis provides a logical source for GCT, especially for farm animals.

Isolation of Donor Germ Cells

Procedures for isolation of testis cells vary among laboratories, depending on the target cell types and the donor species. Two-step enzymatic digestion has been widely applied to isolate both gonocytes and SSCs in many species. In the first digestion step, collagenase and hyaluronidase enzymes are usually used to largely remove testis interstitial cells. As a second step, trypsin-EDTA (with or without additional enzymes) is used to break down seminiferous cords/tubules, while DNase is added to prevent cellular aggregation [64]. Using two-step digestion usually results in a maximum of 10% gonocytes/SSCs in the freshly isolated testis cells [62, 63, 65–70]. As outlined above, the proportion of SSCs can be increased using physically or genetically modified donors [58–61].

After a systematic evaluation of several potential factors affecting germ cell isolation, we recently developed a novel three-step strategy (combining vortexing and digestion) to isolate porcine testis cells with a gonocyte proportion of ~40%, (among fresh cells and before applying enrichment methods) [71] as compared with the conventional two-step enzymatic digestion resulting in collection of ~7% gonocytes.

Enrichment/Purification of Donor Germ Cells

Depending on the donor cells, diverse strategies can be used to enrich (but rarely purify) SSCs [72]. These strategies are generally based on fluorophore-labeled antibody separation of testis cells using fluorescent activated cell sorting (FACS) [51, 65, 68, 73–75], magnetic activated cell separation (MACS) [57, 65, 75–78], forward/side scatter measurements in FACS [51, 68, 79], density gradient centrifugation [43, 65, 67, 74, 80,81], or differential plating [43, 65, 67, 74, 81]. Using these approaches, SSCs have been enriched to as high as 75% in the population of donor testis cells from farm animals [43, 65, 67, 74]. However, work on enrichment of gonocytes, as opposed to SSCs, has been limited to a few reports in rodents and pigs [69, 82–84]. We recently assessed the efficiency of porcine gonocyte enrichment using density gradient and differential plating strategies. We found that gonocytes can be enriched to more than 80% using either Nycodenz density gradient or differential plating (with fibronectin and poly-D-lysine coatings), and to a purity of more than 90% by combining the two strategies (Yang and Honaramooz, unpublished data).

Preservation of Donor Testis Tissue and Cells

Different from the situation for GCT in rodents, preparation of the required high numbers of germ cells from testes of donor farm animals for same day transplantation could be a time-management challenge.

Aside from the time needed for collection of donor testes from farm animals, the high volume of the tissue and presence of dense connective tissue make the process of digestion time consuming and often requiring the tissue or cells to be stored overnight before GCT [32, 39, 40, 43, 74]. If the time required for enrichment of germ cells followed by their transgenesis is added, the preparation time could be longer, and the need for preservation of the tissue/cells is even greater.

Cryopreservation of isolated germ cells allows their storage for extended periods of time; however, not only is it not suitable for short-term preservation, it can also damage cells, as cryopreservation of bovine germ cells resulted in cell survival rates of ~50–70% [85]. We also showed the feasibility of cryopreserving fragments of porcine testis tissue [86, 87] resulting in a postdigestion cell survival of ~55–88% while maintaining the in vivo developmental potential [86].

Short-term preservation of testis cells and tissue, on the other hand, is necessary and could be more suitable for immediate applications such as in GCT and for shipment of cells/tissue between collaborating laboratories. Hypothermic temperatures (above freezing point but below the body temperature) cause a decrease in cellular metabolism rate, oxygen demand, and energy consumption and therefore prolong cell viability. Ice-cold storage of testis tissue for 1 or 2 days was suggested to improve donor-derived spermatogenesis after xenografting [87, 88]. Testis tissue stored at refrigeration temperature for 3 days maintained its structural integrity [89], but cell viability starts to decrease [87]. We recently showed that using proper media, isolated cells from donor piglets could be maintained even at room temperature for at least 24 hours and up to 6 days at refrigeration temperature, resulting in up to 88% after-storage cell viability, and without changing the germ cell proportions or cell culture properties [89, 90].

Identification of Donor Cells after Transplantation

The availability of donor models providing cells with visual markers was critical for original development of GCT technique in mice [1, 2], because they allowed monitoring of the long-term fate of donor cells. Similar donor models are not readily available for use in farm animal GCT. Therefore, to track donor cells, researchers largely rely on fluorescence labeling of donors cells (although only traceable for a short period of time) [32, 39, 43] or use genetic identification of donor-derived cells/sperm. As a proof-of-principle study, we transplanted testis cells from transgenic donor goats into testes of wild-type recipient goats, resulting in production of donor-derived sperm and subsequently transgenic progeny [34]. Microsatellite detection has also been used to identify donor-derived sperm DNA in the semen of recipient rams [44]. Alternatively, transplantation of normal testis cells into recipients with genetic aberrations such as the immotile short-tail sperm syndrome has been used to facilitate detection of normal pig sperm in the semen of recipient pigs as indication of GCT success [37].

Insertion of Genes into Donor Germ Cells

All adult stem cells have the ability to self-renew and to produce differentiated cells; however, SSCs are unique because they produce a lifetime supply of sperm in adults with the potential to contribute genes to progeny. Therefore, if SSCs are incorporated with genes of interest prior to transplantation, their resultant sperm will carry the transgene in the recipient. The desired genes for example can include those of visual markers to facilitate GCT studies and to serve as a step toward generating transgenic farm animals through GCT. Methods of DNA delivery into cells include chemical, lipofection, electroporation, and viral vectors. Compared with nonviral methods, recombinant viral vectors generally have very high cell transfection efficiency rates, and some are able to integrate the transgene into the SSC genome for stable expression. However, construction of the desired viral vectors is more involved and their use requires a facility with a higher biosafety level. Nonviral alternatives, on the other hand, are relatively easy to use and pertain virtually no biosafety risk to the operator or the public but their efficiency rates are usually much lower.

The work in transgenesis of germ cells for farm animal GCT is at early stages. Electroporation of bovine testis tissue in vitro resulted in transfection of SSCs shown after xenografting into the back of immunodeficient mice [91]. Transfection of pig germ cells was also reported after injection of plasmids mixed with a lipofection reagent into busulfan treated testes; however, it was unclear from the report whether SSCs were indeed transfected [92].

In a preliminary study, we used a recombinant adenoassociated virus (rAAV) containing the GFP reporter gene and CMV promoter to transfect isolated pig testis cells in vitro and observed GFP expression in cultured cells and in spermatogenic colonies for several months after GCT into recipient testes [93]. Subsequent use of rAAV vectors carrying the GFP for transfection of goat testis cells prior to GCT into recipient goats led to long-term expression of GFP in recipient testes and presence of transgenic sperm in 35% of the ejaculates. When semen from these recipient goats was used for in vitro fertilization, 10% of embryos were transgenic, showing germline transmission [27]. These results indicate that transgenesis via GCT in farm animals is a promising approach to generate transgenic animals.

POTENTIAL APPLICATIONS OF MALE GERM CELL TRANSPLANTATION IN FARM ANIMALS

Although technically still at an experimental level, there are significant potential applications for GCT in farm animals. This includes genetic modification of farm animals through transplantation of genetically altered male germ cells for improving productivity traits or producing transgenic farm animals. As such, GCT would be an alternative strategy to the currently inefficient and costly methods of generating transgenic farm animals [94, 95]. The development of transgenic pigs, for instance, is of interest because of its potential to provide tissues and organs for xenotransplantation to humans and as a model for biomedical research [96]. Genetically altered dairy goats, sheep, and cows are also of significant economic value for the production of biopharmaceutical proteins in their milk [95, 96]. It has also been proposed that GCT can be used as an alternative way to artificial insemination for dissemination of elite sire bull genetics in extensive beef cattle grazing systems where animal handling is a limiting factor [35, 97]. Another important potential application of GCT is to restore fertility by cryopreservation followed by transplantation of genetic material from immature males (as shown for testis tissue grafting [86]) of rare or valuable livestock breeds that die while they are premature or from horses that undergo early castration but display superior traits later in life. The advantage of using SSCs for genetic dissemination or fertility restoration is that SSCs can be harvested, cultured, propagated, cryopreserved, or transfected and still preserve the potential to colonize the recipient testes [1, 27, 28, 32, 34, 98–102]. Since SSCs can both self-renew and produce a lifetime supply of sperm in adults, they have tremendous potential in modifying the male germ line as compared with, for example, the use of a finite amount of frozen semen from a given donor.

PRODUCTION OF LIVE PROGENY AFTER MALE GERM CELL TRANSPLANTATION

The birth of offspring carrying the donor haplotype after mating of a recipient can be viewed as the most convincing evidence for any successful GCT. In the initial report of GCT in mice, some of the infertile recipients produced enough donor-derived sperm to allow them to sire progeny [1]. As summarized in Table 1, among nonrodent species, live progeny has so far been produced following GCT in only goats and sheep, with an efficiency of ~7–10% [34, 40]. The field application of this new technology for farm animals relies upon the efficient production of donor-derived offspring in the end. Therefore, the feasibility and efficiency of live offspring production via GCT in farm animals need to be investigated further and improved (Figure 1).

CONCLUSIONS AND FUTURE DIRECTIONS

In a short period of time since the first reports in 2002-2003 [32–34, 36, 42], GCT in farm animals has shown great potential and promising initial results. Currently the percentage of donor-derived sperm in the semen of recipients after GCT is rather low, but evidence indicates that the efficiency can be improved. As we move beyond the stage of proof-of-principle studies, it is expected that the research in this area will focus more on improving a number of factors related to the success rate of the technique and on making it a viable option for downstream applications. These improvements are especially needed for obtaining higher numbers and purity of SSCs in the donor populations of cells. Another area of high potential is work on increasing the efficiency of nonviral transfection of germ cells, particularly if the ultimate transgenic animals are to be considered for generating products for human consumption. There are several advantages in pursuing farm animal transgenesis through GCT. For instance, the time from GCT into prepubertal recipient farm animals to first detection of transgenic sperm in the ejaculate is only a few months. Therefore, the time required to start collecting transgenic sperm may be reduced by one generation to about one half of that required by current methods. This time saving factor alone can significantly reduce the maintenance cost and accelerate the generation of a transgenic herd needed for large-scale production.

ACKNOWLEDGMENTS

The authors thank the University of Saskatchewan Colleges of Graduate Studies and Veterinary Medicine for scholarships (to Y. Yang), and the Natural Sciences and Engineering Research Council (NSERC) of Canada for grants (to A. Honaramooz) to support the recent work from the current laboratory summarized in this paper.

REFERENCES

1. R. L. Brinster and M. R. Avarbock, "Germline transmission of donor haplotype following spermatogonial transplantation," Proceedings of the National Academy of Sciences of the United States of America, vol. 91, no. 24, pp. 11303–11307, 1994.
2. R. L. Brinster and J. W. Zimmermann, "Spermatogenesis following male germ-cell transplantation,"Proceedings of the National Academy of Sciences of the United States of America, vol. 91, no. 24, pp. 11298–11302, 1994.
3. M. Nagano, M. R. Avarbock, and R. L. Brinster, "Pattern and kinetics of mouse donor spermatogonial stem cell colonization in recipient testes," Biology of Reproduction, vol. 60, no. 6, pp. 1429–1436, 1999.

4. H. Ohta, K. Yomogida, S. Yamada, M. Okabe, and Y. Nishimune, "Real-time observation of transplanted 'green germ cells': proliferation and differentiation of stem cells," Development Growth and Differentiation, vol. 42, no. 2, pp. 105–112, 2000.
5. F.-X. Jiang and R. V. Short, "Male germ cell transplantation in rats: apparent synchronization of spermatogenesis between host and donor seminiferous epithelia," International Journal of Andrology, vol. 18, no. 6, pp. 326–330, 1995.
6. T. Ogawa, I. Dobrinski, and R. L. Brinster, "Recipient preparation is critical for spermatogonial transplantation in the rat," Tissue and Cell, vol. 31, no. 5, pp. 461–472, 1999.
7. R. L. Brinster, "Germline stem cell transplantation and transgenesis," Science, vol. 296, no. 5576, pp. 2174–2176, 2002.
8. R. L. Brinster, "Male germline stem cells: from mice to men," Science, vol. 316, no. 5823, pp. 404–405, 2007.
9. D. E. Clouthier, M. R. Avarbock, S. D. Maika, R. E. Hammer, and R. L. Brinster, "Rat spermatogenesis in mouse testis," Nature, vol. 381, no. 6581, pp. 418–421, 1996.
10. T. Ogawa, I. Dobrinski, M. R. Avarbock, and R. L. Brinster, "Xenogeneic spermatogenesis following transplantation of hamster germ cells to mouse testes," Biology of Reproduction, vol. 60, no. 2, pp. 515–521, 1999.
11. I. Dobrinski, M. R. Avarbock, and R. L. Brinster, "Transplantation of germ cells from rabbits and dogs into mouse testes," Biology of Reproduction, vol. 61, no. 5, pp. 1331–1339, 1999.
12. Y. Kim, V. Selvaraj, I. Dobrinski, H. Lee, M. C. Mcentee, and A. J. Travis, "Recipient preparation and mixed germ cell isolation for spermatogonial stem cell transplantation in domestic cats," Journal of Andrology, vol. 27, no. 2, pp. 248–256, 2006.
13. I. Dobrinski, M. R. Avarbock, and R. L. Brinster, "Germ cell transplantation from large domestic animals into mouse testes," Molecular Reproduction and Development, vol. 57, no. 3, pp. 270–279, 2000.
14. M. Nagano, J. R. McCarrey, and R. L. Brinster, "Primate spermatogonial stem cells colonize mouse testes," Biology of Reproduction, vol. 64, no. 5, pp. 1409–1416, 2001.

15. M. Nagano, P. Patrizio, and R. L. Brinster, "Long-term survival of human spermatogonial stem cells in mouse testes," Fertility and Sterility, vol. 78, no. 6, pp. 1225–1233, 2002.
16. T. Shinohara, K. E. Orwig, M. R. Avarbock, and R. L. Brinster, "Restoration of spermatogenesis in infertile mice by Sertoli cell transplantation," Biology of Reproduction, vol. 68, no. 3, pp. 1064–1071, 2003.
17. I. Dobrinski, T. Ogawa, M. R. Avarbock, and R. L. Brinster, "Computer assisted image analysis to assess colonization of recipient seminiferous tubules by spermatogonial stem cells from transgenic donor mice," Molecular Reproduction and Development, vol. 53, no. 2, pp. 142–148, 1999.
18. A. Honaramooz, A. Snedaker, M. Boiani, H. Schöler, I. Dobrinski, and S. Schlatt, "Sperm from neonatal mammalia testes grafted in mice," Nature, vol. 418, no. 6899, pp. 778–781, 2002.
19. A. Honaramooz, M.-W. Li, M. C. T. Penedo, S. Meyers, and I. Dobrinski, "Accelerated maturation of primate testis by xenografting into mice," Biology of Reproduction, vol. 70, no. 5, pp. 1500–1503, 2004.
20. S. Schlatt, S. S. Kim, and R. Gosden, "Spermatogenesis and steroidogenesis in mouse, hamster and monkey testicular tissue after cryopreservation and heterotopic grafting to castrated hosts,"Reproduction, vol. 124, no. 3, pp. 339–346, 2002.
21. J. M. Oatley, J. J. Reeves, and D. J. McLean, "Establishment of spermatogenesis in neonatal bovine testicular tissue following ectopic xenografting varies with donor age," Biology of Reproduction, vol. 72, no. 2, pp. 358–364, 2005.
22. R. Rathi, A. Honaramooz, W. Zeng, R. Turner, and I. Dobrinski, "Germ cell development in equine testis tissue xenografted into mice," Reproduction, vol. 131, no. 6, pp. 1091–1098, 2006.
23. R. Rathi, W. Zeng, S. Megee, A. Conley, S. Meyers, and I. Dobrinski, "Maturation of testicular tissue from infant monkeys after xenografting into mice," Endocrinology, vol. 149, no. 10, pp. 5288–5296, 2008.
24. L. Arregui, R. Rathi, S. O. Megee et al., "Xenografting of sheep testis tissue and isolated cells as a model for preservation of genetic material from endangered ungulates," Reproduction, vol. 136, no. 1, pp. 85–93, 2008.

25. J. Ehmcke and S. Schlatt, "Animal models for fertility preservation in the male," Reproduction, vol. 136, no. 6, pp. 717–723, 2008.
26. M. Nakai, H. Kaneko, T. Somfai et al., "Production of viable piglets for the first time using sperm derived from ectopic testicular xenografts," Reproduction, vol. 139, no. 2, pp. 331–335, 2010.
27. A. Honaramooz, S. Megee, W. Zeng et al., "Adeno-associated virus (AAV)-mediated transduction of male germ line stem cells results in transgene transmission after germ cell transplantation," FASEB Journal, vol. 22, no. 2, pp. 374–382, 2008.
28. M. Nagano, C. J. Brinster, K. E. Orwig, B.-Y. Ryu, M. R. Avarbock, and R. L. Brinster, "Transgenic mice produced by retroviral transduction of male germ-line stem cells," Proceedings of the National Academy of Sciences of the United States of America, vol. 98, no. 23, pp. 13090–13095, 2001.
29. F. K. Hamra, J. Gatlin, K. M. Chapman et al., "Production of transgenic rats by lentiviral transduction of male germ-line stem cells," Proceedings of the National Academy of Sciences of the United States of America, vol. 99, no. 23, pp. 14931–14936, 2002.
30. B.-Y. Ryu, K. E. Orwig, J. M. Oatley et al., "Efficient generation of transgenic rats through the male germline using lentiviral transduction and transplantation of spermatogonial stem cells," Journal of Andrology, vol. 28, no. 2, pp. 353–360, 2007. · ·
31. L. R. França, T. Ogawa, M. R. Avarbock, R. L. Brinster, and L. D. Russell, "Germ cell genotype controls cell cycle during spermatogenesis in the rat," Biology of Reproduction, vol. 59, no. 6, pp. 1371–1377, 1998.
32. A. Honaramooz, S. O. Megee, and I. Dobrinski, "Germ cell transplantation in pigs," Biology of Reproduction, vol. 66, no. 1, pp. 21–28, 2002.
33. A. Honaramooz, E. Behboodi, S. Blash, S. O. Megee, and I. Dobrinski, "Germ cell transplantation in goats," Molecular Reproduction and Development, vol. 64, no. 4, pp. 422–428, 2003.
34. A. Honaramooz, E. Behboodi, S. O. Megee et al., "Fertility and germline transmission of donor haplotype following germ cell transplantation in immunocompetent goats," Biology of Reproduction, vol. 69, no. 4, pp. 1260–1264, 2003. · ·

35. M. Herrid, S. Vignarajan, R. Davey, I. Dobrinski, and J. R. Hill, "Successful transplantation of bovine testicular cells to heterologous recipients," Reproduction, vol. 132, no. 4, pp. 617–624, 2006.
36. F. Izadyar, K. den Ouden, T. A. E. Stout et al., "Autologous and homologous transplantation of bovine spermatogonial stem cells," Reproduction, vol. 126, no. 6, pp. 765–774, 2003.
37. M. Mikkola, A. Sironen, C. Kopp et al., "Transplantation of normal boar testicular cells resulted in complete focal spermatogenesis in a boar affected by the immotile short-tail sperm defect,"Reproduction in Domestic Animals, vol. 41, no. 2, pp. 124–128, 2006.
38. Y. Kim, D. Turner, J. Nelson, I. Dobrinski, M. McEntee, and A. J. Travis, "Production of donor-derived sperm after spermatogonial stem cell transplantation in the dog," Reproduction, vol. 136, no. 6, pp. 823–831, 2008
39. J. R. Rodriguez-Sosa, J. D. Silvertown, R. A. Foster, J. A. Medin, and A. Hahnel, "Transduction and transplantation of spermatogonia into the testis of ram lambs through the extra-testicular rete,"Reproduction in Domestic Animals, vol. 44, no. 4, pp. 612–620, 2009.
40. M. Herrid, J. Olejnik, M. Jackson et al., "Irradiation enhances the efficiency of testicular germ cell transplantation in sheep," Biology of Reproduction, vol. 81, no. 5, pp. 898–905, 2009.
41. S. Schlatt, G. Rosiepen, G. F. Weinbauer, C. Rolf, P. F. Brook, and E. Nieschlag, "Germ cell transfer into rat, bovine, monkey and human testes," Human Reproduction, vol. 14, no. 1, pp. 144–150, 1999.
42. H. Joerg, F. Janett, S. Schlatt et al., "Germ cell transplantation in an azoospermic Klinefelter bull,"Biology of Reproduction, vol. 69, no. 6, pp. 1940–1944, 2003.
43. J. R. Rodriguez-Sosa, H. Dobson, and A. Hahnel, "Isolation and transplantation of spermatogonia in sheep," Theriogenology, vol. 66, no. 9, pp. 2091–2103, 2006
44. S. Stockwell, M. Herrid, R. Davey, A. Brownlee, K. Hutton, and J. R. Hill, "Microsatellite detection of donor-derived sperm DNA following germ cell transplantation in cattle," Reproduction, Fertility and Development, vol. 21, no. 3, pp. 462–468, 2009.

45. Z. Zhang, M. B. Renfree, and R. V. Short, "Successful intra- and interspecific male germ cell transplantation in the rat," Biology of Reproduction, vol. 68, no. 3, pp. 961–967, 2003
46. M. Kanatsu-Shinohara, N. Ogonuki, K. Inoue et al., "Allogeneic offspring produced by male germ line stem cell transplantation into infertile mouse testis," Biology of Reproduction, vol. 68, no. 1, pp. 167–173, 2003
47. T. Shinohara, K. E. Orwig, M. R. Avarbock, and R. L. Brinster, "Germ line stem cell competition in postnatal mouse testes," Biology of Reproduction, vol. 66, no. 5, pp. 1491–1497, 2002.
48. A. Honaramooz, E. Behboodi, C. L. Hausler et al., "Depletion of endogenous germ cells in male pigs and goats in preparation for germ cell transplantation," Journal of Andrology, vol. 26, no. 6, pp. 698–705, 2005.
49. J. M. Oatley, A. Tibary, D. M. De Avila, J. E. Wheaton, D. J. McLean, and J. J. Reeves, "Changes in spermatogenesis and endocrine function in the ram testis due to irradiation and active immunization against luteinizing hormone-releasing hormone," Journal of Animal Science, vol. 83, no. 3, pp. 604–612, 2005.
50. T. Shinohara, K. E. Orwig, M. R. Avarbock, and R. L. Brinster, "Remodeling of the postnatal mouse testis is accompanied by dramatic changes in stem cell number and niche accessibility," Proceedings of the National Academy of Sciences of the United States of America, vol. 98, no. 11, pp. 6186–6191, 2001.
51. T. Shinohara, K. E. Orwig, M. R. Avarbock, and R. L. Brinster, "Spermatogonial stem cell enrichment by multiparameter selection of mouse testis cells," Proceedings of the National Academy of Sciences of the United States of America, vol. 97, no. 15, pp. 8346–8351, 2000
52. T. Shinohara, M. R. Avarbock, and R. L. Brinster, "β1- and α6-integrin are surface markers on mouse spermatogonial stem cells," Proceedings of the National Academy of Sciences of the United States of America, vol. 96, no. 10, pp. 5504–5509, 1999.
53. F.-X. Jiang, "Male germ cell transplantation: promise and problems," Reproduction, Fertility and Development, vol. 13, no. 7-8, pp. 609–614, 2001.

54. M. Kanatsu-Shinohara, N. Ogonuki, T. Iwano et al., "Genetic and epigenetic properties of mouse male germline stem cells during long-term culture," Development, vol. 132, no. 18, pp. 4155–4163, 2005

55. R. A. J. Tegelenbosch and D. G. de Rooij, "A quantitative study of spermatogonial multiplication and stem cell renewal in the C3H/101 F1 hybrid mouse," Mutation Research, vol. 290, no. 2, pp. 193–200, 1993

56. C. Huckins, "The spermatogonial stem cell population in adult rats. I. Their morphology, proliferation and maturation," Anatomical Record, vol. 169, no. 3, pp. 533–557, 1971.

57. A. Buageaw, M. Sukhwani, A. Ben-Yehudah et al., "GDNF family receptor alpha1 phenotype of spermatogonial stem cells in immature mouse testes," Biology of Reproduction, vol. 73, no. 5, pp. 1011–1016, 2005

58. T. Shinohara and R. L. Brinster, "Enrichment and transplantation of spermatogonial stem cells,"International Journal of Andrology, Supplement, vol. 23, no. 2, pp. 89–91, 2000.

59. A. M. M. van Pelt, A. R. Morena, F. M. F. van Dissel-Emiliani et al., "Isolation of the synchronized A spermatogonia from adult vitamin A-deficient rat testes," Biology of Reproduction, vol. 55, no. 2, pp. 439–444, 1996.

60. T. Ogawa, I. Dobrinski, M. R. Avarbock, and R. L. Brinster, "Transplantation of male germ line stem cells restores fertility in infertile mice," Nature Medicine, vol. 6, no. 1, pp. 29–34, 2000

61. A. M. M. Van Pelt, F. M. F. Van Dissel-Emiliani, I. C. Gaemers, M. J. M. van der Burg, H. J. Tanke, and D. G. De Rooij, "Characteristics of a spermatogonia and preleptotene spermatocytes in the vitamin A-deficient rat testis," Biology of Reproduction, vol. 53, no. 3, pp. 570–578, 1995.

62. K. E. Orwig, B.-Y. Ryu, M. R. Avarbock, and R. L. Brinster, "Male germ-line stem cell potential is predicted by morphology of cells in neonatal rat testes," Proceedings of the National Academy of Sciences of the United States of America, vol. 99, no. 18, pp. 11706–11711, 2002

63. H. Li, V. Papadopoulos, B. Vidic, M. Dym, and M. Culty, "Regulation of rat testis gonocyte proliferation by platelet-

derived growth factor and estradiol: identification of signaling mechanisms involved," Endocrinology, vol. 138, no. 3, pp. 1289–1298, 1997.

64. A. R. Bellve, J. C. Cavicchia, and C. F. Millette, "Spermatogenic cells of the prepuberal mouse. Isolation and morphological characterization," Journal of Cell Biology, vol. 74, no. 1, pp. 68–85, 1977.

65. M. Herrid, R. J. Davey, K. Hutton, I. G. Colditz, and J. R. Hill, "A comparison of methods for preparing enriched populations of bovine spermatogonia," Reproduction, Fertility and Development, vol. 21, no. 3, pp. 393–399, 2009. · ·

66. D. G. de Rooij and A. M. M. van Pelt, "Spermatogonial Stem Cell Biology," Annual Review of Biomedical Sciences, vol. 5, pp. 105–114, 2003.

67. J. Luo, S. Megee, R. Rathi, and I. Dobrinski, "Protein gene product 9.5 is a spermatogonia-specific marker in the pig testis: application to enrichment and culture of porcine spermatogonia," Molecular Reproduction and Development, vol. 73, no. 12, pp. 1531–1540, 2006

68. K. C. Lo, V. M. Brugh III, M. Parker, and D. J. Lamb, "Isolation and enrichment of murine spermatogonial stem cells using rhodamine 123 mitochondrial dye," Biology of Reproduction, vol. 72, no. 3, pp. 767–771, 2005

69. F. M. F. van Dissel-Emiliani, D. G. De Rooij, and M. L. Meistrich, "Isolation of rat gonocytes by velocity sedimentation at unit gravity," Journal of Reproduction and Fertility, vol. 86, no. 2, pp. 759–766, 1989.

70. J. M. Orth, J. Qiu, W. F. Jester Jr., and S. Pilder, "Expression of the c-kit gene is critical for migration of neonatal rat gonocytes in vitro," Biology of Reproduction, vol. 57, no. 3, pp. 676–683, 1997.

71. Y. Yang, M. Yarahmadi, and A. Honaramooz, "Development of novel strategies for the isolation of piglet testis cells with a high proportion of gonocytes," Reproduction, Fertility and Development, vol. 22, no. 7, pp. 1057–1065, 2010.

72. H. Khaira, D. McLean, D. A. Ohl, and G. D. Smith, "Spermatogonial stem cell isolation, storage, and transplantation," Journal of Andrology, vol. 26, no. 4, pp. 442–450, 2005.

73. N. R. Moudgal, M. R. Sairam, H. N. Krishnamurthy, S. Sridhar, H. Krishnamurthy, and H. Khan, "Immunization of male bonnet monkeys (M. radiata) with a recombinant FSH receptor preparation affects testicular function and fertility," Endocrinology, vol. 138, no. 7, pp. 3065–3068, 1997.

74. F. Izadyar, G. T. Spierenberg, L. B. Creemers, K. den Ouden, and D. G. de Rooij, "Isolation and purification of type A spermatogonia from the bovine testis," Reproduction, vol. 124, no. 1, pp. 85–94, 2002.

75. H. Kubota, M. R. Avarbock, and R. L. Brinster, "Culture conditions and single growth factors affect fate determination of mouse spermatogonial stem cells," Biology of Reproduction, vol. 71, no. 3, pp. 722–731, 2004

76. G. Giuili, A. Tomljenovic, N. Labrecque, M. Oulad-Abdelghani, M. Rassoulzadegan, and F. Cuzin, "Murine spermatogonial stem cells: targeted transgene expression and purification in an active state,"EMBO Reports, vol. 3, no. 8, pp. 753–759, 2002

77. K. Gassei, J. Ehmcke, and S. Schlatt, "Efficient enrichment of undifferentiated GFR alpha 1+ spermatogonia from immature rat testis by magnetic activated cell sorting," Cell and tissue research, vol. 337, no. 1, pp. 177–183, 2009

78. V. von Schönfeldt, H. Krishnamurthy, L. Foppiani, and S. Schlatt, "Magnetic cell sorting is a fast and effective method of enriching viable spermatogonia from djungarian hamster, mouse, and marmoset monkey testes," Biology of Reproduction, vol. 61, no. 3, pp. 582–589, 1999

79. H. Kubota, M. R. Avarbock, and R. L. Brinster, "Spermatogonial stem cells share some, but not all, phenotypic and functional characteristics with other stem cells," Proceedings of the National Academy of Sciences of the United States of America, vol. 100, no. 11, pp. 6487–6492, 2003.

80. C. Marret and P. Durand, "Culture of porcine spermatogonia: effects of purification of the germ cells, extracellular matrix and fetal calf serum on their survival and multiplication," Reproduction Nutrition Development, vol. 40, no. 3, pp. 305–319, 2000.

81. G. Dirami, N. Ravindranath, V. Pursel, and M. Dym, "Effects of stem cell factor and granulocyte macrophage-colony stimulating factor on survival of porcine type a spermatogonia cultured in

KSOM," Biology of Reproduction, vol. 61, no. 1, pp. 225–230, 1999.

82. T. J. Moore, M. de Boer-Brouwer, and F. M. F. van Dissel-Emiliani, "Purified gonocytes from the neonatal rat form foci of proliferating germ cells in vitro," Endocrinology, vol. 143, no. 8, pp. 3171–3174, 2002.

83. R. van den Ham, A. M. M. van Pelt, M. P. de Miguel, P. J. S. van Kooten, N. Walther, and F. M. F. van Dissel-Emilani, "Immunomagnetic isolation of fetal rat gonocytes," American Journal of Reproductive Immunology, vol. 38, no. 1, pp. 39–45, 1997.

84. S. Goel, M. Sugimoto, N. Minami, M. Yamada, S. Kume, and H. Imai, "Identification, isolation, and in vitro culture of porcine gonocytes," Biology of Reproduction, vol. 77, no. 1, pp. 127–137, 2007

85. F. Izadyar, J. J. Matthijs-Rijsenbilt, K. Den Ouden, L. B. Creemers, H. Woelders, and D. G. De Rooij, "Development of a cryopreservation protocol for type A spermatogonia," Journal of Andrology, vol. 23, no. 4, pp. 537–545, 2002.

86. M. Abrishami, M. Anzar, Y. Yang, and A. Honaramooz, "Cryopreservation of immature porcine testis tissue to maintain its developmental potential after xenografting into recipient mice," Theriogenology, vol. 73, no. 1, pp. 86–96, 2010.

87. W. Zeng, A. K. Snedaker, S. Megee et al., "Preservation and transplantation of porcine testis tissue,"Reproduction, Fertility and Development, vol. 21, no. 3, pp. 489–497, 2009.

88. K. Jahnukainen, J. Ehmcke, S. D. Hergenrother, and S. Schlatt, "Effect of cold storage and cryopreservation of immature non-human primate testicular tissue on spermatogonial stem cell potential in xenografts," Human Reproduction, vol. 22, no. 4, pp. 1060–1067, 2007.

89. Y. Yang, J. Steeg, and A. Honaramooz, "The effects of tissue sample size and media on short-term hypothermic preservation of porcine testis tissue," Cell and Tissue Research, vol. 340, no. 2, pp. 397–406, 2010.

90. Y. Yang and A. Honaramooz, "Effects of medium and hypothermic temperatures on preservation of isolated porcine testis cells,"

Reproduction, Fertility and Development, vol. 22, no. 3, pp. 523–532, 2010.

91. J. M. Oatley, D. M. de Avila, J. J. Reeves, and D. J. McLean, "Spermatogenesis and germ cell transgene expression in xenografted bovine testicular tissue," Biology of Reproduction, vol. 71, no. 2, pp. 494–501, 2004

92. J.-H. Kim, H.-S. Jung-Ha, H.-T. Lee, and K.-S. Chung, "Development of a positive method for male stem cell-mediated gene transfer in mouse and pig," Molecular Reproduction and Development, vol. 46, no. 4, pp. 515–526, 1997

93. A. Honaramooz, et al., "Use of adeno-associated virus for transfection of male germ cells for transplantation in pigs," Theriogenology, vol. 1, no. 59, p. 536, 2003.

94. H. Niemann and W. A. Kues, "Transgenic farm animals: an update," Reproduction, Fertility and Development, vol. 19, no. 6, pp. 762–770, 2007.

95. C. L. Keefer, "Production of bioproducts through the use of transgenic animal models," Animal Reproduction Science, vol. 82-83, pp. 5–12, 2004.

96. H. Niemann and W. A. Kues, "Application of transgenesis in livestock for agriculture and biomedicine," Animal Reproduction Science, vol. 79, no. 3-4, pp. 291–317, 2003.

97. J. R. Hill and I. Dobrinski, "Male germ cell transplantation in livestock," Reproduction, Fertility and Development, vol. 18, no. 1-2, pp. 13–18, 2006

98. M. R. Avarbock, C. J. Brinster, and R. L. Brinster, "Reconstitution of spermatogenesis from frozen spermatogonial stem cells," Nature Medicine, vol. 2, no. 6, pp. 693–696, 1996.

99. M. Nagano, M. R. Avarbock, E. B. Leonida, C. J. Brinster, and R. L. Brinster, "Culture of mouse spermatogonial stem cells," Tissue and Cell, vol. 30, no. 4, pp. 389–397, 1998.

100. M. Nagano, T. Shinohara, M. R. Avarbock, and R. L. Brinster, "Retrovirus-mediated gene delivery into male germ line stem cells," FEBS Letters, vol. 475, no. 1, pp. 7–10, 2000.

101. T. Shinohara, M. Kato, M. Takehashi et al., "Rats produced by interspecies spermatogonial transplantation in mice and in vitro microinsemination," Proceedings of the National Academy of

Sciences of the United States of America, vol. 103, no. 37, pp. 13624–13628, 2006

102. E. Goossens, V. Frederickx, G. De Block, A. C. Van Steirteghem, and H. Tournaye, "Reproductive capacity of sperm obtained after germ cell transplantation in a mouse model," Human Reproduction, vol. 18, no. 9, pp. 1874–1880, 2003.

Citations

CHAPTER 1

Ching-Shwun Lin, Advances in Stem Cell Therapy for Erectile Dysfunction, doi: 10.1155/2014/140618.

CHAPTER 2

Antonio Mancini, Roberto Festa, Sebastiano Raimondo, et al., "Biochemical Alterations in Semen of Varicocele Patients: A Review of the Literature," Advances in Urology, vol. 2012, Article ID 903931, 6 pages, 2012. doi:10.1155/2012/903931.

CHAPTER 3

Takashi Yuasa, Yuri Nagasawa, Katsumasa Osanai, et al., "Induction of a bZIP Type Transcription Factor and Amino Acid Catabolism-Related Genes in Soybean Seedling in Response to Starvation Stress," Journal of Botany, vol. 2013, Article ID 935479, 8 pages, 2013. doi:10.1155/2013/935479.

CHAPTER 4

Marion Mehlis and Theo CM Bakker, Male reproductive traits of full-sibs of different age classes in three-spined sticklebacks (Gasterosteus aculeatus), doi:10.1186/2193-1801-2 175.

CHAPTER 5

Ganapati D. Yadav and Jyoti B. Sontakke (2013). Methods for Separation, Recycling and Reuse of Biodegradation Products, Biodegradation - Engineering and Technology, Dr. Rolando Chamy (Ed.), ISBN: 978-953-51-1153-5, InTech, DOI: 10.5772/56241.

CHAPTER 6

J P Mulhall, M S Anderson, T Lubrano, and T V Shankey, Peyronie's disease cell culture models: phenotypic, genotypic and functional analyses, doi:10.1038/sj.ijir.3900874.

CHAPTER 7

Divyaswetha Peddinti, Bindu Nanduri, Abdullah Kaya, Jean M Feugang, Shane C Burgess, and Erdogan Memili, Comprehensive proteomic analysis of bovine spermatozoa of varying fertility rates and identification of biomarkers associated with fertility, doi: 10.1186/1752-0509-2-19.

CHAPTER 8

Alaa S. Abou-Elhamd, Ahmed O. Salem, and Aziza A. Selim, "Histomorphological Studies on the Prostate Gland of Donkey Equus Asinus during Different Seasons," Journal of Histology, vol. 2013, Article ID 643287, 19 pages, 2013. doi:10.1155/2013/643287.

CHAPTER 9

Rajes Mandal, Damodar Badyakar, and Jitamanyu Chakrabarty, Role of Membrane Lipid Fatty Acids in Sperm Cryopreservation, http://dx.doi.org/10.1155/2014/190542.

CHAPTER 10

J. M. Morrell and H.Rodriguez-Martinez "Practical Applications of Sperm Selection Techniques as a Tool for Improving Reproductive Efficiency,"Veterinary Medicine International, vol. 2011, Article ID 894767, 9 pages, 2011. doi:10.4061/2011/894767.

CHAPTER 11

Ali Honaramooz , and Yanfei Yang, "Recent Advances in Application of Male Germ Cell Transplantation in Farm Animals," Veterinary Medicine International, vol. 2011, Article ID 657860, 9 pages, 2011. doi:10.4061/2011/657860.

Index

R

S

T

U